For Florrie and Sid, of course

This paperback edition published in 2009 by Collins

First published as *Vegetables* in 2006 by Collins
an imprint of HarperCollins
77–85 Fulham Palace Road
London W6 8JB
www.collins.co.uk

Collins is a registered trademark of
HarperCollins Publishers Ltd

14	13	12	11	10	09
6	5	4	3	2	1

Text © Sophie Grigson 2006
Photography © William Shaw 2006

Editor: Susan Fleming
Art direction: Mark Thomson
Design: Emma Ewbank
Photographer: William Shaw
Food stylist: Sam Squires
Stylist: Rosie Dearden

A catalogue record for this book is available
from the British Library.

ISBN 978-0-00-728958-5

Printed and bound at Printing Express, Hong Kong

The Vegetable Bible

Sophie Grigson

Collins

Contents

Introduction

I have no choice but to make this introduction relatively short. I've used up my space allowance several times over already, and the book has grown royally in length since its original inception. The trouble with writing about vegetables is that there are just so many, so much to say about each one, so many enticing ways to prepare them. This is also the joy of writing about them and more importantly of cooking and eating them.

When I compiled my original list of vegetables that I wanted to include in this book, I decided to concentrate on those that could be bought relatively easily in this country, with just a handful of exceptional rarities (such as chervil root or wild asparagus) thrown in for good measure. The original 60 vegetables have increased to over 70, ranging from the familiarity of the carrot or potato, to the more unexpected taste of oca or jicama. And still I have not shoehorned them all into these pages. Devotees of Chinese arrowheads or waterchestnuts, Indian tindoori or drumsticks or bitter gourds will be disappointed. My daughter complained that there were no recipes for palm hearts, and remains barely mollified by my excuse that I've only once bought them fresh, in Spain, and canned vegetables have no place on these pages.

Vegetables have long been something of a passion of mine. This is my second book on vegetables, coming over a decade after the first. I'm still learning about them, coming across new ones, delighting in new and old ways of cooking homely vegetables. I remain fascinated by their differences, their similarities, the way they take starring role, or blend comfortably into the chorus, the way they contrast, the way they add subtlety, the wonderful colours, the rich earthy tones, the sweetness and the textures, the forms, the connection with the land we live in, or with the magic of foreign worlds. I like the notion that the onion is virtually ubiquitous, that other cooks all over the world chop them and fry them just as I do, I love the exoticness of oca, so strange and new in Europe, but as old as the hills of the Andes where they are used without a second thought. Even familiar territory harbours magic discoveries – like the white sprouting broccoli of Leicestershire, or the dramatic purple carrots of Mallorca.

To make the book easier to use (and write) I've grouped vegetables together with the cook in mind. This may occasionally make botanists blench, and from them I beg indulgence. To me it makes more sense to slot beansprouts alongside asparagus and cardoons in the 'shoots and stems' section, than to keep them with beans and peas. Globe artichokes caused endless arguments, but in the end we kept them next to cardoons to which they are so closely related, even though no-one could ever argue that they are either shoot or stem.

One repetitive refrain runs through the following pages. With almost all vegetables, freshness makes a marked difference in flavour. With some it is more apparent than others. Newly picked spring greens are sensational, for instance, as are peas eaten straight from the pod out in the vegetable garden or allotment where they are grown. These are the kind of simple pleasures we should all have access to. Unfortunately so many of the vegetables sold in our shops have been held in storage for too long, or have been flown so far, that they have lost their brand new sparkle. They will still be in notionally good condition, but no longer in their prime.

This is why I like to buy locally grown vegetables when I can. If they are organic, so much the better. I'm no puritan – I eat cherry tomatoes in the middle of winter from time to time because I can't bear the thought of going totally without fresh tomatoes for nine months of the year. I regularly forget which day of the month my local farmers' markets fall on, but when I do get it right, both I and the environment around me reap the benefits. The more we support our local producers, the more opportunities there will be to buy locally grown crops and the more choice we will have.

Above all, however, the message of this book is to make the most of the incredible richness of the vegetable world. This is no health manual, but we all know that vegetables are good for us and we should be eating more of them. It's not difficult if you give them a chance. Buy widely; choose wisely; cook exuberantly.

Sophie Grigson

Author's acknowledgements

My initial encounters with vegetables were, without exception, positive, thanks to my mother, the late Jane Grigson, who cooked them with care and love. I have her to thank for making vegetable-eating a pleasure right from the start, and for encouraging me to experiment with both familiar and new vegetables in later years. More recently, the regular weekly box of vegetables from Riverford Organics has shown me what an extraordinary difference genuine freshness makes to even the most pedestrian vegetables.

I would also like to acknowledge the debt I owe to so many of my friends, who have put up with me moaning about how long it has taken to pen this book, and above all to my editor, Denise Bates, and all of her team at HarperCollins, for their extraordinary patience and forbearance. The wonderful Susan Fleming has fitted copy-editing around the piecemeal delivery of the various sections of the book without a murmur of annoyance, at least in my hearing.

Once again I have been lucky enough to work with William Shaw, one of my favourite photographers (despite his appalling jokes), backed up by a wizard team consisting of the blessed Sam Squire on food and the long-suffering Rosie Dearden on styling – a real diamond, even though she doesn't like cheese. Weird.

A big thank you to Zoltan and the cheery gang that run the coffee machine at Esporta in Oxford, which is where I retreat to write in relative peace. Annabel Hartog and Leslie Ball have helped me test recipes at home, while Sarah and Jennine have kept house, children and admin running smoothly. Last, but by no means least, a big thank you to the two most important people in my life, Florrie and Sid, who make me laugh, shout, get up in the morning, listen to Radio 1, and question almost every assumption I've ever made. They are also pretty good at eating vegetables. What more could a mother hope for?

Publisher's acknowledgements

Thank you to North Aston Organics for their help with photography of vegetables, and The Conran Shop and Harrods for the loan of props.

Cook's notes

There is one important element of vegetable preparation that I have omitted from the individual entries for fear of tedious repetition: unless they are to be peeled, all vegetables should be rinsed before use. Beautiful earthy potatoes and other roots will obviously need to be scrubbed as well, so a vegetable brush is an essential piece of equipment. A nail brush fits the purpose well enough, but make sure that everyone in your house knows and respects the fact that it is only to be used for vegetables, and not to scrub engine oil or paint off soiled hands.

In most instances, precise measuring of ingredients is not absolutely necessary. Take vegetable quantities as rough guidelines. Unless you are making something like the carrot cake on page 28 or the potato cakes on page 73, a little more or a little less will not ruin a dish. There is no point wasting a quarter of a potato, when following a recipe for mash, for instance.

On the whole, it makes sense to stick with either imperial or metric measurements. It makes life simpler, if nothing else. I often suggest using handfuls of this or that. Some people find this frustratingly vague, but it allows whoever is using the recipe to make their own decisions about the final strength of flavours in a dish. Ingredients, particularly herbs and vegetables, vary greatly from one batch to another, from one season to another. As cooks, we have to take this in our stride, adding a little bit more here, a little bit less there in order to compensate for fluctuations in flavour.

Unless otherwise specified, eggs are always free range and always large. Spoon measurements are rounded. I use a standard 15 ml tablespoon, 10 ml dessertspoon and 5 ml teaspoon. Recipes that include olive oil will taste better if made with extra virgin olive oil. Herbs are all fresh, with the exception of bay leaves (good fresh or dried) and dried oregano (use the fabulous Greek rigani, dried wild oregano, if you can get it), which is more exciting than fresh. Pepper and nutmeg should always be freshly ground to maximise spicy impact.

Finally, remember that suggested cooking times are not absolutes. Every oven has its own individual quirks, and settings vary. Similarly the width and make-up of saucepans will affect cooking times. So, check foods regularly as they cook, and if they look done, smell done, taste done, they probably are.

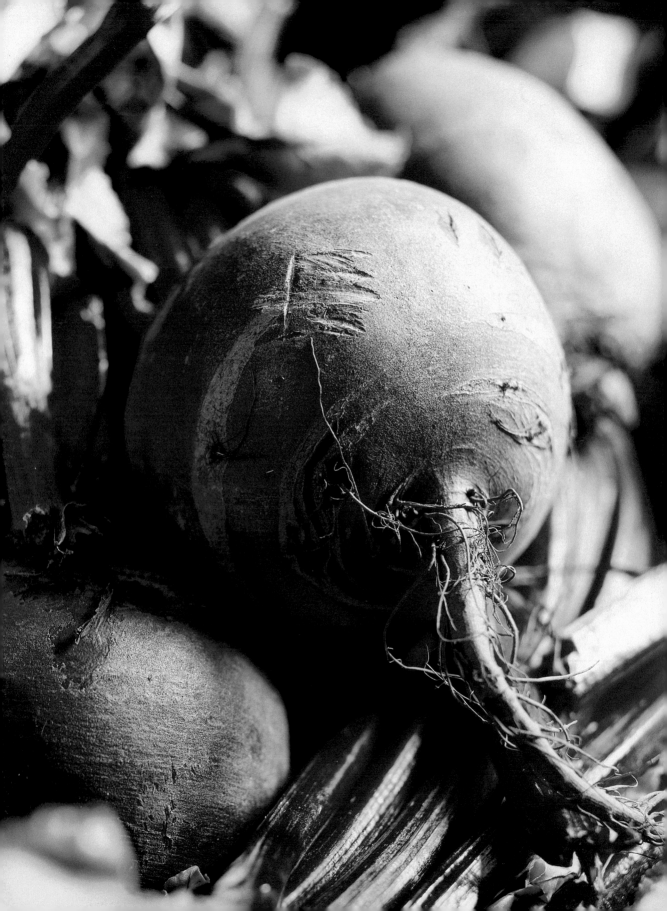

Roots

* *

Beetroot Carrots **Celeriac**
Chervil root **Hamburg parsley**
Jerusalem artichokes **Jicama**
Kumara **Oca** Parsnips
Potatoes Radishes **Salsify**
and Scorzonera Swede
Sweet potatoes Turnips
Yams

* *

Beetroot

* * *

I'd like to serenade the beetroot. Thank your lucky stars then that this is a book, and you can't hear me try. Tunefulness was never my strong point. The fact is, though, that beetroot is a miraculous vegetable. Despite extraordinary maltreatment (what else would you call boiling the poor things in vats of malt vinegar?) the beetroot has re-emerged in recent years as something of a star. It features on the menus of the most elevated of restaurants, and it appears regularly in the smartest recipe books, regaining its rightful reputation as a truly delicious, unique vegetable. What other vegetable can offer the combination of full sweet, earthy flavour together with the rich purple-red of a classic beetroot?

If the foregoing leaves you bewildered, it may just be that you have never tasted beetroot at its finest. In other words, home-roast beetroot, cooked slowly to preserve its true flavour. Sure, you can save time and buy it ready-cooked in neat little vacuum packs, but it will have already lost so much to the processing that it is hardly worth the bother. Sure, you can save time and boil your beets in a large pan of water, but again, so much flavour flows out that you end up with a dumbed-down version.

The **classic dark purple**, staining beetroot is not the only form of the vegetable in existence. The colourways can vary from the **palest white** spattered with rose, to the summery hue of **golden beetroot**. Although both occasionally wander on to the shelves of smart greengrocers, or even the better supermarkets, they are hardly common fare. You are more likely to come across them at a farmers' market. Or, of course, you could grow them yourself and enjoy them pulled straight from the ground, golf-ball sized. Is the taste of these golden beets different? A little, I think, though not radical enough to make headline news. The colour is the main attraction plus the fact that the juice doesn't stain clothing to anything like the same extent.

Practicalities

BUYING If possible, buy beetroot by the bunch, complete with leaves. The leaves are the best indicator of freshness. When they are crisply firm, squeaky in their perfection, you know that the beetroot has come out of the ground recently. As it happens, these telltale leaves are also rather good to eat. Like some earthily rich form of spinach, they can be stir-fried or blanched and served up with a knob of butter melting over them, or Italian-style with a slick of olive oil and plentiful freshly squeezed lemon juice. Or, chop fine and use in a stuffing for ravioli. They're good, too, treated like kale, blanched and fried up with crisp, salty bacon.

As for the beets themselves, only buy them if they are firm with taut skins. Any suggestion of softness or wrinkles tells you that they are older than they should be. It's one thing for you to keep them hanging around in your vegetable drawer for a few days, but it's not on for the retailer to palm off old stock on you. It is rare to have much option over size, but if you do, choose medium-sized ones over large, for a gentler, but never wimpy, taste. Snap up teensy beetroots whenever you get the chance, for these are the choicest of all, with a marvellous sweetness and silky-smooth texture when cooked.

COOKING Although it is not the only way to cook beetroot, by far the best general method is to roast them, guarding all their juiciness and flavour. For most purposes, the process is as follows: wash the beetroots well (but don't scrub brutally, which will rupture the skin) and trim off the leaves, leaving about 2 cm (¾ in) of stalk in place to minimise bleeding. Do not trim off the root. Wrap each beetroot individually in foil, place in a roasting tin or ovenproof dish and slide into a preheated oven. For the finest results the temperature should be fairly low – say around 150°C/300°F/Gas 2. You should allow 2–3 hours for the beetroots to cook. They will still turn out well at a higher temperature if you want to speed matters up a little, or have something else cooking in the oven – anything up to 200°C/400°F/Gas 6 will do nicely. To test, unwrap one of the larger beetroot and scrape gently at the skin near the root. When it comes away easily, the beetroots are done. Take them out and cool slightly, then unwrap and skin each one.

I don't boil beetroot, although many people would cook it no other way. Boiling introduces a wateriness that diminishes the joy of good beetroot.

If you want to speed up the cooking process, then I would suggest that you think of peeling and cutting up raw beetroot into smaller pieces (say 2–3 cm/1 in cubes), then roasting in a hot oven, tossed with a little olive oil, salt, pepper and some whole garlic cloves and sprigs of thyme, or a good sprinkling of fennel seeds or dill seeds. As with most roast vegetables, they'll need some 40–60 minutes in the oven – cook uncovered, turning occasionally and adding a little water or orange juice if you think they look worryingly dry. It may be necessary to cover the dish with foil towards the end of the cooking time if the chunks of beetroot are still not quite tender. Sautéed beetroot is also surprisingly delicious – make the cubes a little smaller, say 1–1.5 cm (½ in) across, and sauté them in olive oil or sunflower oil until tender.

PARTNERS Despite, or perhaps even because of, its distinctive presence, beetroot has an affinity with a remarkable number of other ingredients. In eastern Europe, where it is used most famously to create borscht – beetroot soup in several different forms – beetroot is often combined with aniseed flavours (fennel seed, aniseed, dill and so on) and with soured cream. Try serving cubes of hot cooked beetroot tossed with fresh dill and butter, or fry it briefly with cubes of eating apple and bruised fennel seeds, then serve topped with a spoonful of soured cream (or stir crème fraîche, not soured cream, which will split, into the pan to make a light sauce). Cooked beetroot (puréed or finely diced) is also a brilliant addition to mashed potato, turning it a startling bright pink, which will wow children as much as it amuses parents.

It is, perhaps, in salads that beetroot scores most noticeably, but not the kind of horrorscape of bleeding beetroot lying supine and flabby against miserably limp lettuce leaves, stained gorily with streaks of dark red. No, a good beetroot salad needs a little care in its creation, so that the colour works for it rather than against. Dress the beetroot with vinaigrette while still hot, so that it absorbs some of the tastes, then set aside until ready to plate up with other ingredients. In salads, classic beetroot partners are orange, apple, potato, celery and walnuts in particular. Salty additions also work well – crisp bacon, black olives and anchovy, for instance. On the whole I think it best not to muddle the beetroot with too many partners. The idea should be to highlight its delights, not to mask.

Raw beetroot makes a handsome addition to salads in moderation.

The most famous example of this is the French salade nantaise: frisée or blanched dandelion leaves and/or tender lamb's lettuce (a.k.a. mâche or corn salad), tossed with coarsely grated shreds of raw beetroot and a warm dressing made with bacon frizzled in its own fat and a touch of oil, garlic and red wine vinegar. A gorgeous treat of a salad. I also use raw beetroot with sweet cos lettuce and grapefruit tossed in an animated oriental-toned dressing (see page 381), to totally different effect.

* *

Australian market beetroot dip

The main markets in both Melbourne and Adelaide are thrilling. Bustling and vibrant, they offer superb produce, ranging from fruit and veg, through cheeses, wines, meats and breads, not forgetting dazzling deli stands where you can choose from impressive ranges of freshly made pestos and dips. The brilliant pink of one dip made us pause, then inspired a picnic built around it. The natural sweetness of beetroot balanced by a touch of sourness from the cream and lemon and a waft of spice is very good – eat it with warm pitta bread or batons of cucumber, pepper, carrot and celery.

Serves 6

3 medium fresh beetroots, roughly
   300–350g (11–12oz)
1 teaspoon cumin seeds
1 teaspoon coriander seeds

250g (9oz) soured cream or thick
   Greek-style yoghurt
1–2 tablespoons lemon juice
salt and pepper

Trim each beetroot, leaving about 3cm (1¼in) of stalk and the root in place. Wrap each one in foil, place in a baking dish and roast (see above) until tender. Dry-fry the cumin and coriander seeds in a heavy frying pan over a moderate heat until the scent curls temptingly round the kitchen. Tip into a bowl or a mortar and leave to cool, then grind to a powder.

   As soon as they are cool enough to handle, skin the beetroots. Set half of one aside; cut up the rest roughly and toss into a food processor. Add all the other ingredients, including the ground spices, and process until smooth.

Grate the reserved beetroot or chop finely (messy, I know, but if you want that rather attractive, not-quite-perfectly-smooth texture, it has to be done) and stir into the mixture. Taste and adjust the seasonings.

Serve at room temperature with warm pitta bread, and sticks of carrot, celery, pepper or cucumber.

* *

Beetroot, clementine and pine nut salad with orange dressing

Beetroot and orange work prettily and tastefully together, in every sense of the word. Serve this as a side dish or as a first course. You can make it more substantial by adding big flakes of hot-smoked salmon or trout. Alternatively, tear up a brace of buffalo mozzarella and add them, carefully so that they don't stain, after the salad has been dished up.

Serves 4–6

4 beetroots, roasted, skinned and cut into wedges	**Dressing**
	5 tablespoons extra virgin olive oil
4 clementines or ortaniques	grated zest of 2 clementines
a good handful of flat-leaf parsley leaves	2–3 tablespoons rice vinegar or cider
3 small shallots, thinly sliced into rings	vinegar
3 tablespoons pine nuts, toasted	salt and pepper

To make the dressing put the oil and zest into a pan and infuse over a very low heat for 20 minutes. Strain and cool. Whisk the vinegar with salt and pepper, then gradually whisk in the orange oil. Taste and adjust seasonings.

As soon as the beetroot is cooked and cut up, toss with a little of the dressing, then leave to cool. Peel the clementines and slice thinly. Just before serving, toss the clementine discs with the parsley leaves, shallots, pine nuts and the remaining dressing, then arrange in a casual but artful way in a serving dish or on individual plates with the beetroot.

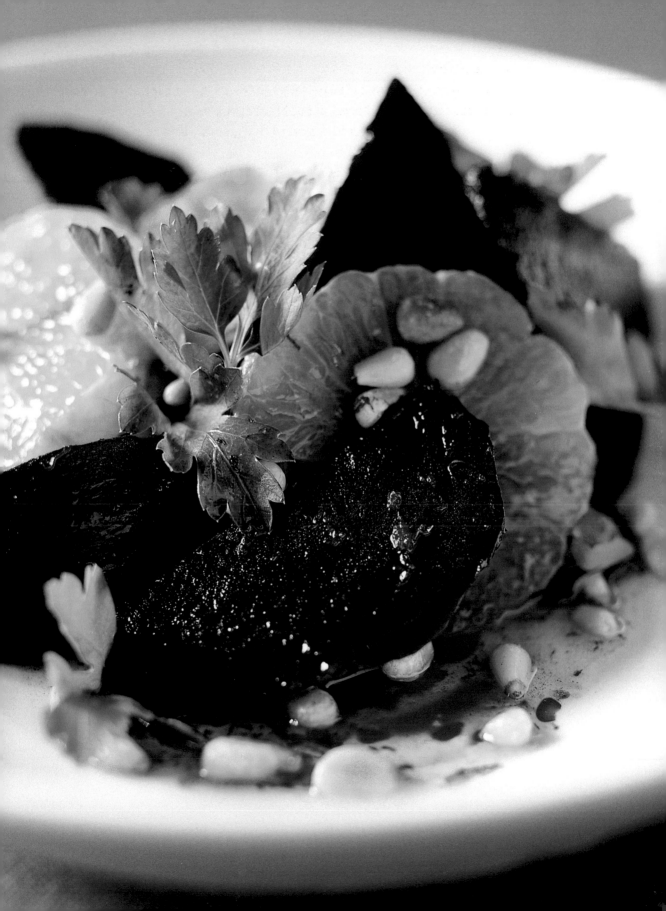

* *

Blushing dauphinoise

This is a dish of heavenly decadence, laden with cream, spiked gently with a touch of horseradish. Like a standard potato dauphinoise, it is something for special occasions only, and there is no point even thinking about making it if you are trying to cut down on fat. I would actually be quite happy to gorge on this as a main course, but more conventionally, it sits well with roast feathered game, or a fine joint of beef.

Allow plenty of time for the dauphinoise to cook – this is not a dish to be rushed. Too high a heat will curdle the cream and blacken the top without ever achieving the melting texture you are aiming for.

Serves 6–8

15 g (½ oz) butter
300–450 ml (10–15 fl oz) whipping cream
300 ml (10 fl oz) crème fraîche
3 tablespoons creamed horseradish
550 g (1¼ lb) slightly waxy maincrop potatoes, such as Cara or larger Charlottes, peeled and very thinly sliced

500 g (1 lb 2 oz) beetroot, peeled and thinly sliced
8 canned anchovies, roughly chopped (optional)
salt and pepper

Preheat the oven to 150°C/300°F/Gas 2. Grease an ovenproof gratin dish thickly with the butter. Beat the whipping cream into the crème fraîche along with the horseradish.

Lay about one-third of the potato slices over the bottom of the buttered dish. Season with salt and pepper, then cover with half the beetroot and sprinkle over half the anchovies, if using. Season again, then pour over enough of the cream mixture to come up to the level of the beetroot. Repeat the layers and then finish with the last third of the potato. Pour over the remaining cream, topping up with more whipping cream if necessary, so that the cream fills all the gaps and rises until about level with the top of the potatoes. Season again.

Bake, uncovered, for about 2 hours, until the potatoes and beetroot are tender all the way through, and the top is richly browned with traces of purple-pink cream bubbling up at the sides. Serve hot or warm.

* *

Carrots

* * *

I like carrots. You like carrots. Everyone likes carrots. No point analysing their success – we know that they do a brilliant job bobbing up time and again on plates the world over. Naturally, there are carrots and then there are carrots. And by that I mean that some carrots have the most exquisite sweet carroty flavour, so good you should really just gobble them up raw, and then sadly, other carrots are dull and lacklustre, providing, one hopes, vitamins and other good-health requirements, if not a great deal in realms of pleasure.

There is no telling before the first bite, which makes buying carrots the tamest form of Russian roulette going. There are people who swear blind that organic carrots taste better than non-organic, and often they do. But no one has yet managed to convince me that it is their organicness that makes the difference. No, I reckon that it's a lot more to do with variety, conditions in the field, freshness and luck, as well as good husbandry.

You may also not be aware that the orange carrot is a comparatively modern phenomenon, and not one that occurs in the wild. The true colour of the carrot is **off-white** in the case of the Mediterranean native, or **purple** or **red** when growing in more exotic places like Afghanistan, though one imagines that there aren't many left growing in the wild there. You can, however, find **purple** carrots closer to home in more hospitable surroundings. They are still eaten on the island of Mallorca – a trip to the excellent covered market in the heart of Palma is all it takes to track them down. The difference in taste is minimal but the colour is sheer drama.

Practicalities

BUYING
A happy carrot is firm from tip to stem, no bruising or discoloration, with a pleasing light carroty smell. The slightest hint of flabbiness spells disaster, and slimy ends or rotting soft spots are to be avoided like the plague.

Buying carrots in bunches, with a duster of fluffy green leaves, is the only way you can be sure that they are newly tugged from the earth, but since they store rather well (especially with a dusting of soil still protecting them) freshness is not the critical issue it is with so many other vegetables. Take advantage of it when bunched carrots are on offer, and for the rest of the year pick out carrots of similar size to each other so that they cook evenly. Really small mini carrots, cute though they are, often taste of very little. Costwise it makes sense to go for larger carrots, which should have developed more depth of flavour. The swelling of ginormous carrots, on the other hand, may be partially due to too much water, so they have a tendency to dullness. These are crude generalisations, so there will always be exceptions, but they are the best I can offer as guidelines.

Store carrots either in an airy, dry, cool spot, or in the vegetable drawer of the fridge.

COOKING Peeling or scraping or just a quick scrub? All three have their supporters, but personally I go for the peeling unless my carrots are pristine organic roots of impeccable freshness. Scraping is a messy business, I find, and slower than peeling. I know that peeling is wasteful, but you could save the peelings for the stockpot, or the compost, or even get yourself a back-yard pig to feed them to. There is no doubt that commercially grown carrots must be either peeled or scraped in order to eliminate pesticide residues. When it comes to organic carrots, by definition free from pesticides, you might well consider that a good wash is sufficient.

Raw carrots are under-used. I love them in salads, coarsely grated and dressed perhaps with a mustardy vinaigrette, studded with raisins or currants and toasted pine nuts or walnuts. Or to give a more exotic air, try tossing them with lemon juice, rosewater, a little sugar, salt and a touch of sunflower oil, Moroccan-style. Grated carrots make a handsome addition to a sandwich, too, especially with cheese or hummus.

There are times when **'over'-cooked** carrots are wonderful – in a stew, say, where they've donated some of their sweet flavour to the other ingredients in exchange for some of theirs. However, carrots that have been left to boil in plain water for too long have received nothing in compensation but water, ergo they taste of very little. **Simmered** or **boiled** or **steamed** carrots do not take long to cook – the thickness of the pieces dictates exactly how long, but think in terms of 4–6 minutes. That should be long enough for the heat to have developed the flavour, but not so long that it all leaches out. If you know that the carrots you are about to cook are not very sweet, try adding a teaspoonful or two of sugar to the cooking water.

Boiled perfectly, a good carrot retaining just the right degree of firmness is a pleasure to eat plain, but even nicer with a gloss of melted butter, or fragrant lemon olive oil. In the summer I add a speckling of chopped lemon balm or mint; in the winter thyme or savory enhances the flavour.

Although boiling or steaming will always remain the principal way we cook carrots, once in a while have a go at **frying** (see the salad recipe overleaf) or stir-frying them, cut into slender batons. **Roasted** carrots should become part of your regular repertoire, if they aren't already. They taste divine, and are sooo very easy. Just peel the carrots and halve or quarter lengthways if they are huge, then toss them into a roasting tin with a little extra virgin olive oil, a handful of garlic cloves (no need to peel), a few chunky sprigs of thyme or rosemary and a scattering of coarse salt. Roast in a hot oven (200–220°C/400–425°F/Gas 6–7) for around 40–45 minutes, stirring once or twice, until patched with brown and extremely tender.

PARTNERS Since carrots are so amiable, there are few tastes that don't marry well with them. I don't much like the idea of canned anchovies or chocolate with carrots, but I'm hard pressed to think of much else to avoid. Carrots love to be cooked with spices, with herbs, with garlic and chilli, in sweet dishes (such as carrot cake), in pickles, with meat or fish, with cheeses, and of course with other vegetables. This, I imagine, is one of the reasons that you bump up against carrots wherever you eat in the world. And this is also why we should value them more than we do.

* *

Fried carrot salad with mint and lemon

I've been making this salad for years and years and it still seems just as fabulous as it did way back in the mists of time. It comes down to taking a bit of time over the frying, so that the carrots soften as their inner sugars caramelise and every mite of flavour in them concentrates itself. Add plenty of fresh lemon and lots of breathy mint and you have a small miracle of a salad on your hands. If you don't believe me, have a go.

Incidentally, if you prefer, you can roast the carrots in a hot oven (around 220°C/425°F/Gas 7) with a generous dousing of good olive oil for some 30–40 minutes, until browned and tender.

Serves 4

450 g (1 lb) carrots (smaller rather than
   larger)
3 tablespoons extra virgin olive oil
juice of ½ lemon
2 tablespoons chopped mint
salt and pepper

If using small carrots, top and tail them, then halve lengthways and cut each piece in half. Treat medium-sized carrots in much the same way, but quarter them lengthways.

Heat the oil in a wide, heavy frying pan and add the carrots. Fry slowly, shaking and turning every now and then, until the carrots are patched with brown and tender. This should take about 15 minutes. Tip into a bowl and mix with the lemon juice, mint, salt and pepper. Leave to cool and serve at room temperature.

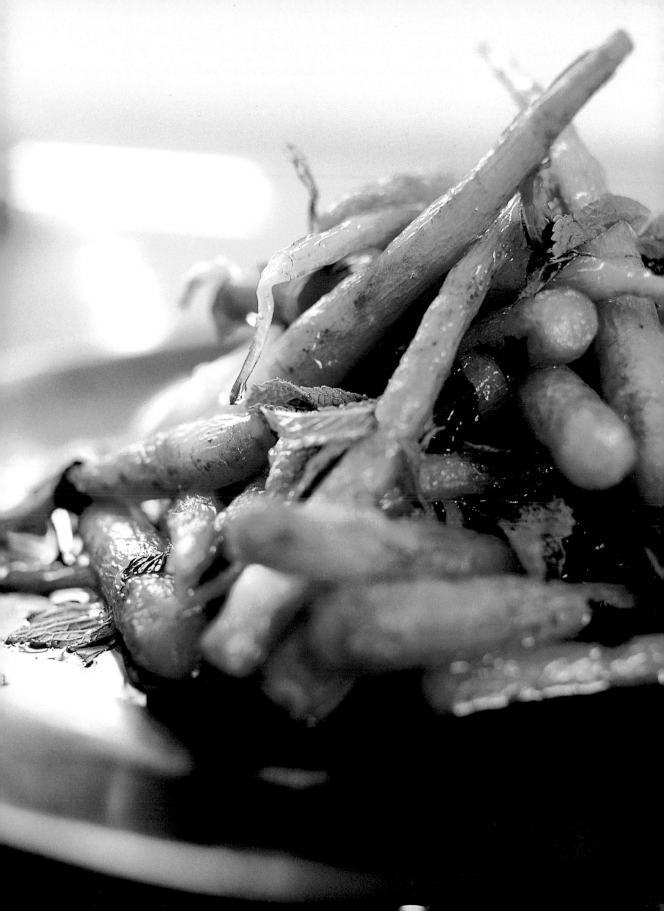

* *

Carrot and pickled pepper soup

For this soup I use small, round, sweet-sharp pickled red peppers with a bit of a kick to them, to throw a shot of excitement into a comforting carrot soup. If you can't find any good red pickled peppers, then you could replace them with pickled jalapeño peppers – but go gently, as the heat can be more intense and the colour is less attractive.

Serves 4–6

1 onion, chopped
500 g (1 lb 2 oz) carrots, sliced
1 bouquet garni (3 sprigs lemon thyme,
   1 sprig tarragon, 2 sprigs parsley,
   1 bay leaf), tied together with string
2 tablespoons extra virgin olive oil
2 tablespoons pudding rice
4 hot or 6 mild pickled red peppers, roughly
   chopped

1.5 litres (2 ¾ pints) light chicken or
   vegetable stock
lemon juice
salt and pepper

To serve
a little soured cream (optional, but good)
roughly torn coriander or parsley leaves
4–6 pickled red peppers, sliced

Sweat the onion and carrots with the bouquet garni and oil for 10 minutes in a covered saucepan over a gentle heat. Now add the pudding rice and the peppers and stir until the rice is glistening with the oily juices. Add the stock, salt and pepper and bring up to the boil, then reduce the heat and simmer for 10–15 minutes, until the rice and carrots are tender. Draw off the heat and cool slightly, then liquidise in several batches. Add a little more stock or water if the soup is too thick for your taste, and stir in a couple of squeezes of lemon juice. Taste and adjust seasoning. Reheat when required.

To serve, ladle into soup bowls, add a few small dollops of soured cream and then top with the coriander or parsley and sliced peppers.

* *

Carrot falafel with tomato and carrot salad

The best falafel I've eaten over the decades have almost invariably been bought from street stalls and eaten on the hoof, jostling for space with tomato, cucumber and lettuce in the cavity of a warm pitta bread.

Back at home, lacking the ambience of the bustling street, I resort to making my own falafel, lightened with the natural sweetness of grated carrot, and served as a first course with a fresh and invigorating salad. They've not got the street–stall shimmer, but the taste is terrific, nonetheless.

In terms of culinary notes, the most important is that you should never ever even think of using tinned chickpeas for making falafel. They have to be made with dried chickpeas, soaked overnight, to get the right texture and firmness. No debate on this one. The second, a follow-on from the first, is that you mustn't rush the cooking. If the temperature of the oil is too high, the falafel will never cook through to the centre.

Serves 4–6

125 g (4 1/2 oz) dried chickpeas, soaked
  overnight
6 spring onions, trimmed and roughly
  chopped
1 large clove garlic, chopped
2 carrots, grated (about 200 g/7 oz)
30 g (1 oz) parsley leaves, roughly chopped
1 teaspoon ground cumin
1/2 teaspoon baking powder
sunflower and olive oil for frying
salt and pepper

To serve
leaves from a small bunch of coriander
18 mini plum tomatoes, halved
1 shallot, halved and thinly sliced
1 carrot, coarsely grated
juice of 1/2 lemon
2 tablespoons extra virgin olive oil
3–4 tablespoons thick Greek-style yoghurt

To make the falafel, drain the chickpeas and place in the bowl of a food processor with the spring onions, garlic, carrots, parsley, cumin, baking powder, salt and pepper. Process to a smooth paste. You should be able to roll it into balls that hold together nicely – not too soft and soggy, nor irritatingly crumbly.

Take a little of the mixture and fry in a little oil. Bite into it and consider whether the seasoning needs to be beefed up. Act upon your thoughts immediately. Now, scoop out dessertspoonfuls of the mixture and roll into balls, then flatten gently to a thickness of around 1.5 cm (⅝ in). Cover and set aside until needed.

Shortly before serving, heat up a 1cm (½ in) depth of sunflower oil, or mixed sunflower and olive oils, in a saucepan. When good and hot, add a few of the falafel and fry for some 3 minutes on each side, until crustily browned and cooked through. You may have to try one to check that you're getting the timing just right. What a pity – just don't try too many.

While they are in the pan, mix the salad ingredients – coriander, tomatoes, shallot, carrot, lemon juice and oil – and divide among plates (or pile into one big bowl). Serve the hot falafel with the salad and a dollop of thick yoghurt on the side.

* *

Braised pheasant (or guinea fowl) with carrots, Riesling and tarragon

This is, in essence, a smart pot-roast, with the carrots and Riesling flavouring the natural cooking juices of the birds. If you have a brace of pheasants, there should be enough to feed six comfortably, but a guinea fowl will probably not satisfy more than four. Either way, the finished result is smart enough to grace a dinner party, but easy enough to serve as a good supper dish when you need something of a boost.

Serve the birds and their sauce with steamed or boiled new potatoes and some sort of green vegetable, to counterpoint the tender sweetness of the carrots.

Serves 4–6

15 g (½ oz) butter
1 tablespoon sunflower oil
2 pheasants or 1 plump guinea fowl
1 onion, chopped
3 cloves garlic, sliced
500 g (1 lb 2 oz) carrots, cut into batons
4 sprigs tarragon
150 ml (5 fl oz) dry Riesling
100 ml (3 ½ fl oz) double cream
salt and pepper

Heat the butter with the oil in a flameproof casserole large enough to take the birds and all the carrots. Brown the pheasants or guinea fowl in the fat, then remove from the casserole. Reduce the heat, then stir the onion and garlic into the fat and fry gently until tender. Add the carrots and tarragon and stir around for a few minutes, then return the pheasants or guinea fowl to the pot, nestling them breast-side down in amongst the carrots. Pour over the Riesling and season with salt and pepper. Bring up to the boil, then cover with a close-fitting lid. Turn the heat down low and leave to cook gently for 1 hour, or a little longer if necessary, turning the pheasants or guinea fowl over after about half an hour.

Once the birds and carrots are tender, lift the birds out on to a serving plate and keep warm. Stir the cream into the carrots and juices and simmer for 2 minutes or so, then taste and adjust seasoning. Spoon around the birds and serve immediately.

* *

Carrot cake

Everyone knows that carrot cake is a very good thing, indeed. What a cheery thought it is that you can have your cake and eat vegetables at the same time.

This is the recipe I return to regularly, after playing away with less successful variations. I'm not usually a big fan of baking cakes or pastry with wholemeal flour, but for once it makes absolute sense, absorbing some of the moisture that the carrot provides, and giving the substance the cake needs.

Serves 8–12

250 g (9 oz) light muscovado sugar
250 ml (9 fl oz) light olive oil or sunflower oil
4 large eggs
2 tablespoons milk
250 g (9 oz) wholemeal flour
2 rounded teaspoons baking powder
60 g (2 oz) ground almonds
2 tablespoons poppy seeds
125 g (4 1/2 oz) shelled walnuts,
   roughly chopped

250 g (9 oz) carrots, grated

Frosting
200 g (7 oz) cream cheese
200 g (7 oz) butter, softened
250 g (9 oz) icing sugar, sifted
1 teaspoon vanilla extract
12 walnut halves to decorate

Preheat the oven to 180°C/350°F/Gas 4. Base-line two 20 cm (8 in) round cake tins with baking parchment and grease the sides. Whisk the sugar with the oil, eggs and milk. Mix the flour with the baking powder, ground almonds, poppy seeds, walnuts and carrots. Make a well in the centre and add the sugary liquids, scraping the last of the sugar from the bowl. Mix the ingredients thoroughly.

Scrape into the two prepared cake tins and bake for 40–45 minutes until firm to the touch – check by plunging a skewer into the centre. If it comes out clean, then the cake is cooked. While the cake is baking, beat the cream cheese with the softened butter, icing sugar and vanilla extract to make the frosting.

Let the cakes cool in their tins for 5 minutes, then turn them out on to a wire rack. Leave to cool completely, then sandwich together with about one-third of the frosting. Spread the remaining frosting over the top and down the sides, then decorate with the walnut halves.

* *

Celeriac

* * *

Perhaps the most brutish-looking of vegetables (swede competes for the title, and it's hard to decide which merits the crown most), celeriac is a form of celery with an absurdly swollen rootstock, known technically as a corm. Both celeriac and celery share the Latin name *Apium graveolens*, even though they look so very different. When the stems are left on celeriac, sticking up like a brush, the connection is more obvious. The stems are slender, but topped with the same leaves, as if someone had squeezed hard on the broad succulent stems of a head of celery, forcing all the liquid back down into the root to puff it up like a balloon. The odd thing is that celeriac doesn't taste at all like celery. Celeriac tastes of nothing but itself. Most people love it, and many people find it infinitely preferable to celery.

So, discount the exterior and concentrate on the firm, cream-hued interior. Solid and dense and generously proportioned, it is a remarkably delicious vegetable. I've never really understood why we don't use it more: over in France it is the substance of one of their favourite mainstream salads, sold in every charcuterie and supermarket, as popular as and infinitely better than, most of the coleslaw consumed here. Yet here it is still considered something of an outsider, idly hovering on the fringes of popularity. How much longer before it breaks through to become a household name?

Oddly enough, celeriac sales were boosted by the vogue for the Atkins diet. Celeriac is, apparently, very low in carbohydrate. What a godsend for those who missed potatoes. Here was a great substitute, particularly when mashed with shedloads of cream and butter. Now that the Atkins diet is no longer as fashionable as it once was, I hope that the celeriac habit endures – it is far too engaging a vegetable to drop the minute the diet is over.

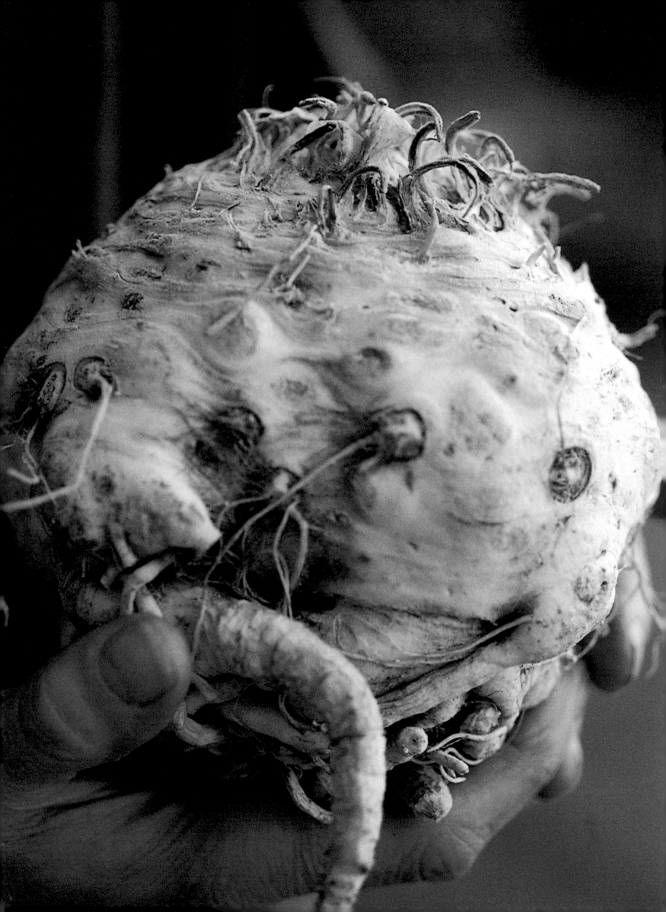

Practicalities

BUYING Celeriac is always big, but don't buy the most colossal ones, as these may have swelled up so far that the centre has become spongy or hollow. Be satisfied with plain big. Choose celeriac that is firm and heavy with no soft, bruised spots. Store it in the vegetable drawer of the fridge, where it will keep happily for a week or more.

COOKING Celeriac can be cooked in a number of ways, but before that you have to take off the outer layer and the gnarled tangle of roots at the base. I usually slice the celeriac thickly then discard the roots and cut away the skin around the edge of each disc. If I'm boiling the celeriac, I then hack it into big chunks, ready to drop into the pan. If not used immediately, celeriac discolours, so once cut drop it into a bowl of water acidulated with the juice of ½ lemon or a dash of wine vinegar.

The most cherished way to serve celeriac is **mashed**, either à la Atkins, in other words pure celeriac and lots of rich cream and butter, or – rather nicer, both in texture and flavour – mashed with equal quantities of potato, a large knob or two of butter and some milk. Either way it begs for plenty of salt and a good scraping of nutmeg. Another fine variation that I make occasionally, especially as Christmas approaches, is a mash of celeriac and chestnuts – true, the colour is muddy, but the taste is divine. Unless you are saintly, use vacuum-packed cooked chestnuts, and mash with double the quantity of celeriac, butter and cream. Nutmeg is essential. Distract from the colour with a sprinkling of chopped chives and a knob of melting butter in the centre of the hot mash.

As with most vegetables, celeriac can be **sautéed** (cut into small cubes) over a lively heat, or **roasted** in the oven, tossed in olive oil. To make celeriac **chips**, parboil thick batons of celeriac (just 2–3 minutes will do the trick), drain well and then deep-fry, or shallow-fry, or toss with oil and roast in a hot oven for 10–15 minutes.

I adore a celeriac and potato **dauphinoise**, rich and creamy. For this one, I usually blanch the slices of celeriac and potato in boiling salted water for a couple of minutes, before layering and baking slowly in the oven until heavenly soft and tender.

Raw celeriac is rather good too. I don't like it grated – a bit slushy – but I do like it cut into juliennes (thin batons), which increases the prep time, but is worth the bother. Remember to toss it with lemon or lime juice as you cut it, to prevent excessive browning. Although there is no reason why it shouldn't be added to any number of salads, the classic is always going to be céleri rémoulade, for which I give a recipe overleaf. Frankly, you just can't beat it.

SEE ALSO CELERY (PAGE 124).

* *

Roast chicken with apple, celeriac and hazelnut stuffing

Celeriac makes a good basis for a stuffing, a strong enough flavour to come through without fighting the taste of the chicken. The celeriac 'chips' around the outside semi-simmer and semi-roast as the bird cooks, absorbing some of the juices from the chicken for extra flavour.

Serves 4

1 plump and happy free-range chicken
a little olive oil
½ celeriac, peeled and cut into 'chips'
salt and pepper

Stuffing
½ celeriac, peeled and finely diced
1 onion, chopped
2 cloves garlic, chopped

30 g (1 oz) butter
8 sage leaves, chopped
1 eating apple, cored and diced small
40 g (1½ oz) shelled, skinned hazelnuts, roasted and chopped
80 g (scant 3 oz) soft white breadcrumbs
1 egg, lightly beaten

Preheat the oven to 200°C/400°F/Gas 6.

To make the stuffing, begin by sautéing the celeriac, onion and garlic together in the butter until tender – take plenty of time over this, say 10 minutes or more, so that their flavours really get a chance to develop. Stir in the sage leaves and cook for a further 30 seconds or so. Now mix the vegetables and buttery juices with the apple, hazelnuts, breadcrumbs,

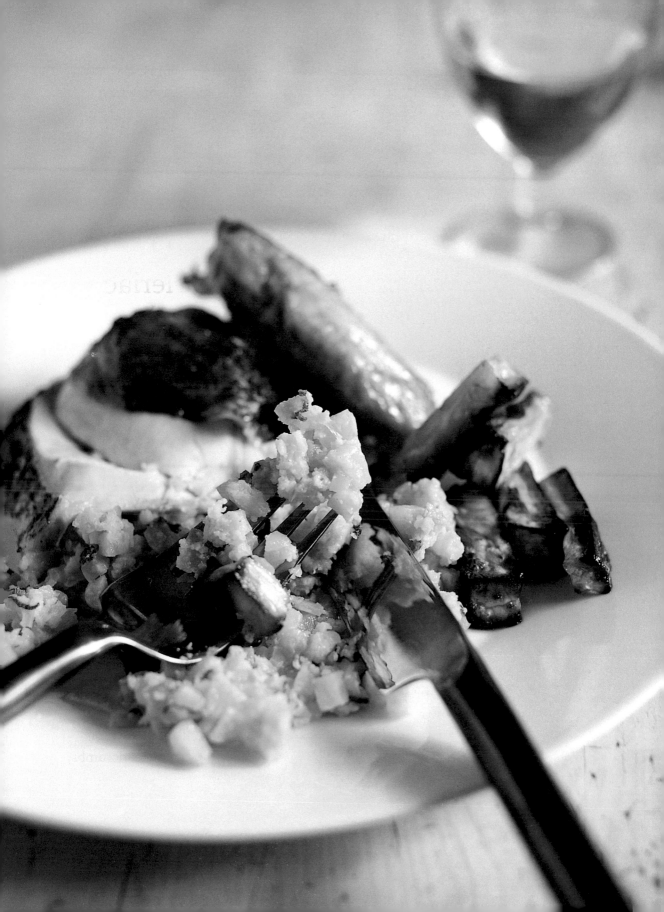

seasoning (be generous with it) and enough beaten egg to bind.

Fill the cavity of the chicken with the stuffing. You'll probably have more than you need, so pack the remainder into a shallow ovenproof dish and bake alongside the bird until browned and hot – it won't taste as good as the stuffing inside the bird, but it gets the crisp crust as a bonus.

Place the stuffed bird in a roasting tin or shallow ovenproof dish and smear a little olive oil over its skin. Season generously with salt and pepper. Pour a small glass of water around the bird and surround with the celeriac chips. Roast for about 1¼ hours, basting the bird occasionally with its own juices (add a little more water if it needs it) and turning the celeriac chips occasionally – they should soften and catch a little brown here and there.

Test to make sure that the chicken is cooked by plunging a skewer into the thickest part of the thigh – if the juices run clear then it is done. If they run pink and bloody, then get the whole lot back into the oven for another 15 minutes and then try again.

Let the chicken rest in a warm place for 20 minutes before serving.

* *

Céleri rémoulade

Whenever we're in France we head straight for the charcuterie to buy garlic sausage and a tub of céleri rémoulade. In this instance 'céleri' is short for 'céleri-rave', in other words, celeriac. 'Rémoulade' indicates that it is tossed in a mustardy mayonnaise, to transform it into one of France's favourite salad dishes. Few French domestic cooks ever make their own – why bother when the shop-bought céleri rémoulade is so good? Outside France it is another matter – especially if you make your own mayonnaise, which takes no time at all in a processor or liquidiser. The celeriac itself is best cut by hand, rather than grated, which inevitably produces an over-fine mushy salad. Soften it to agreeable floppiness by soaking in lemon juice and salt for a while.

Either serve your céleri rémoulade as one amongst a bevy of salads, or make it a first course, perhaps accompanied by some lightly cooked large prawns, or thin slices of salty Parma ham.

Serves 6

1 small celeriac
juice of 1 lemon
2 tablespoons single cream
3 tablespoons home-made mayonnaise
2 teaspoons Dijon mustard
salt and cayenne pepper

Peel the celeriac, removing all those knobbly twisty bits at the base. Now cut the celeriac in half, then cut each half into thin slices – you're aiming roughly at about 3–5 mm (1/8 – 1/4 in) thick, no more. Cut each slice into long, thin strips. Toss the celeriac with the lemon juice as you cut, to prevent browning, then once all done, season with salt and cover with clingfilm. Set aside for half an hour or so to soften.

Drain off any liquid, then toss the celeriac strips with the cream, mayo, mustard, salt and cayenne. Taste and adjust seasoning, then serve.

* *

Speedy mayonnaise

I've given up on making mayonnaise the proper, old-fashioned way. Nowadays, I opt for the quick liquidiser method, which yields up a mayonnaise that is every bit as good and so much less stressful.

Two brief notes. Avoid the temptation to increase the amount of olive oil. In quantity it gives an unpleasant bitterness. The second is the old familiar: as home-made mayonnaise inevitably contains raw egg, do not offer it to the very young, the old, pregnant women, invalids.

Makes roughly 250 ml (9 fl oz)

1 egg
1 tablespoon very hot (but not boiling) water
1 tablespoon lemon juice

250 ml (9 fl oz) sunflower or grapeseed oil
50 ml (2 fl oz) extra virgin olive oil
salt

Break the egg into the goblet of the liquidiser and add the hot water. Whirr the blades to blend, then add the lemon juice and salt. Measure the oils into a jug together. With the motor running, pour the oil into the egg, in a constant stream, until it is all incorporated. By this time, the mayonnaise will be divinely thick and glossy. Taste and adjust the seasoning.

* *

Roast celeriac with Marsala

This is a repeat recipe, originally printed in my book *Taste of the Times*, which is now out of print. It is so good, however, that I have no qualms about including it again here. As the celeriac roasts, it absorbs some of the raisiny flavour of the Marsala (but not the alcohol, which just burns off), whilst caramelising to a golden, sticky brownness. Excellent with game, in particular.

Serves 4

1 medium-large celeriac
a little sunflower oil
a knob of butter
5 tablespoons sweet Marsala
salt and pepper

Preheat the oven to 180°C/350°F/Gas 4. Cut the celeriac into 8 wedges, then trim off the skin as neatly and economically as you can. Toss the wedges in just enough oil to coat. Smear the butter thickly around an ovenproof dish, just large enough to take the celeriac wedges lying down flat (well, flattish, anyway). Lay the celeriac in the dish, season with salt and pepper and pour over the Marsala.

Roast for about 1 hour, turning the wedges and basting every now and then, until richly browned all over and very tender. You may find that you have to add a tablespoon or two of water towards the end to prevent burning.

* *

Chervil root

* * *

The rarity of chervil root is a small tragedy. I have come across them a mere three or four times in my adult life and I regret profoundly that they are not more common, for they are nothing short of delicious. I first discovered them in a market near Orléans in France. This is their home region. However, even in France they remain bemusingly rare. This may partly be due to their appearance. They don't look at all promising. Small, brown, dirty cones, looking for all the world like a pile of rough-hewn, old-fashioned children's spinning tops, they don't exactly shout 'buy me'. It may well be that you or I have strode past them without even noticing their presence. Oh that it weren't so. These insignificant morsels are blessed with a remarkable flavour, something like a cross between a chestnut and a parsnip, and if only you could lay your hands on them, I have no doubt that they would soon become all the rage.

Practicalities

BUYING

There's no point angsting about freshness – just grab hold of them if you are lucky enough to find any. Ideally, they should be pleasingly firm, but personally I'd snap them up even if they were just a mite softer and wrinklier – the taste is still good, though they are harder to peel in this state.

COOKING

Give them a good scrub to remove any dirt (however much elbow grease you employ, the skin will remain unappealingly grubby-looking). The skin is edible, but not especially so. Peel the little darlings before cooking for the best results. They taste fab just **simmered in salted water** until tender (like a parsnip, this is not a vegetable that benefits from the al dente school of cooking), drained well and then finished with a knob of butter. Even more devastatingly divine, however, are **roast** chervil roots. Again peel before cooking, then roast in a little olive oil or oil and butter in the normal fashion, until tender as butter inside, lightly browned and a little chewy outside. Cooked this way, they go spectacularly well with roast beef, or a good steak. I dare say that chervil root has enormous potential and could be mashed, chipped, souped and so on. One day, maybe, I'll get to find out, but that will just have to wait until the day I can source them regularly, and easily. Roll on that day.

* *

Hamburg parsley

* * *

As entries go, this one will be very short. Not because Hamburg parsley doesn't rate, but more because it has become increasingly hard to find. I don't think I've seen it for sale for the best part of a decade, more's the pity. Therefore my aim now is merely to prime you, just in case you stumble across a tray of Hamburg parsley unexpectedly. If you do, please buy some and encourage the seller/grower to spread the word.

Although it looks like a shocked parsnip, colour washed out to ghostly off-white, and is about the same size and shape, Hamburg parsley is actually nothing more unusual than a form of the commonest of herbs, parsley. They share the same Latin name, *Petroselinum crispum*, but the energy flows down to the root of the Hamburg variety, swelling it out to a satisfying girth. Not for nothing is it also known as parsley root. It is far less sweet than a parsnip and does have a distinct parsley zing, which is surprising at first.

Although you could serve it as a straight vegetable, just boiled and buttered, the flavour is strong. In practice, it is more usual to add it in moderation to **stews** and **soups**, cut up into chunks. In this context, it blossoms, imparting something of its parsley scent to the whole, and absorbing other flavours to mollify its own in a most beguiling manner. If you have only one or two roots, you might prefer to **boil** and **mash** them with double or triple quantities of potato and plenty of butter to make excellent, parsley-perfumed mash to accompany some dark, rich, meaty stew.

* *

Jerusalem artichokes

* * *

Once upon a time, many centuries ago, intrepid explorers crossed the Atlantic Ocean at great peril and discovered all sorts of miraculous things. There were potatoes and tomatoes and chocolate and gold. There were chillies to make up for a dismaying lack of black pepper. Less lauded and celebrated, however, was the discovery of the *Helianthus tuberosus*. It belongs to a later period of exploration and intrepidity, when the pioneering spirit of the first settlers in North America led them to the flaps of Native American tepees. This time, along with turkeys and cranberries, they also sampled the delights of one of the windiest vegetables known to man, the knobbly Jerusalem artichoke.

Not as celebrated as potatoes or tomatoes and never exported with quite the same passionate love/hate devotion, nonetheless the Jerusalem artichoke was a significant addition to the greater vegetable repertoire. It has since gone in and out of fashion and now hovers amongst the bevy of vegetables that are almost but not quite popular, but still beloved by many devotees.

I count myself amongst them. Jerusalem artichokes are delicious and special and still remarkably seasonal. This is a crop that belongs to the late autumn and winter, a root vegetable with the gorgeous natural sweetness that slow growth in the darkness of moist earth imparts. Knobbly they may be, but the texture of the cooked tuber is smooth and gently crisp, defying comparison with others.

There is, as the name suggests, a passing resemblance in flavour to globe artichokes but there is no way you could confuse the two. The Jerusalem artichoke is very much its own man. With one half of the name explained, you might then wonder why a native American vegetable has acquired a Levantine moniker. The answer is simple: corruption. Not fraudulent illegal corruption, but verbal. The Jerusalem artichoke is closely related to the sunflower and, like the sunflower, its open-faced flower follows the sun from morning to evening. The Italian for sunflower is 'girasole', translating literally as turning towards the sun. 'Jerusalem' is merely a mispronunciation of this, lending an added exoticism to a vegetable that has travelled far.

Not so exotic is its propensity to flatulence. Theories abound as to how to minimise the after-effects, but to be frank I've never been that bothered. Except once, when I was breastfeeding my first child. A generous helping of Jerusalem artichokes gave rise to a distinctly sleepless night, and a very cranky mother and baby. Lactating mothers apart, I would suggest that you just accept that Jerusalem artichokes will induce wind to some degree, and ignore it. The taste is too good to let a minor inconvenience put you off.

As if to make up for their inherent windiness, Jerusalem artichokes are often grown as windbreaks along the edge of a vegetable garden. They are easy and undemanding, ideal for the not-so-green-fingered gardener, reproducing silently and prolifically underground as the tall stems stretch upwards to protect less hardy plants.

Practicalities

BUYING There are two key things to bear in mind when buying Jerusalem artichokes. The first is that they should be fairly firm with just the slightest give (i.e. not as hard as a potato, but firmer than a tomato). The second is that it is worth spending a few extra seconds sorting through the box to select the least knobbly tubers. Charming and funny though the more knobbly ones look, the fact is that you are going to have to peel the wretched things at some point. Smaller knobbles will just have to be sheared off and discarded; larger ones may ultimately go the same way if you can't be bothered to peel each and every one of them. In other words, you pay for a lot of waste.

COOKING The next issue is when to peel them. My mum always used to peel them after boiling – she thought it easier – but I veer the other way, preferring to peel them before they go into any pan. The first method is probably more economical in that it minimises waste, as the skin just pulls away, but it does mean that reheating will be necessary. Peeling them first means that they can be whisked straight from the pan to the table, which suits me better. Be aware, however, that peeled raw Jerusalem artichokes discolour very quickly. Within minutes they take on a rusty colour as they oxidise. To prevent this (especially if there is to be a time lapse between peeling and cooking) drop the prepared Jerusalem artichokes into a bowl of acidulated water (i.e. water with the juice of ½ lemon, or a tablespoon or two of vinegar, swished in).

Jerusalem artichokes can be cooked in most ways. **Plainly boiled** or **steamed**, tossed with a squeeze or two of lemon and a knob of butter, and served hot is the most obvious. But equally as good (if not better) are **roast** artichokes, bundled into the oven still swaddled in their skins (no choice here), with a small slick of olive oil and a sprinkling of salt. Once cooked it is up to each consumer to decide whether to eat the skins or not.

I've often included Jerusalem artichokes in **stir-fries** (they make a rather good substitute for water chestnuts), where if you get the timings right they retain a slight crunch, alongside the characteristic sweet nuttiness. They go fantastically well with chicken in a creamy **stew**, even better encased in puff pastry to transform the stew into a pie.

PARTNERS Some people like them **raw** in salads. I don't. I do, on the other hand, like them lightly cooked and cooled in a tarragon or chervil-flecked dressing, to stand as a salad on their own, or to add to other ingredients. Nut oils – hazelnut or walnut – bring out the natural nutty taste of the vegetable. Prawns (or lobster if you fancy something really smart) and Jerusalem artichokes on a bed of watercress or rocket make a most appetising starter or main course in the middle of the cooler months. Grill or bake a rasher or two of pancetta or dry-cured bacon until crisp, perch it on top and you're heading towards perfection.

SEE ALSO GLOBE ARTICHOKES (PAGE 139).

* *

Jerusalem artichoke broth

I have fond memories of my mother making Palestine soup way, way back, in the cubbyhole of a kitchen in our holiday home in France. As a name for Jerusalem artichoke soup it now strikes one as a distinctly tasteless joke, but to be fair it pre-dates the creation of Israel in 1948. When I came to look up the soup in her *Vegetable Book* (Michael Joseph, 1978) it turns out to be a puréed cream of a soup, and not at all the clear broth studded with knobbles of sweet, semi-crisp artichoke that I thought I recalled. Memory plays strange tricks…

This is how I now prefer to make the soup, the intensity of slow-cooked vegetable sweetness shot through with a balancing measure of white wine vinegar. All in all, it is a deceptively simple creation, obviously at its best when simmered in a home-made stock, but still more than palatable when a decent instant vegetable bouillon is substituted.

Serves 6

1 large onion, halved and sliced
675 g (1½ lb) Jerusalem artichokes, peeled, halved and sliced
2 tablespoons extra virgin olive oil
4 good sprigs thyme
1 bay leaf
1 litre (1¾ pints) chicken or vegetable stock
2 tablespoons white wine vinegar

2 tablespoons roughly chopped parsley
salt and pepper

To serve (optional)
6 thick slices baguette
150 g (5 oz) single Gloucester, mature Cheddar or Gruyère cheese, coarsely grated

Put the onion, artichokes and oil into a pan and add the thyme and bay leaf, tied together with string. Cover and sweat over a low heat for some 15 minutes, stirring occasionally. Now add the stock, vinegar, salt and pepper (be generous with the pepper, please) and bring up to the boil. Simmer for 10 minutes, then taste and adjust seasoning. Discard the thyme and bay leaf and serve, sprinkled with parsley.

If using the bread and cheese, toast the baguette lightly on both sides under the grill. Then, just before serving, top with grated cheese and slide back under the grill to melt. Float a slice of cheese on toast in each bowl of soup as you serve.

Chicken and Jerusalem artichoke pie

Jerusalem artichokes impart an enormous depth of flavour to any sauce or stock they are simmered in, which is what makes this otherwise fairly classic chicken pie so appetising. For a dish like this, I use a mixture of breast and leg meat, cut into large chunks. The darker flesh stays moister throughout the double cooking.

Serves 8

500 g (1 lb 2 oz) puff pastry
plain flour
1 egg, lightly beaten

Filling
1 onion, chopped
2 cloves garlic, chopped
30 g (1 oz) butter
500 g (1 lb 2 oz) Jerusalem artichokes, peeled and cut roughly into 1.5 cm ($^5/_8$ in) thick chunks

finely grated zest of 1 orange
150 ml (5 fl oz) dry white wine
2$^1/_2$ tablespoons plain flour
300 ml (10 fl oz) chicken stock
700 g (1 lb 9 oz) boned chicken, cut into 3–4 cm (1$^1/_2$ in) chunks
150 ml (5 fl oz) double cream
salt and pepper

Begin with the filling. Fry the onion and garlic gently in the butter until tender without browning. Now add the Jerusalem artichokes, orange zest and white wine and boil down until the wine has virtually disappeared. Sprinkle over the flour and stir for a few seconds so that it is evenly distributed. Gradually stir in the stock to make a sauce. Season with salt and pepper, then stir in the chicken. Now cover and leave to simmer away quietly for some 10 minutes or so, stirring occasionally. Then uncover and simmer for 5 minutes, until the sauce has thickened. Stir in the cream and cook for a final 3 minutes. Taste and adjust the seasoning. Spoon into a 1–1.5 litre (1$^3/_4$–2$^1/_2$ pint) pie dish and leave to cool.

Roll out the pastry thinly on a floured board. Cut out a couple of long strips about 1 cm ($^1/_2$ in) wide. Brush the edge of the pie dish with the beaten egg. Lay the strips of pastry on the edge, curving to fit and cutting so that they go all the way around but don't overlap. Brush them with egg, then lay the remaining pastry over the top. Trim off excess, and press the pastry down all around the edge to seal. Use the pastry trimmings to make leaves or flowers or whatever takes your fancy, and glue them in place with the egg wash. Make a hole in the centre so that steam can escape. Chill the pie in the fridge for half an hour.

Preheat the oven to 220°C/425°F/Gas 7. Brush with egg wash and place in the oven. After 10–15 minutes, when the pastry is golden brown, reduce the heat to 190°C/375°F/Gas 5. Continue baking for a further 20–25 minutes. Serve hot.

* *

Jicama

* * *

Sometimes the best place to hide something is in a place so obvious that no-one but those in the know think to look there. Jicama is just such a cleverly hidden secret, for sale openly in our towns and cities, if only you know where to look. No point asking for it in supermarkets, in farm shops, in greengrocers, in farmers' markets. No point in asking for it by this name, either, even if you have the finest South American accent – 'hee-kah-ma'. You must, instead, replace it with a far duller name: yam bean. This is odd because it is neither yam, nor bean, and bears no resemblance to either.

It looks something like a chunky turnip, with a matt mid-brown skin. In other words, it has a thoroughly undistinguished appearance, which makes hiding it all the easier. The place to look, in this innocent game of vegetable hide and seek, is in the vegetable racks of a Chinese supermarket, where you are virtually guaranteed to discover a plentiful supply of jicama/yam bean.

Apart from the fun of the game, there is a point to tracking down a jicama or two. The point is that they are so good to eat, and so different to most other vegetables. Under the worthy brown skin, the flesh is a clean pure white. It tastes, when raw, something like green peas, and has the consistency of a large radish, juicy and crunchy and refreshing.

Practicalities

BUYING If a choice is to be had, opt for medium-sized jicama – larger ones will have begun to develop a mealier texture, which though not unpleasant is less enticing. They should be firm all over, with a matt brown skin. The skin should be unbroken – cuts or bruises suggest that rot may have set in.

In the vegetable drawer of the fridge, a jicama will last for up to a week, even when cut (cover the cut edge with clingfilm to prevent drying out). To use, you need do no more than cut out a chunk, pare off the fibrous skin, and slice or cube the white flesh.

COOKING Raw jicama is a brilliant addition to a summer salad, but my favourite way to eat it is **Mexican style**. In other words, dry-fry equal quantities of coriander and cumin seeds, grind to a powder and add cayenne to taste. Arrange the sliced jicama on a plate, squeeze over lime juice and sprinkle with the spice mixture and a little salt, before finishing with a few coriander leaves. That's it. When they are at their ripest, I add slices of orange-fleshed melon to the jicama, which makes it even more luscious. Batons of **raw** jicama are an excellent addition to a selection of crudités served with hummus or other creamy dips.

Jicama responds well to **stir-frying**, too, again on its own with just garlic and ginger to spice it up, or with other vegetables. It needs 3–4 minutes in the wok to soften it partially, without losing the sweet crunchiness entirely.

* *

Kumara

* * *

It isn't too clever to sell two different vegetables by the same name, even when they look virtually identical. However, for many years that is just what has been happening. When I was a child, the sweet potatoes that my mother brought home as an occasional treat were always white fleshed and we just adored them: roasted in their jackets until tender, then eaten slathered with salted butter.

More recently sweet potatoes have turned orange and soggy. In truth it is not a miraculous transformation, just that one (in my opinion slightly inferior) variety has replaced t'other. For a few transitionary years, you had no idea which you were buying, unless you scratched away the skin to inspect the underlying colour. Anyone with the slightest bit of sense would have seen that these vegetables should be called by different names, and at last that seems to have happened, with the happy reintroduction of the white-fleshed sweet potato, a.k.a. the kumara, to this country.

The word 'kumara' comes from the Maori name for the white-fleshed *Ipomoea batatas*. They are, as you might well infer from this, extremely popular in New Zealand, and indeed in many places around the Pacific. Their country of origin is thought to be Mexico, where roast kumara are sold by street vendors, to be anointed with condensed milk and eaten as a pudding rather than a vegetable. Try it some time and see how good it is.

Kumara is also the sweet potato used widely in the Caribbean for making pies and dumplings. The orange-fleshed sweet potato is not a good substitute here, as the flesh is too watery and lacks the necessary starch to bind ingredients together.

So the point that I'm trying to make is this: kumara are downright gorgeous and you really should try them if you haven't already. They are still not exactly commonplace but at least one of the larger supermarket chains is importing them regularly, and you may well find them in Caribbean food stores. Go search and you will be well rewarded.

Practicalities

BUYING If you have the choice, pick out kumara that are on the larger side, with firm, smooth, dark pink-brown skin. Bruises and soft patches, as always, warn you to steer clear. Cut ends will be a dirty greyish colour, but don't let this bother you – it's just a spot of oxidisation, not a sign of something disturbing.

Kumara like to be kept in a cool, airy, dark spot, which is not the fridge. Over-chilled kumara develop a tougher centre, at least that's what producers say. In practice, I've found that a day or two in the fridge doesn't make any noticeable difference to the texture once cooked, which is handy if you don't happen to have a cool, airy, dark spot to hand. Better the fridge, I find, than a warm kitchen where they are likely to start sprouting.

Longer term storage (they should keep nicely for up to a fortnight) and you really ought to treat them as they prefer – try wrapping them individually in a couple of sheets of newspaper to exclude light and absorb any humidity in the air.

COOKING In terms of preparation, remarkably little is required. Give them a rinse, trim off discoloured ends and voilà, one kumara ready for the pot.

Or the oven. Which is exactly where you should start if you have never eaten kumara before. Just don't stall there, as many people do. Yes, **baked** kumara are delicious, but that's first base. You bake them just as if they were ordinary potatoes, in other words, prick the skin and then put them straight into the oven at somewhere around 180–200°C/350–400°F/Gas 4–6. Size will dictate how long they take to cook, but think in the region of 45–60 minutes. Split them open and serve with salted butter, or flaked Parmesan or Cheddar, or a great big dollop of Greek-style yoghurt. Remember that if you are eating them with the main course, you will need to partner them with something salty – I find that they are rather good with bacon, or even with tapenade. Excellent, too, with sausages.

Americans and New Zealanders like to surmount their baked kumara with other sweet things like pineapple, grated apple or dates (hmmm), or drizzle orange juice over them, which makes far more sense to me.

So, once you've done the oven experience, it's time to move on. Kumara

Roots . 47

can be cooked in most of the ways that suit potatoes, i.e. **sautéed, chipped, roast, mashed** or **boiled** (a bit dull, frankly). Additionally, kumara can even be eaten **raw**, or transformed into **pudding**. I've tried it raw, grated into a salad. It's okay, but not something to write home about. Pudding, on the other hand, is a natural end for the chestnutty kumara. Think that's odd? Just try making a kumara fool (see recipes) and then tell me that it's not pretty impressive.

PARTNERS In recent days, I've sautéed cubes of kumara with diced spicy chorizo, which was very successful, and then taken more sautéed kumara and tossed it with rocket and feta and a vigorous lime juice, chilli and sunflower oil dressing to serve as a first course. Mashed kumara are good on their own, seasoned fully to balance the sweetness, or speckled with finely chopped spring onion or coriander. I rather fancy a smoked haddock fish cake held together with cooked kumara (slightly more smoked haddock than kumara, I think), though I haven't tried it yet.

Also good, and I say this from experience, is a kumara **cake** – just substitute grated kumara for the carrot in the recipe on page 28. Fantastic.

SEE ALSO SWEET POTATOES (PAGE 91).

* *

Smoky Parmesan roasted kumara cubes

Just damn gorgeous, these are. They're wolfed down by one and all whenever I make them. There is something utterly irresistible about the combination of sweet kumara with a salty, crisp cheesy crust and a hint of hot smoke from the Spanish pimentón. They probably should go with something (a real burger, perhaps, or roast pheasant) but you might just make them as a snack when the right moment comes.

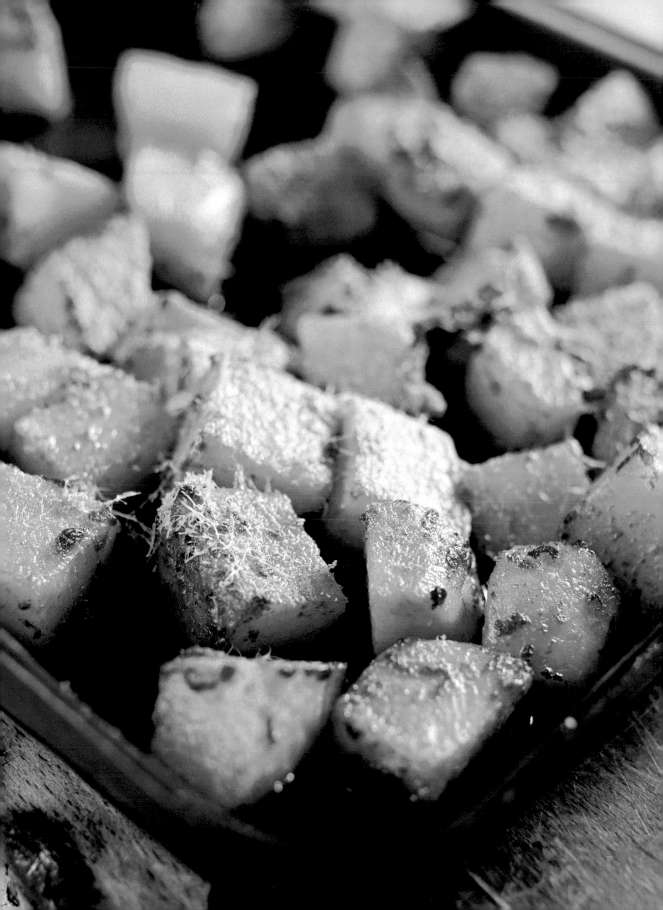

Serves 6

600 g (1 lb 5 oz) kumara
30 g (1 oz) Parmesan, freshly grated
1 heaped teaspoon Spanish smoked
 paprika (pimentón)
3 tablespoons olive oil
salt

Preheat the oven to 200°C/400°F/Gas 6. Cut the kumara into 2 cm (scant 1 in) cubes. Blanch in boiling salted water for 4 minutes, then drain thoroughly. Toss with the Parmesan, paprika, salt and oil.

Put a roasting tin or baking tray in the oven for 5 minutes to heat through really well. Take out of the oven and quickly tip the kumara on to the hot tray. Spread out in a single layer, then dash it back into the oven before the tray loses any more heat. Roast for 20 minutes, turning once, until golden brown and tender. Eat while still hot, but not so hot that they burn your mouth.

* *

Kumara crème brûlée

The Brits tend to like their kumara and sweet potato served along with the main course, salted and savoury, but they are in fact sweet and suave enough to work nicely in puddings. And if you don't believe me, just give this one a try.

Mashed with cream and eggs, kumara become as smooth as butter. Add a little heat and they bake to form a tender custardy mixture that is perfect topped with a crisp crust of sugar. Although many traditional recipes partner them with cinnamon and other warm spices, I prefer to add vanilla to highlight their chestnut-like taste.

Serves 6–8

1 kg (2¼ lb) kumara, give or take
30 g (1 oz) unsalted butter
30 g (1 oz) caster sugar
1 teaspoon vanilla extract

200 ml (7 fl oz) whipping cream
4 egg yolks

To finish
caster sugar

Bake the kumara in their skins just as if they were potatoes, or peel and boil until tender and drain thoroughly.

Preheat the oven (or reduce the temperature if you've baked the kumara) to 140°C/275°F/Gas 1. Weigh out 350g (12oz) of the hot kumara flesh, then mash with the butter and sugar until smooth. Now stir in the vanilla, cream and egg yolks. Divide among 6–8 ramekins. Stand them in a roasting tin and pour enough water into the tin to come about 2cm (scant 1in) up the sides of the ramekins. Place in the oven and leave to cook for about 40 minutes until just firm. Take out of the oven and lift the ramekins out of the hot water, then cool, cover and chill in the fridge.

Up to 2 hours before eating, preheat the grill thoroughly. Sprinkle the surface of each baked kumara custard with a thick layer of caster sugar, then place under the grill. Don't get them too close to the heat – as with any crème brûlée, they need to be close enough for the heat to melt the sugar, but not so close that it burns before it liquefies and caramelises. As the sugar begins to melt, turn the custards every few minutes so that they caramelise fairly evenly. Take out and leave to cool and set. Eat with a little whipped cream.

* *

Kumara fool

Make as for the crème brûlées above, but leave out the egg yolks and beat in a little more cream. Don't cook the mixture – just spoon into bowls and serve as it is.

* *

Oca

* * *

Will the oca ever make it big in Europe? It ought to. It could…and I for one will be cheering when it does. This small tuber grows well enough here, but its real home is far, far away, up in the chilly heights of the Andes. And in Bolivia, Ecuador and Peru it is rated almost as highly as its compatriot, the potato. I first came across oca in a market north of Quito, the capital of Ecuador. It was the last stop of our holiday, so back came my haul of oca in the suitcase (smuggled in, if you must). We ate some, we grew some. We loved them. Almost end of story.

In fact that would have been the end, if I hadn't spotted oca for sale here at home a couple of times in the past decade. If you are blessed enough to stumble across a rare basket of oca up for grabs, take them at once. The flavour of the fresh tuber lies somewhere between that of a new potato and a tart green apple, with a mealy, soft texture. Very good and just unusual enough to be interesting, without being weird.

The tart, appley tang comes courtesy of a splash of oxalic acid. If this sounds dismaying, reflect that this same acid gives rhubarb its distinctive sourness, far more astringent than the humble oca. Mind you, there are literally hundreds of varieties of oca grown down the backbone of the Andes and they vary from highly acidic to incredibly mild. The sharper varieties are not eaten fresh, but given a 'soleado', or a sunning. Left out in the sunshine for up to two weeks, the acidity dampens right down and starches turn to sugars. The result is an even smaller tuber, but with a startling sweetness closer to a sweet potato than any mouth-puckering stem of pink rhubarb. Dehydrated and frozen oca, known as 'chaya', are stashed away for leaner times.

The oca has travelled less than many vegetables, but it has at least dashed across the oceans to New Zealand where it is grown commercially in a small way. Here it is known simply as the New Zealand yam, despite not being a yam at all, or Maori potato, or more interestingly, as 'uwhikaho', or 'uwhi' for short.

Practicalities

BUYING The commonest of oca, the ones that I've come across, are relatively small – say about 10 cm (4 in) long – have a waxy reddish skin and a crinkled form. In fact, they look a little like pink fir apple potatoes. Unlike most vegetables, freshness is not critical. Smooth skinned, plump oca will be gifted with a more distinct note of acidity than those that are beginning to shrivel a little having had time to develop more sweetness. In other words, this is a two-in-one vegetable, which is a rare and delightful gift from Mother Nature. So, as long as they have been stored well, wrinkles are not to be derided. Soft damp patches or worse still, a hint of mould, are not good things on the other hand. However, since you are not likely to come across oca frequently, you can't really afford to be too choosy. Just throw out any that are beyond saving.

Oca, as you may well have inferred, keep well in the right conditions. The vegetable drawer in the fridge is just fine, but if the sun is shining, you might prefer to spread them out on trays outside (cover with muslin if you have some to hand, to protect from flies) to sweeten up a little. You can even freeze them – not a bad idea if you've found a rare clutch of oca for sale. As with any other vegetable, damp is destructive, so keep them dry.

COOKING Oca can be eaten **raw**, especially the sweeter sunned ones, say in a salad, or cut into strips to dip into a chillied tomatoey dip perhaps. I prefer them cooked, exactly as you would a potato. In other words, rinse them, trim off ends, but don't even attempt to peel. Then **boil** them in salted water until tender. They can also be **roasted** in the oven, coated in a little olive oil to prevent drying out, or **steamed**, or **sautéed**. They make heavenly **crisps**, but perhaps that is something to save for a time when oca have hit the big time and are as widely available here as they are in the highlands of Ecuador.

Parsnips

* * *

The parsnip is an honest vegetable. No airs and graces, no pretensions to grandeur, no fancy frills and ribbons. It has a solid sunny nature, the kind that one can rely on time and time again. You can trust a parsnip – trust it to come out well, to cook up nicely, to sit comfortably alongside most winter dishes. Your parsnip doesn't fade into the background – there's no doubting its presence – just takes a comfortable stance amongst the other elements on a plate.

I like parsnips a lot, saving them for the colder months of the year, which in the past was the only time when you ever got them. Until recently, no parsnip was worth eating if it hadn't been touched by a frost or two. Now we get them all year round. That's modern varieties for you. So maybe I'm being a stick-in-the-mud when I ignore summer parsnips, invariably perfectly shaped and clean as a whistle. Although I know that you can, for instance, make a handsome salad with lightly cooked parsnips, I'm really not that interested when the sun is hot, or even tepid, in the way of so many summer days.

Parsnip is a comfort vegetable, one that rides to the rescue when the courgettes have long since swelled to marrows. Plain buttered parsnip is nice, mashed parsnip good, parsnip crisps excellent and roast parsnips totally irresistible. Frosts may no longer be crucial to the success of the parsnip, but nature has a habit of getting things right. Parsnips are definitely better adapted to cold weather, natural fodder for us humans when the cold weather sets in, but well out of kilter with the warmth of summer.

Practicalities

BUYING Most of my adult life, I've bought parsnips from either a greengrocer, or from the supermarket, clean as a whistle and ready to cook. I've never been disappointed. Until recently. Until I signed up for a weekly veg box and began to receive the occasional helping of dirty parsnips amongst other vegetables. They have been something of a revelation, inducing retrospective disappointment for all those parsnips that have fallen short of these paragons over the years. Yes, I am now convinced that it is worth scrubbing the jacket of earth off those long ivory roots, just for the exquisite flavour that lies underneath. These have been the best parsnips I have ever encountered, putting all others in the shade. That mucky soil coating does indeed keep flavour locked in, just like my mum always said (actually, she was usually talking about potatoes, but the theory is the same). Look out for the muckiest roots you can find next time you visit a winter farmers' market and leap on them with glee. As long as the dirt is not there to mask stale parsnips pulled far too long before from the ground, I have no doubt that you will notice the improved taste.

The trouble with this, of course, is that nice, neat, scrubbed parsnips will begin to disappoint. Nothing to be done about that. If you can't buy them dirty, buy them clean and be sure to pick out roots that are firm and not too heavily blemished. They'll keep for a few days, but not as long as carrots, I find. Flabby, aged parsnips are not only dull in taste, but also a complete pain to prepare. Put them in the compost bin and vow not to forget about good parsnips again.

COOKING I like my parsnips peeled, but with organic ones this is not strictly necessary, especially if you have very small parsnips that can be cooked whole. What is necessary with sizeable parsnips is the disposal of the woody core. Cut the fatter parts of the parsnips in quarters lengthways and lop out the white heart – another candidate for the compost bin – before cooking.

Most recipes for parsnips begin with a spell in **boiling** water (just long enough to soften, but not so long that they go mushy) but after that they will almost certainly demand something more. 'Kind words butter no parsnips' is an old saying, distinctly out of vogue in the 21st century when kind words are considered essential to the development of children, dogs and houseplants. But way back when it was heard tripping from the tongues of the wise and wealthy, toughness was an altogether more praiseworthy quality for training the young and the wayward. The point here is the essential buttering of those parsnips. There is no debate on this issue.

Parsnips, lovely vegetables that they are, are magically enhanced by lashings of butter or good oil, or dripping, or cream: butter on boiled parsnips, cream and/or butter in mashed parsnips, goose fat or oil and a touch of butter for roast parsnips.

The soft, starchy nature of parsnips makes them candidates for any sort of **mashing** or **puréeing**. Straight parsnip mash is perhaps too intensely sweet for most tastes – I find it nicer mashed with, say, half the volume of cooked potatoes, as well, of course, as butter, milk or cream, salt and a heavy dose of freshly grated nutmeg, or a few pinches of cinnamon. Parsnip and potato mash makes a fine topping for old-fashioned cottage, shepherd's or fish pie.

Alternatively, you could **purée** the parsnip with plenty of thick béchamel sauce, again softening the total parsnip essence. This mixture can be turned into a **gratin** of sorts, by mixing in an egg or two, spreading out thickly in an ovenproof dish, scattering the top with freshly grated Parmesan mixed with equal quantities of breadcrumbs plus a few dots of butter and then sliding the whole lot into a hot oven to cook until browned and bubbling. Very good indeed.

Parsnip **soups** are terrific too, made along classic soup lines, pepped up with curry (see recipes) or with fresh root ginger, cut half in half with apple or pear, or aromatised with lemon thyme. Croûtons or crisp grilled bacon or pancetta are excellent with parsnip soups.

My mother occasionally treated us to Saratoga **chips**. 'Saratoga chips' was the original name for potato crisps, supposedly invented by a disgruntled chef in the town of Saratoga, but my mother's Saratoga chips were proper British chips, made with parsnip. Great name, great treat. Par-boil 'chips' of parsnip, being really, really attentive so that they don't overcook to a pap. Drain well and dry, then deep-fry until golden brown and serve sprinkled with grains of salt. So good. Parsnip **fritters** are pretty appealing too – again parboil pieces of parsnip, then dip into either a beer batter or a tempura batter and deep-fry until crisp and golden brown. Serve with wedges of lemon, and salt flavoured with crushed toasted cumin. For a smarter starter fritter, cube par-cooked parsnip and stir into the beer batter along with roughly chopped small shelled prawns or shrimps, then fry spoonfuls in hot oil until golden brown.

I often add parsnips to **stews**, just 20 minutes or so before the stew finishes cooking so that they have time to absorb some of the flavours, but not so long that they collapse. They are good in a chicken stew, but even better in an earthy beef stew.

And finally, try baking a parsnip **cake** – replace the carrots with grated parsnips in the recipe on page 28. You'll be amazed at how good the cake is, and you can keep your family and friends guessing the mystery ingredient for hours.

* *

Tortilla-wrapped refried parsnips

Tortilla night at Hacienda Grigson, but madre mia, no beans to refry!!! And then we thought – wait a moment, hold on, but wouldn't the starchy texture of parsnips work rather well as a substitute? And you know what, they were better than a mere substitute, bringing a welcome new vigour to what has become one of my family's favourite suppers.

The parsnips, incidentally, can be cooked and mashed with their spices and onion way before they are needed, then gently reheated just before serving. The salsa positively benefits from being made an hour or so in advance, leaving time for the flavours to meld and develop.

Serves 4

750 g (1 lb 10 oz) parsnips
2 teaspoons cumin seeds
1/2 teaspoon ground turmeric
4 tablespoons extra virgin olive oil
1 small onion, chopped
1 clove garlic, crushed
salt and pepper

Salsa
250 g (9 oz) sweet tomatoes, deseeded and
  finely chopped
1 shallot, finely chopped
1 clove garlic, crushed

1–2 red chillies, deseeded and finely
  chopped
1/2 teaspoon dried oregano
2 tablespoons chopped coriander leaves
juice of 1 lime

To serve
8 corn tortillas
125 g (4 1/2 oz) feta cheese, crumbled
6 crisp young lettuce leaves, shredded
pickled jalapeño chillies
1 avocado, peeled, sliced and tossed in a
  little extra lime juice
150 ml (5 fl oz) soured cream

For the salsa, merely mix all the ingredients together, then set aside at room temperature.

Prepare the parsnips as normal and cut into big chunks. Bring a pan of water to the boil (not too big, please) and stir in half the cumin seeds, all the turmeric and some salt. Now add the parsnip pieces and cook until tender. Drain, reserving some of the cooking water.

Heat the olive oil in a frying pan and fry the onion with the garlic and remaining cumin seeds until tender. Pile in the parsnips and, as they sizzle in the oil, mash them up roughly with a large fork. After about 3–4 minutes, add 3 tablespoons of the cooking water to moisten them, and carry on frying and mashing for a few more minutes until you end up with a thick, fragrant, rough mash, golden and appetising.

Just before serving, wrap the corn tortillas in foil and heat through in a low oven, or alternatively wrap in clingfilm and heat through in the microwave (check packet for timings). Put all the other extras into separate bowls and place them on the table, along with the salsa. Spoon the parsnips into a bowl and place on the table along with the hot tortillas.

It's all ready to go now. Each diner takes a tortilla and adds a big spoonful of parsnip mash, spreading it roughly down the diameter of the tortilla, then tops it with as much cheese, salsa, lettuce, extra chillies, avocado and soured cream as they fancy. Then that lucky person just rolls it all up and takes a great big bite.

Parsnip and ham gratin

This is a terrific supper dish. Ham and parsnip are happy bedfellows, but need a good dose of spiky mustard in the sauce to bring them to life.

Serves 4

8 wee parsnips, or 4 big chunky parsnips
15 g (½ oz) butter
8 slices very nice cooked ham indeed
30 g (1 oz) Parmesan, freshly grated

Sauce
30 g (1 oz) butter
30 g (1 oz) plain flour
600 ml (1 pint) milk
2 tablespoons coarse-grain or Dijon
  mustard
salt, pepper and freshly grated nutmeg

Preheat the oven to 200°C/400°F/Gas 6.

Peel the parsnips. Boil small ones whole until just tender. With great big boys, you'll need to quarter them lengthways and cut out the tough cores, before boiling them until just tender. As soon as the parsnips are cooked, drain, run under the cold tap and then drain again, really, really thoroughly.

To make the sauce, melt the butter and stir in the flour. Stir over a gentle heat for about 1 minute, then draw off the heat. Gradually stir in the milk, just a slurp at a time until you have a thick, smooth cream, then add more generously, stirring it in well each time. Bring back to the boil, stirring and scraping the bottom and sides of the pan. Let the sauce simmer genteely now, for a good 5–10 minutes, stirring occasionally, until thickened pleasingly. Mix in the mustard, salt, pepper and a keen grating of nutmeg. Taste and adjust the seasoning.

Butter a baking dish with a little of the 15 g (½ oz) butter, and spoon a little of the sauce into the dish. Wrap the small parsnips individually in slices of ham. With the larger, quartered ones, wrap two quarters together in each slice of ham. Lay the rolls of ham and parsnip side by side in the dish, then pour over the remaining sauce. Sprinkle the Parmesan evenly over the top, dot with the remaining butter and slide into the oven. Bake for about 20 minutes, until golden brown and bubbling. Serve straightaway.

Thai-curried parsnip soup

Many moons ago, sometime in the 1970s, my mother, the food writer Jane Grigson, came up with a great idea – curried parsnip soup. It's an idea that has gone mainstream, with variations and personalisations aplenty. This is my homage to her brilliant and innovative concept. As with her original, the wonderful sweetness of parsnip is balanced and beautified by the use of spices – this time round it's ginger and lemongrass, aided by frisky doses of lime and fish sauce.

Serves 3–4

2 tablespoons sunflower or vegetable oil
2 fresh red chillies, deseeded and chopped
500 g (1 lb 2 oz) parsnips, peeled, roughly cut up and cored if necessary
1 onion, chopped
2 cloves garlic, chopped
2.5 cm (1 in) piece fresh root ginger or galangal, peeled and chopped
2 stems lemongrass

300–450 ml (10–15 fl oz) vegetable or chicken stock
2 tablespoons fish sauce
1 x 400 ml can coconut milk
juice of 1 lime
a handful of coriander leaves
a handful of Thai or Mediterranean basil leaves
a handful of mint

Put the oil, chillies, parsnips, onion, garlic and ginger (or galangal) into a fairly large pan. Cut off and discard the top of each stem of lemongrass, leaving the lower, fatter 10 cm (4 in) or so. Using either a meat mallet, the end of a rolling pin or the flat of a wide-bladed knife (press down on it firmly with your fist), semi-flatten the lemongrass stems so that they stay more or less in one piece, but are sufficiently damaged to release their extraordinary flavour. Add them to the pan. Give the contents a quick stir, then cover and place over a gentle heat. Leave to sweat gently, checking once, for about 10 minutes.

Now add the lower quantity of stock and the fish sauce. Bring up to the boil, then simmer quietly, uncovered, for 10–15 minutes until the parsnip is very tender. Fish out the lemongrass and stir in the coconut milk, then liquidise the soup, adding some or all of the remaining stock if you find the soup too thick.

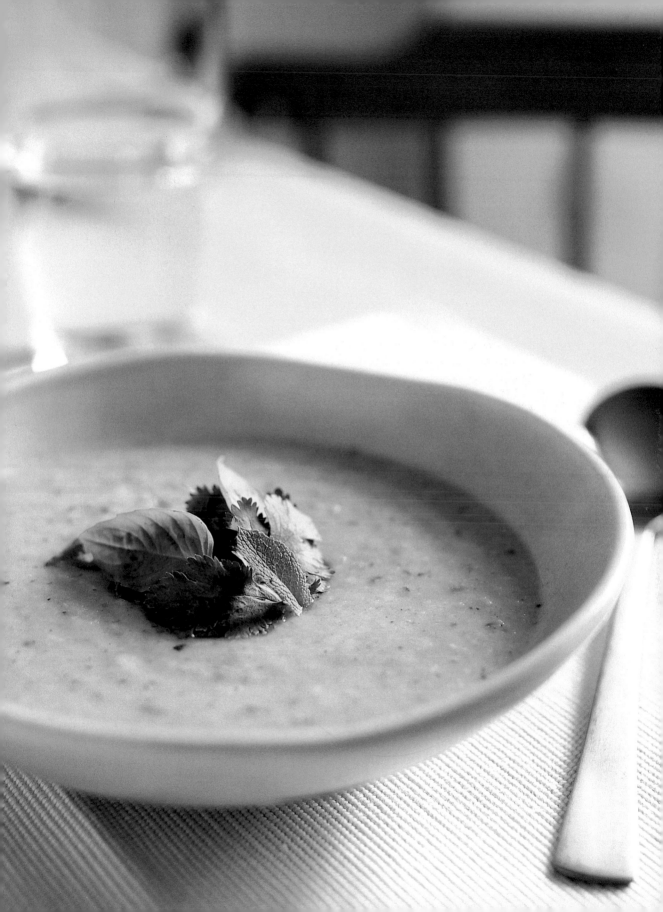

When nearly ready to eat, reheat the soup. Stir in the lime juice, then taste and adjust the seasoning, adding more fish sauce if it tastes under-salted. Mix the fresh herbs together, roughly tearing up larger leaves of basil or mint. As you serve the hot soup, top each bowlful with a small mound of fresh herbs.

* *

Potatoes

* * *

Some vegetables go in and out of fashion. The potato just stays put, miraculously straddling fashion and permanence without stumbling. Rather like Shakespeare, but with a far broader fan-base. It has a fascinating but well-documented history which I shall skate over blithely: originating in the Andes, hitting Europe in the 16th century, greeted with deep suspicion but eventually taking root big time, both literally and metaphorically, unwitting cause of the Irish famine. I would go into more detail, but as a subject the potato deserves a book of its own, and many excellent tomes have already been written on the subject. Search one out, read and marvel at this most extraordinary of commonplace items.

Practicalities

BUYING Much of what follows will be well known to anyone who cooks or eats, but read on if you have time, for hidden away amongst the general knowledge you may find a few useful hints.

More and more, in farm shops and the few remaining specialist greengrocers, sellers are having the courtesy to let us know the varietal name of the potatoes they sell. This is a good thing, and supermarkets have done their best to emulate it. Why shouldn't we choose potatoes in the way that we choose apples? Sure, we may not be able to hold the specific attributes of ten different types of potato in our head at all times, but there's pleasure to be had in stumbling across a favoured variety, that we know tastes good, and pleasure to be had in discovering that whilst one variety is fluffy and dry fleshed, another is smoother and waxier and has a distinct undertone of almonds.

Broadly speaking potatoes fall into two main categories, each more suited to certain styles of cooking than others. The dominant category is that of the **maincrop** potatoes, larger to very large, with a drier, mealy flesh, in season from late summer onwards into the cold months. Smaller but highly valued are the **waxy** potatoes, a group that includes junior new potatoes as well as what are known as 'salad potatoes' which retain their dense waxy texture right into maturity. The rightful season of the new potato is from late spring through to midsummer by which time they are tipping from adolescence into maincrop adulthood. Salad potatoes are harvested later, from maybe July on into the autumn.

Of course, these seasons for potatoes are now all but obliterated. Modern farming methods, imports and long storage mean that we can and do enjoy any sort of potato at any time of the year. And yet... there is a natural harmony (as always) in the old-fangled seasons. In winter we crave all those warm, caressing comfort dishes that can only be made with maincrop potatoes – steaming jacket potatoes, creamy mash, crisp-coated roasties or finger-burning fresh-fried chips. Then as the ground warms, food lightens and new and salad potatoes are in the ascendant, so exactly right with a piece of poached salmon, or grilled chicken breast, or thick slices of ham with a zesty salad. Nothing then supersedes the rightness of a good potato salad, critical side dish at a barbecue, on a picnic and at a summer wedding.

Choosing the right potato for the job in hand is important, although all rules are made to be broken. Just get to know them first, before you attempt flagrant breaches. In other words use chunky maincrop potatoes for: baking, mashing, boiling, roasting, deep-frying, sautéing, adding to doughs to lighten them (e.g. in potato bread, or potato scones), gratins and so on. Save new potatoes for: boiling, salads, sautéing, gratins, and roasting whole. Yes, there are overlaps, but the results will differ with the potato variety used.

I've had to concede, reluctantly, that my mother was right when she insisted that one should always buy dirty potatoes. A thin jacket of dried-on muck does indeed seem to preserve flavour to some extent. Not critical, but a bonus if you are prepared to spend a couple of extra minutes at the sink scrubbing them clean. Dirt or no dirt, glance over potatoes as you pick them out to ensure that they are free from bruised machinery gashes, mouldering patches (a sign of poor storage), sprouting shoots, and above all patches of green. That charming green coloration tells you that the potatoes have been exposed to light for too long, thus developing poisonous toxins. Not a good thing.

Maincrop and salad potatoes can be kept for some time in the right conditions (a dark, cool, dry place) but new potatoes have a short shelf life. Eat them within a few days of purchase to enjoy them at their best. Don't leave either sort of potato in a closed plastic bag for any longer than is necessary – moisture will gather in its folds, and sooner or later your potatoes will start to rot.

Don't keep potatoes in the fridge, or at least not for more than a day or two. In the icy claustrophobic atmosphere, the starches in the potato mutate into sugars, which, while not cataclysmic, is not really appropriate for most potato dishes.

COOKING   With their light flavour, and engaging textures, there is no end to the ways in which one can use potatoes. Potato recipes abound right around the globe, in each region gilding the basic lily with characteristic local ingredients to mould them into the local cuisine. They are just so darned versatile, a word that I loathe, but which is absolutely right in this context. For this reason I'm not going to list a chapter of ideas for how to embellish potatoes. Once you can make silky mash, bake jacket potatoes, turn out perfect crisp roast potatoes, sauté diced potatoes, and conjure up a mean potato salad, you will have mastered all the essential techniques you need to create almost any potato dish ever invented. The rest, frankly, is just a question of exercising your curiosity and imagination.

Mash

The marvellous yet confusing thing about making mashed potatoes is that there is no absolute one-and-only ideal recipe. I happen to think that perfect mashed potatoes are as smooth as silk, not quite runny, but nowhere near stiff, with plenty of nutmeg and butter to boot. You may disagree. Once you are in control of the basics, however, you can adjust method, ingredients and quantities endlessly to suit your own credo.

My mum always baked potatoes for mash and so do I – the flesh is drier and has a more distinct flavour. Microwaved potatoes are good too. Boiling comes next in line, as long as you use evenly sized potatoes and boil them in their skins. As soon as they are drained, cover with a clean tea-towel and leave to steam-dry for 5–10 minutes before peeling off the skins. Don't peel potatoes and cut into chunks before boiling – they will just get waterlogged and lose much of their taste to the water, producing a dull, flat-tasting mash.

Good varieties for mashing are King Edward, Maris Piper, Golden Wonder, and Kerr's Pink (my favourite), amongst others.

Mashed potatoes are a perfect receptor for all kinds of extra, zippy ingredients – try stirring in some coarse-grain mustard or a spoonful of creamed horseradish. The Irish love to add chopped spring onions softened in butter or cooked cabbage, or you could go ultra modern and mix in roughly chopped rocket leaves and the finely grated zest of a lemon.

Serves 4

1 kg (2 1/4 lb) floury maincrop potatoes
115 g (4 oz) butter, at room temperature
150–300 ml (5–10 fl oz) hot milk, or a mixture
  of milk and cream
salt and freshly grated nutmeg

Either bake or boil the potatoes in their skins (see above). Halve baked potatoes while still warm and scoop their flesh out into a bowl. Save skins for making crisp-roast potato skins (see page 75). Peel boiled potatoes while still warm and place in a bowl. Add the butter.

Now the mashing itself. For a really smooth mash use one of the following methods:

  a) push the potato little by little through a potato ricer

  b) rub the potato through a vegetable mill (mouli-légumes)

  c) mash roughly with a fork, then whisk with a hand-held electric whisk until light and fluffy

  d) mash roughly with a fork, then rub through a sieve.

Scrape the puréed potato into a saucepan and place over a gentle heat. Add plenty of seasoning and about a third of the hot milk (or milk and cream). Beat hard with a wooden spoon, gradually adding more milk until the mash hits the kind of consistency that sets your mouth watering. Taste and adjust seasoning, and serve.

* *

Sage and onion mash

Chop 1 onion and fry in a little butter or oil until golden brown. Cover 10 leaves of fresh sage with boiling water (to release more flavour). Drain immediately, dry the leaves and chop roughly. Stir sage and onions into a bowl of hot mash made as above.

* *

Roast potatoes

Perfect roast potatoes with a crackling crisp crust masking a melting, fluffy interior are rarer than they should be. The method is not hard, but it requires some forethought. The potatoes must be par-cooked in advance, then roughed up in order to develop that irresistible golden brown, crusty exterior.

If you are cooking a roast, don't tuck the potatoes around the meat, but roast them in a separate tin, large enough to spread the potatoes out in an even single layer, not jam-packed in tightly.

The best fats to use are melted lard or dripping (without the jelly), olive oil or sunflower oil or, best of all, goose fat (available in cans and jars). I prefer to use either Cara potatoes, which have a smooth texture, or end-of-season large new potatoes, but for a fluffier interior head for the old faithfuls – King Edward, Maris Piper, Désirée, Estima and their kin.

Serves 4

1.3 kg (3 lb) large potatoes
6 tablespoons goose fat,
  lard, olive oil or sunflower oil
salt

Preheat the oven to 200°C/400°F/Gas 6.

Peel the potatoes and cut into medium-sized chunks – say about 5 cm (2 in) across. Cook in boiling salted water until three-quarters cooked – around 5–6 minutes. Drain thoroughly. Use a fork to scratch criss-cross lines all over the surfaces of each chunk of potato, roughing up the exterior so that it crisps perfectly.

Put the fat in a large roasting tin and slide into the oven. Heat through for 5–8 minutes. Quickly take the tin out and add the potatoes. Turn so that they are all coated in hot fat. Return immediately to the oven. Roast for about 40–50 minutes, turning the potatoes after the first 25 minutes and then again once or twice more, until they are browned and crisp all over.

Serve straightaway.

* *

Chips

Who doesn't love chips? And the best chips of all are those you make at home, from scratch. Frying up a batch of real chips is not something you will want to do every day, but as an occasional treat they're worth every moment of standing over a hot pan.

Chips are fried twice, the first time at a gentle heat to just soften them right through to the centre, the second time at a higher heat to brown the outside. You can do the first batch of frying ahead of time, but leave the second hot, hot, hot session until just before serving. If you use an electric deep-fryer the temperatures are easy to gauge. If you don't then it is worth investing in a food thermometer.

Good varieties for chips include King Edward, Maris Piper and Désirée. Cara give a slightly waxier texture which I love but if you prefer a fluffier centre stick with one of the first three.

Serves 3–4

3 large potatoes
sunflower or vegetable oil for deep-frying
salt

Peel the potatoes and cut into slices about 1 cm (½ in) thick. Cut lengthways into batons of about the same thickness. Cover with cold water to prevent browning, until you are almost ready to cook them.

Set the oil to heat up. The right heat for the first fry is 150°C/300°F. Drain the potatoes then dry them thoroughly on kitchen paper or clean tea-towels. Deep-fry in several batches so that the temperature of the oil is not lowered too much, allowing them to cook for about 4 minutes, without browning, until tender right through. Drain on kitchen paper and leave to cool.

Just before serving, reheat the oil, this time to 180°C/350°F. Deep-fry the chips, again in batches, until golden brown.

The only thing you need to do now is drain and salt the chips. The best way to do this is in a large brown paper bag. Yes, honestly. Tip the chips into the bag, add plenty of salt, fold over the top and shake – the bag absorbs excess fat, and the salt gets evenly distributed. If you don't have a brown paper bag to hand, drain the chips briefly on a triple layer of kitchen paper, then sprinkle with salt. Serve straightaway while still good and hot.

* *

Baked potatoes

Baked potatoes are fabulous comfort food, and so easy. Just pop them into a hot oven when you get home from work, go and have a bath or a glass of wine, or whatever unwinds you after a hard day, then an hour later they emerge, steaming hot, crisp outside and gorgeously tender inside. Whether you dish them up as the main part of a meal with a sumptuous topping, or as a side order, baked potatoes are warming and reassuring, and of course, they taste just fine too.

For each person you need one large baking potato – any large maincrop potato will do the job nicely. Prick the skin all over with a fork to prevent it bursting during cooking. Now you have choices to make. You can a) leave the potato just as it is, or b) dampen it and rub salt into the skin – this gives a deliciously salty skin – or c) rub oil all over the skin, to make the skin crisper, or d) go for both oil and salt or e) wrap the potato in foil for a tender, soft-skinned potato.

Once you've reached a decision and finished preparing your potato, bake for 50–60 minutes or until tender right through. Test by pushing a skewer into the centre. Once the potato is cooked, cover with a cloth and let it sit for 5 minutes before cutting open – this makes the flesh fluffier and lighter.

One final point – if you're rushed for time, push a skewer lengthways through the centre of the potato before putting it into the oven. The skewer conducts heat directly to the centre of the potato so that it cooks more quickly.

* *

Roast new potatoes with thyme and lemon

Little new potatoes are delicious roasted in the oven. They cook to a wonderful, melting tenderness that is just irresistible. The sharpness of the lemon pieces is particularly good with them.

Serves 4

1 kg (2¼ lb) small new
   potatoes
6 sprigs thyme
1 lemon
4 tablespoons extra virgin
   olive oil
salt

Preheat the oven to 220°C/425°F/Gas 7. Put the potatoes and thyme in a roasting tin or ovenproof dish – it should be large enough to take them all in a single layer. Cut the lemon into 8 wedges, then cut each wedge into 3 pieces. Add them to the potatoes then drizzle over the olive oil and sprinkle with salt. Turn the potatoes and lemon until all are coated in oil.

Bake for 40–45 minutes, stirring twice during that time, until the potatoes are patched with brown and very tender. Serve hot.

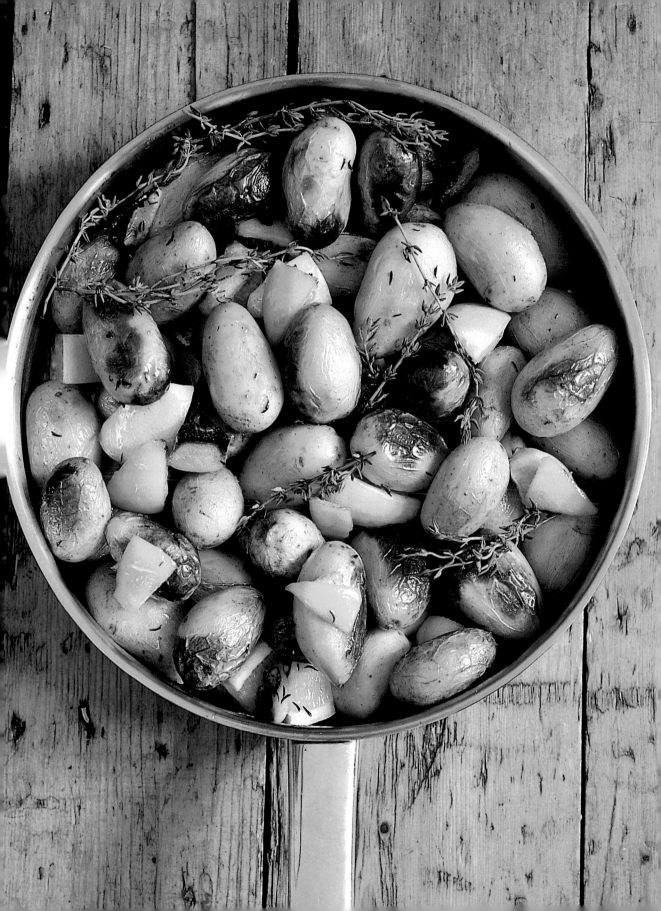

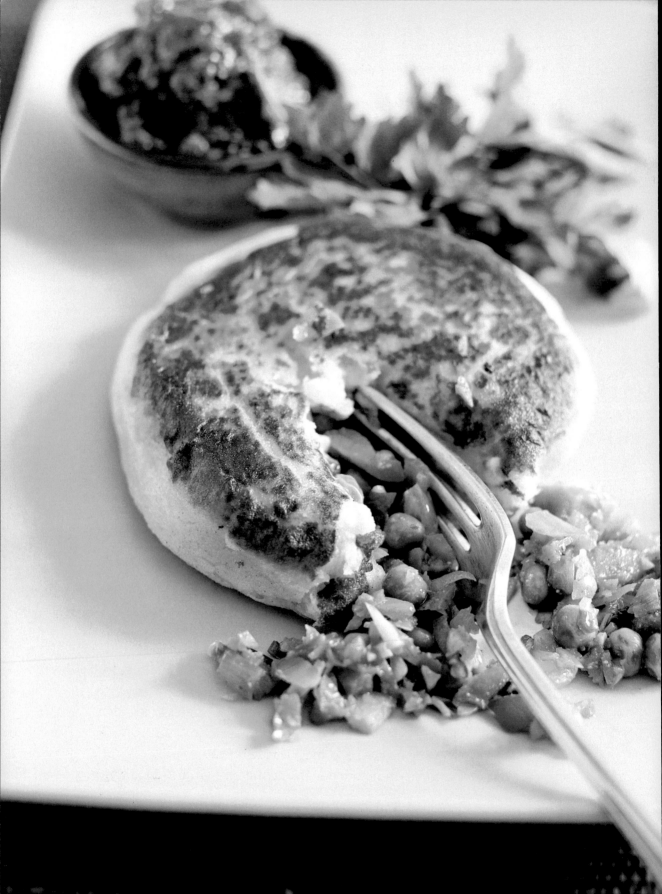

Indian stuffed potato cakes

Wow – these Indian potato cakes are so utterly wonderful, yet they are made with the most ordinary of vegetables: potatoes, carrots, peas and onions. Clever spicing is all it takes, that and a little ingenuity. They are easy to make, look good, and taste even better. I like them just as they are, but if you want to dress them up a little more, adding another beguiling layer of taste, make the sweet sour tamarind and date sauce overleaf to serve with them.

Serves 4 as a main course, 8 as a starter

650 g (1 lb 7 oz) floury potatoes
40 g (1½ oz) plain flour
½ teaspoon salt
vegetable oil for frying

Filling
115 g (4 oz) lightly cooked fresh peas or
 frozen peas, thawed
115 g (4 oz) carrots, roughly chopped
1 onion, chopped

1 red or green chilli, deseeded and chopped
2 cm (¾ in) piece fresh root ginger, grated
1 large clove garlic, chopped
1½ tablespoons sunflower or vegetable oil
1 teaspoon ground cinnamon
1 teaspoon ground cumin
juice of ½ large lime
2 tablespoons chopped coriander leaves
salt

First boil the potatoes in their skins until tender. Drain, then pull off the skins and mash the potatoes thoroughly. Work in the flour and salt to form a malleable 'pastry'. Divide into 16 pieces. Oil your hands lightly. Take one of the pieces of potato dough, roll into a ball, then flatten it to form a circle that's roughly 8 cm (3 in) in diameter. Repeat with the rest of the portions and then cover with a tea-towel until needed.

While the potatoes are cooking, make the filling. Pile all the vegetables, chilli, ginger and garlic into the processor and pulse until finely chopped, but not so fine that they form a purée. Heat the oil in a frying pan and add the chopped veg. Stir over a moderate heat for about 5 minutes, then stir in the cinnamon and cumin. Continue cooking for another 5 minutes or so, then season with salt. Take off the heat, cool slightly, then stir in the lime juice and coriander. Taste and adjust seasoning. Divide into 8.

Take one of the circles of potato dough, mound an eighth of the filling in the centre, then cover with a second disc of potato. Pinch the edges together to seal. Roll back into a ball, then flatten slightly to form a potato cake that's roughly 2.5 cm (1 in) thick. Repeat with the remaining dough and filling.

Heat 2 tablespoons oil in a heavy frying pan over a moderate heat. Lay the potato cakes in the pan, without overcrowding. The oil should sizzle as they come into contact with it. If it is too cool, the cakes will stick to the pan. Leave them to cook – without moving around – for 3–4 minutes, then turn and brown the other side.

Serve while still hot on their own, or with the tamarind and date relish below.

* *

Tamarind and date relish

This is a sweet sharp relish that goes well with all kinds of spicy foods. And with a slice of good cooked ham or a gammon steak. Not spicy, not Indian at all, but a happy match.

Serves 6–8

40 g (1½ oz) tamarind pulp,
  or 4 tablespoons ready-made
  tamarind purée
85 g (3 oz) stoned dried dates

1 teaspoon ground cumin
1 teaspoon ground coriander
½ teaspoon salt

Put the tamarind pulp, if using, in a bowl and pour over 150 ml (5 fl oz) boiling water. Let it sit and soften for about 20 minutes, then stir and break up. Rub through a sieve and discard pips and fibres.

Put the dates into a saucepan with 300 ml (10 fl oz) water and simmer for 10 minutes or until very soft. Sieve the dates and their water to make a thick purée.

Mix with the cumin, coriander, tamarind purée and salt and stir in enough water to make a thick sweet and sour sauce. Taste and adjust seasoning.

* *

Oven-baked potato skins with soured cream, garlic and chive/coriander dip

I like to eat the skin of my baked potatoes, but many people just scoop out the inside. Don't let the skins go to waste, particularly if they still have a little potato flesh clinging to them. Coated lightly in oil and baked in a hot oven they crisp up to make a treat of a snack. Restaurants charge a hefty price for the privilege of eating fried potato skins and dips, but at home you can make something just as good for next to nothing.

Serves 2

roughly 200 g (7 oz) leftover potato skins
2 tablespoons sunflower oil
salt

Dip
100 ml (3 ½ fl oz) soured cream
2 tablespoons finely chopped chives or
    coriander
1 clove garlic, crushed
salt

Preheat the oven to 220°C/425°F/Gas 7.

Cut the potato skins into wide strips or long tapering triangles. Toss with the oil, making sure that they are evenly coated. Spread out on a baking sheet and bake for 10–15 minutes, turning once, until crisp. Check them regularly as they lurch from perfectly done to burnt all too swiftly.

Meanwhile mix all the dip ingredients together. Scrape into a bowl and place on the table. Serve the hot, crisp potato skins as soon as they come out of the oven, with the soured cream dip.

* *

Cypriot potatoes with red wine and coriander

'Patates spastes' is a rather remarkable way of cooking potatoes – and extraordinarily delicious. First the potatoes are cracked open, then deep-fried and then, finally, finished with fragrant coriander seeds and red wine. The result is so good that they are worth cooking and eating just for a snack, though of course they are excellent with any red meat dish.

Serves 4

750 g (1 lb 10 oz) small new potatoes, scrubbed
sunflower or vegetable oil for deep-frying
1 tablespoon extra virgin olive oil

1 heaped tablespoon coriander seeds, coarsely crushed
130 ml (4½ fl oz) red wine
salt and pepper

Bash each potato with a wooden mallet or the end of a rolling pin, to crack open. Take it easy at first until you get the impact just heavy enough to do the job, without smashing each one to smithereens.

Heat a 4–5 cm (1½ in) depth of sunflower or vegetable oil in a saucepan, over a moderate heat. It's hot enough when a cube of bread dropped into it fizzles gently and browns within 1 minute. Wipe the potatoes dry, then deep-fry in batches until golden brown, about 4 minutes. Drain on kitchen paper.

Now get a clean saucepan, and add the olive oil. Set over a low heat and when the oil is warm add the potatoes, coriander, salt and pepper, then at arms' length, pour over the wine. Stir so that everything is nicely mixed, then cover tightly and leave to cook gently for another 17–20 minutes until the potatoes are tender and the wine has all been absorbed. Shake the pan once in a while, to prevent sticking, and turn the potatoes after about 10 minutes so that they each get a chance to sit in the wine.

Eat the wine-soaked potatoes while still hot and fragrant.

* *

Radishes

* * *

There are two ways to look at radishes. The first is as one of life's more pleasing incidentals, a healthy pre-meal nibble that goes on the table alongside a bowl of olives or crisps or tortilla chips or whatever it is that you present when friends come round to eat. The other is as proper vegetables. Both are valid.

Crisp, peppery little **summer radishes** are indeed the perfect way to kick-start a meal, bold enough to set the gastric juices flowing, yet barely denting the appetite. They look handsome too, like miniature pink torpedoes, tipped in some instances with a flash of white. These small radishes are just the tip of the iceberg, however. **Winter radishes** are massive in comparison, and fiery in flavour. Look out for them in markets and farm shops – usually black-skinned and dusty with soil, chunky of girth, tapering to a point, like a shadowy parsnip or carrot. They can be eaten raw, but are not for the faint-hearted. Cooking subdues the peppery power, turning them into a pleasant, juicy vegetable, with a taste reminiscent of turnip minus the brassica tang of sulphur.

Then there are the **oriental radishes**, typified by the incredibly lengthy, white-skinned **mooli** or **daikon**. If you have a yen for Japanese food, then this is the vegetable that is shredded into long crisp threads and piled alongside sushi and sashimi. It is believed to aid digestion, and is used widely throughout Japan. Though you are unlikely to find them in shops, other members of this group can be extraordinarily beautiful. They may not look anything special, but this is a beauty that is more than skin-deep. Cut them in half and you will reveal flashes and circles of stunning pink and purple in many different designs. Usually mild enough to use in salads, these are the radish supermodels. Like human supermodels they are rare and need to be nurtured and supported selflessly. In other words, you will probably have to grow your own, if you want a chance to discover the ultimate potential of the humble radish.

Practicalities

Flabbiness is as big a no-no for a radish as it is for a supermodel. Career ended just like that, new model steps in. The whole raison d'être for a radish is crispness and freshness and vitality. The peppery spice is the added bonus, and that too is spoiled by flabbiness, swiftly developing a nasty sulphurous undertow (radishes are related to cabbages and mustards). One good reason to buy small radishes in bunches is that the leaves give you an instant freshness reading. Do they look lively and bright? Or are they wilting and curling in on themselves? If the latter is the case, they are already past their zenith, heading down the road to flabby doldrums and perhaps there already. The big winter and oriental radishes are rarely sold with leaves, and have a far longer shelf life. They should still be firm, however, without signs of flab or bruising.

Use up small radishes within a day or two of buying. To prepare, cut off the leaf (which can be cooked and eaten like spinach) and scrape away the papery flakes of skin around the stalk end. Rinse well and pop into a bowl of cold water. Keep in the fridge until ready to eat, then drain, dry and put out on the table. In France, they are accompanied by a pat of unsalted butter, and a little pot of coarse salt. Smeared with a dab of butter and dipped in salt they are extra good. Alternatively, mix crumbled flaky sea salt with crushed cumin and coriander and dip radishes into the mix to add extra savour.

Small radishes also have a place in the salad bowl. Halve them or slice them, before scattering over fresh summer salads of all sorts. They are particularly good in a potato salad, instead of finely chopped onion, where they add a hint of fire and colour. To cook as a vegetable, either sauté or stir-fry, or braise whole in barely enough water or stock to cover, adding a knob of butter.

The black-skinned winter radish is the one to use for more determined cooking. It needs to be peeled before cooking, then sliced thickly or cut into chunks. It can simply be simmered in boiling salted water, but is best, I find, added to meaty, chunky stews and braised gently in the savoury juices.

Oriental radishes may need to be peeled (nibble a little bit first to see if the skin is palatable or not), then they can be sliced or shredded thinly for salads, both western and Asian style. They are also good stir-fried, mixed with other vegetables, or added to stews.

* *

Sea bass with rosemary and radish stuffing

Finely chopped radishes add a gentle peppery touch to a piquant stuffing for roast sea bass.

Serves 4

1 sea bass, weighing around 1–1.5 kg
   (2¹/₄–3¹/₄ lb), scaled and cleaned
olive oil
2 cloves garlic, finely chopped
2 tablespoons finely chopped rosemary
salt and pepper

Stuffing
8 summer radishes, trimmed and chopped
1 shallot, chopped
1 slice Parma ham or other prosciutto
   crudo, chopped
1 generous tablespoon olive oil
3 tablespoons slightly stale breadcrumbs
2 teaspoons rinsed capers, roughly chopped
1 tablespoon parsley

To serve
lemon wedges

Preheat the oven to 170°C/325°F/Gas 3.

To make the stuffing, fry the radishes, shallot and ham gently in the olive oil until tender. Mix with all the remaining ingredients, plus some salt and pepper. Brush the insides of the fish with a little olive oil, season lightly and fill with the stuffing. Lay in an oiled ovenproof dish.

Heat 4 tablespoons olive oil over a low heat and add the garlic. Cook until the garlic is lightly coloured. Draw off the heat and strain the oil over the fish. Season with salt and pepper and sprinkle with the chopped rosemary. Bake in the preheated oven for about half an hour until the fish is just cooked through. Check the fish once or twice as it cooks and if it is looking dry, baste with its own juices, or drizzle with a little extra oil.

Serve piping hot with lemon wedges and citrus radish confit (see below).

* *

Citrus radish confit

If you have never tasted cooked summer radishes before, then there is no better recipe to start with than this. It is based on a recipe that I came across years ago in a French magazine. The confit is a sweet, sharp and slightly peppery relish, with a glorious pink colour. Try it with fish, with meat (lovely with lamb) and even with bread and cheese. Make double quantities if you have plenty of radishes to hand, and reheat the remainder the next day.

Serves 4

250 g (9 oz) summer radishes, trimmed
finely grated zest and juice of ½ lemon
finely grated zest and juice of ½ orange
2 tablespoons granulated or caster sugar
20 g (¾ oz) butter
salt and pepper

Slice the radishes into discs about 5 mm (¼ in) thick. Put into a wide shallow pan with all the remaining ingredients and enough water to almost cover. Bring up to the boil, then reduce the heat and simmer gently for about 30 minutes, stirring from time to time, until all the liquid has reduced down to a few tablespoons of rich buttery syrup, and the radishes are very tender.

Serve warm (it reheats beautifully).

* *

Salsify and Scorzonera

* * *

Salsify and scorzonera are kissing cousins, often confused but virtually indistinguishable at heart. If you haven't met either of them before, that's hardly surprising. Although we have a long history of cultivating and growing them, they are no longer in vogue. I can't remember the last time I spotted either in a greengrocery (they do still exist, you know), let alone a supermarket. To find them you will either have to grow them yourself, or head off in search of some extremely upmarket food emporium (I'm thinking Harrods, maybe) or an extremely classy greengrocer.

What you are looking for when you arrive are long, slender taproots – say around a foot long (that's 33 cm) – almost invariably clad in a healthy dusting of earth. True salsify has off-white skin under the dirt, but most of the time what is sold as salsify is actually scorzonera, which has black skin. Since they taste much the same, I guess it doesn't matter much whether the label is technically correct.

The taste of salsify/scorzonera is light and delicate, the texture smooth and tender. I adore them, but some people just find them bland. Each to his own. If you are a first timer with salsify, make a bit of a fuss about them and handle them with respect. Don't expect fireworks, but do anticipate a genteel pleasure with a distinctly old-fashioned and rather soothing aura about it.

Practicalities

BUYING The long roots of salsify (and from now on I'm using that to cover both salsify and scorzonera) should always be firm. Root droop and flabbiness means they are on their way out, fit only for the compost heap. Crying shame, really. Good, earthy, firm roots are the ones to bear home in triumph. Store them in a cool, dark, airy place (or the vegetable drawer of the fridge) for up to 4–5 days.

COOKING To prepare them, begin by rinsing thoroughly. The skin, most likely black but possibly whitish, can be scrubbed off or peeled. Alternatively, you may prefer to blanch the salsify in their skins, then pull the skin off after cooking. My ma was a great one for the post-pan peeling session – it's less wasteful and if you are going to reheat them later or use them in a composite dish, then it makes sense. Obviously if you are going to take them straight from the pan to the dinner table, then you will need to peel them before they are cooked. They oxidise fairly swiftly, so if you need to keep them hanging around after peeling, submerge them in cold water with the juice of ½ lemon.

In most instances, salsify are cut into convenient lengths and **boiled** or **steamed** before use. Keep an eye on them and drain as soon as they are tender and before they overcook to a soggy mush. Say 7–8 minutes in simmering water, though that will vary with thickness.

Serve them hot from the pan, with a knob of butter melting over them and perhaps a stippling of finely chopped parsley. Or, if you prefer, reheat them by frying in butter until lightly patched with brown.

PARTNERS One of my childhood favourites was the chicken and salsify pie my mother made once in a while (substitute lightly cooked salsify for the Jerusalem artichokes in the pie on page 43), and indeed salsify works very well with chicken. And with cream. And with butter. And with anything gentle and soothing. It is not a vegetable that takes gleefully to big flavourings such as chilli, or garlic, or tomato, or anchovies and so on. They drown out the taste of the salsify itself.

Salsify can be excellent in salads, dressed while still warm with a classic vinaigrette, then married with milder green salad leaves (little gem, cos, mâche, spinach and the yellow heart of a frisée lettuce), beans (green or cannellini type), leeks, prawns or chicken or eggs.

If you have only a smallish amount of salsify, then one of the best ways of showing it off is to transform it into fritters to serve as a first course. Dip lengths of lightly cooked salsify into a light fritter batter or tempura batter, and deep–fry until crisp and golden brown. Serve instantly, with wedges of lemon.

* *

Phil Vickery's oil-braised salsify

This is how the chef Phil Vickery likes to cook salsify, braised gently to a tender richness in olive oil, then fried until the exterior is browned just before serving. It's a distinctly restaurant technique (most of the cooking achieved in advance, requiring only a couple of minutes to finish), but one that adapts well to a home kitchen, especially when you are cooking for a dinner party and want to minimise last-minute kitchen shenanigans.

When Phil and I were talking vegetables, he also mentioned that this method works brilliantly with swede.

salsify
olive oil to cover
salt

Preheat the oven to 140°C/275°F/Gas 1. Scrub and peel the salsify. Cut into 10 cm (4 in) lengths. Place in an ovenproof dish that will take them in a close-fitting single layer – don't use a dish that is way too big, or you'll have to use way more oil.

Pour over enough oil to just cover the salsify. Slide into the oven and leave to braise gently for around 1 hour until tender. Leave to cool in the oil.

Just before serving, heat up a frying pan. Take the salsify out of the oil, drain well and fry briskly until browned here and there. Season with salt and serve immediately.

* *

Salsify and flageolet salad

Salsify makes a fine salad all on its own, but I prefer it matched with other ingredients. Nothing too bold and intense, you understand. Pale green flageolets (if you use dried ones, soak 200 g/7 oz overnight, then simmer in unsalted water until tender; drain and dress while still hot), a few extra slender strips of grilled pepper, the sweet, tender leaves of a little gem lettuce. That's much more like it. Try adding the thinnest slivers of Moroccan preserved lemon – delicatessens and some supermarkets sell them, but avoid the lemons preserved with chilli, which are too feisty for this. You will need just half of a normal-sized lemon, or an entire one if they are miniature lemons.

Serves 6

450–500 g (1 lb–1 lb 2 oz) salsify
2 tinned piquillo peppers, or 1 grilled and
   skinned red pepper, deseeded
1/2–1 preserved lemon (optional – see intro)
1 x 400 g can cooked flageolet beans,
   drained and rinsed
1 tablespoon chopped parsley
leaves of 1 little gem lettuce

Dressing
1 tablespoon white wine vinegar
1/2 teaspoon Dijon mustard
a pinch of caster sugar
3–4 tablespoons extra virgin olive oil
salt and pepper

Scrub and peel the salsify, then cut into 5 cm (2 in) lengths and simmer in salted water until tender, but not mushy. Drain thoroughly.

While they are cooking, make the dressing in the usual way. In other words, whisk the vinegar with the mustard, sugar, salt and pepper, then whisk in the oil a spoonful at a time. Taste and adjust the seasoning – it should be fairly sharp to balance the starchiness of the flageolets, and lift the delicate salsify.

As soon as the salsify is drained, but while it is still hot, toss in a little of the dressing and leave to cool down. Cut the pepper(s) into very thin strips. Scrape the inner flesh out of the preserved lemon, if using, and discard. Cut the peel into extremely thin strips and mix with the salsify, peppers, flageolets and parsley, adding the remaining dressing. Set aside. Just before serving toss in the little gem leaves. Serve at once.

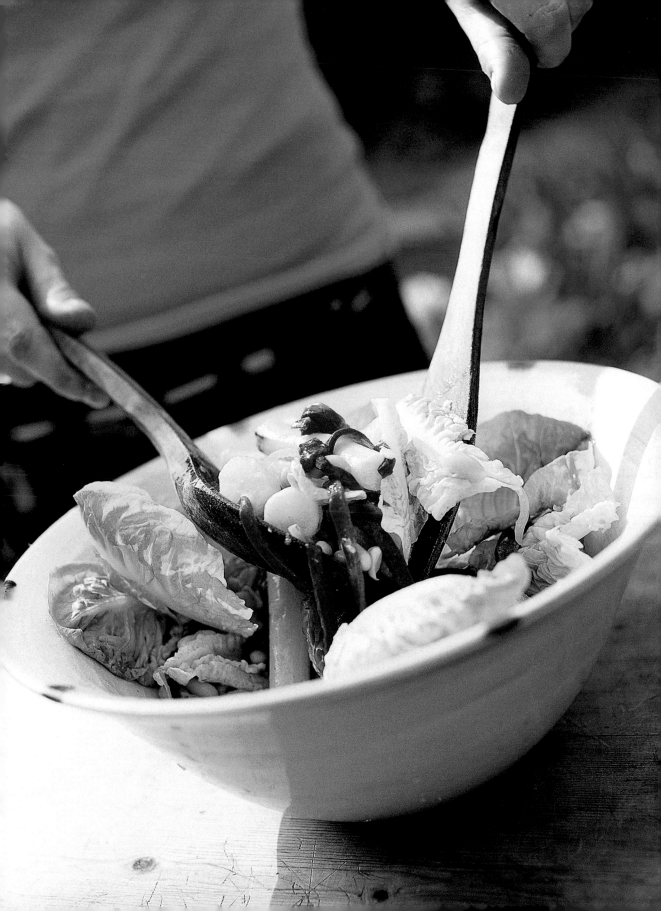

* *

Salsifis à l'estragon

This is a classic French way of dressing up any number of vegetables, but it seems particularly well suited to salsify. They embrace the cream with consummate ease, and the warm aniseed scent of the tarragon brings out the best in them. Very good served with a plain roast chicken.

Serves 4–6

600 g (1 lb 5 oz) salsify
15 g (½ oz) unsalted butter
2 tablespoons dry vermouth
4 tablespoons crème fraîche
leaves from 1 sprig tarragon,
  chopped
salt

Scrub and peel the salsify, then cut into 10 cm (4 in) lengths and simmer in salted water until tender, but not mushy. Drain thoroughly. Melt the butter in a frying pan and when it is foaming add the salsify. Fry for 2–3 minutes until beginning to colour, then add the vermouth. Swirl around and bubble until it is virtually all evaporated. Now add the cream, tarragon and salt and let it all cook down for a few more minutes until the sauce has thickened enough to just coat the salsify lightly. Taste and adjust seasoning, then serve.

* *

Salsifis au curry

As for salsifis à l'estragon, but replace the tarragon with a teaspoon (or two) of good curry paste – a soft korma paste is ideal. The idea is to give a mild hint of curry flavour, but not so much that it overwhelms the flavour of the salsify.

Swede

Swede is an unattractive vegetable. Lumpish, large and arrayed in dull colours, it does little to endear itself to a potential buyer. Beauty, we are told, lies beneath the skin and somewhat reluctantly I have now come to the conclusion that there is a dash of truth to this here. In the case of swede, it is not a startling beauty, but rather a quiet comforting comeliness.

It took a minor spot of focus-grouping amongst friends (thank you, Jess, Jennine et al) to draw me to this conclusion, having successfully ignored the swede for several decades. Now, I realise that, if it is cooked congenially and adequately buttered up (literally), lowly swede is actually rather good. And cheap. Not a bad thing, either. As a new convert, I even found myself defending it when a young friend of my son described it as the vegetable from hell. Which it can be when tarnished with age and presented watery and dull. Such is the stuff of criminal cooking, probably institutional.

Swede-novice that I am, the recipes I've chosen for this section are basic and straightforward. I've not yet got to the stage where I get inventive with swede, and besides I'm not entirely sure that it would be a good idea. There's an underlying whiff of sulphur even in the freshest cannonball swede and it needs to be handled cautiously. Instead of treading roads previously unexplored, I'm playing safe, looking north to Scotland, where swedes are known as turnips or 'neeps', and south to Cornwall. And should you ever come across references to 'rutabaga' in American cookbooks, I hope you won't be too disappointed to be told that this, too, is swede.

Practicalities

BUYING Swede keeps very well without rotting, but I would suggest that you do not attempt to mature your swedes for any length of time. Age brings out the sulphur bitterness, which stops being pleasant the second it is clearly detectable. So, pick out healthy-looking, firm and smooth-skinned spheres and cook them within a week at most.

The ideal storage place, as for most vegetables, is a cool, dry, airy spot, but failing that, the fridge will do nicely. A half-used swede should be covered in clingfilm before returning to the fridge and then used up within a day or two, before it starts tainting milk and butter.

Boiling and **mashing** tend to be the preferred methods of cooking swede. Together they work fine, but if there's one thing to be avoided it is serving great big lumps of watery swede all on their own. The only times whole chunks of simmered swede are even remotely acceptable are when they've been cooked in a flavourful broth (as in Scotch broth) or beef stew. Swede is too doughty for more delicate chicken stews. Friends recommend **roasting** wedges of swede, or **braising** wedges in olive oil (as for Phil Vickery's salsify on page 83), but these are cooking methods for the swede aficionado, not for nervous beginners like me.

* *

Peppery mashed swede and carrot

This is the dish that my guides Jess and Jennine insisted that I should include. They were not in total agreement as to the details, but the main theme was much the same. It is good, I have to admit, as long as there is plenty of butter mashed roughly into the swede, along with terrific quantities of freshly ground black pepper.

Although it goes against my every instinct, I followed Jess's instructions to cook swede and carrot for an extraordinary 40–60 minutes. It turns out that she is right, as it gives a rough mash that is tender but still not totally devoid of texture. The ratio of carrot to swede is another personal foible. You might like to increase the carrot to 50 per cent of the total.

Incidentally, if you replace the carrot with potato (roughly equal quantities with the swede) and add a quartered onion to the pan too, what you end up with is Orkney clapshot.

Serves 6

1 swede, weighing about 675 g (1½ lb),
   peeled and cut into 2 cm cubes
about 250 g (8 oz) carrots, thickly sliced
60 g (2 oz) butter
salt and ginormous amounts of freshly
   ground black pepper

Bring a pan of unsalted water to the boil and add the swede and carrots.
Turn down the heat to give a pleasantly slow simmer, then walk away and
forget about the vegetables for at least 40 minutes, and up to an hour.
Actually, don't ignore them totally – you'll need to check every now and
then that the water level hasn't dropped down too low. If it is disarmingly
low, top up with more boiling water.

   When both vegetables are terrifically soft, drain them well and return
to the pan along with the butter, salt and lots and lots and lots of freshly
ground black pepper. Mash the whole lot together, taste and adjust
seasoning, and serve swiftly

* *

Bashed neeps

Bashed neeps is a variable dish. On an average day it is just mashed 'neeps'
with butter and pepper, and is what posher people might once have called
'turnip purry'. On high days and holidays, however, cream comes into play
along with a generous slug of whisky for those who fancy it.

Serves 6–8

2 swedes, peeled, cubed
   and boiled until tender
30 g (1 oz) butter
80 ml (3 fl oz) double cream
2 tablespoons whisky
3 tablespoons chopped chives
salt and pepper

Drain the swedes thoroughly, then return to the pan with the butter, cream and generous quantities of seasoning. Mash together roughly over a gentle heat until piping hot. Stir in the whisky and most of the chives. Taste and adjust seasoning, then serve with the remaining chives sprinkled over the top.

* *

Cornish pasties

From the south of the country comes one of the finest of recipes embracing swede. I'm not for one moment saying that this is a definitive recipe for a Cornish pasty, but it is something close, with fine steak baked slowly on top of a thin layer of swede and potato. This vegetable layer is essential to soak up the juices from the meat, keeping the pastry crisp on the bottom.

Makes 4

Pastry
500 g (1 lb 2 oz) plain flour
a pinch of salt
160 g (5 ½ oz) butter
60 g (2 oz) lard
icy water
1 egg yolk, beaten, to glaze

Filling
500 g (1 lb 2 oz) rump steak, cut into small
  cubes
1 onion, chopped
1 large potato, peeled and very thinly sliced
1 small swede, peeled and very thinly sliced
salt and pepper

To make the pastry, mix the flour with the salt. Rub in the butter and lard, then add just enough water to mix to a soft but not sticky dough. Wrap in foil or clingfilm and chill for at least half an hour. Bring back to just under room temperature before rolling out.

Mix the steak with the onion and plenty of seasoning. Line a baking sheet with non-stick baking parchment. Divide the pastry into four, and roll out each piece large enough to cut out a 20 cm (8 in) circle (use a side plate as a template).

Arrange one-quarter of the potato in the centre of each pastry circle in an oval shape and season. Lay one-quarter of the swede over that, then mound a quarter of the steak mixture over that, moulding it to cover the potato. Dampen the edges around one half of each pastry circle with a little of the egg glaze, then bring both sides up over the filling, crimping the edges firmly together to form the characteristic pasty shape. Rest in the fridge for half an hour.

Preheat the oven to 220°C/425°F/Gas 7. Brush the pasties with egg glaze, then bake for 15 minutes. Reduce the heat to a lowly 170°C/325°F/Gas 3 and leave the pasties to bake for a further hour. Check regularly and cover with foil if the pastry is browning too rapidly. Serve hot, warm or cold.

* *

Sweet potatoes

* * *

It's the colour that does it for me, every time. It's so damn cheery. Brighter than even a carrot; it's that orange. Not on the outside, of course. No, the skin of a sweet potato is a muted, more sophisticated wine-dregs rose. Remarkably similar, if not identical, to the skin of a kumara (see page 46), the white-fleshed form of the sweet potato, which would be confusing if kumara were more commonly available.

The vibrant orange of the flesh of the sweet potato only develops as the tuber cooks. Raw, the colour of the flesh sends me back to a time when junior aspirins were coloured just that attractive shade of faded, pinky orange. You can, I am assured, eat sweet potatoes raw – grated perhaps into a salad – but I've tried it and I don't think I'll bother again. The moistness of the sweet cooked flesh, with its psychedelic-sweetie hue, is what appeals.

Despite the obvious allure of the sweet potato, it has taken an awfully long time to make headway on this side of the Atlantic. It came back from the Americas with the Spanish Conquistadors, and indeed the very first potato of any kind to be planted on our shores is rumoured to have been an *Ipomoea batatas*, not a true potato (*Solanum tuberosum*) at all. They are not, incidentally, even vaguely related, belonging to different botanical families. Unlike real potatoes, sweet potatoes crave warmth and without it they won't thrive; England's climate is hardly sub-tropical, and the crop was a miserable failure.

Now we've given up growing them in the great outdoors, and finally are importing them in increasing numbers. Sales are swelling, we are slowly taking them to our hearts, and they look like becoming a permanent fixture in the British diet. Hurrah. It's only taken 500 years.

Practicalities

BUYING Taut skin and firm bodies – that's what you're looking for, just like on the beach. At the risk of sounding ageist, wrinkles are to be rejected, and there's no point at all in handing over your cash for a sweet potato that has soft patches. The tips may be slightly discoloured but this is only to be expected – those sweet potatoes have travelled a long way. If I have a choice I pick larger tubers, merely because they are less fiddly to handle.

Stored in a cool place they will last for several weeks, but like most vegetables the sooner you cook them the better they will taste.

COOKING I'll bet you a tenner that most of the sweet potatoes eaten here are **baked** in their jackets. It's the obvious way to cook a sweet potato. None of that sweetness leaching out, and no extra damp creeping in. It makes sense. Treat them just like ordinary potatoes – prick the skin, rub in a little salt if you wish, then bake at around 190°C/375°F/Gas 5 until tender. Time will depend on the size of the potatoes, but we're talking in terms of 45–60 minutes, give or take. Or microwave them, again just as you would an ordinary potato.

Baked sweet potatoes are just great served instead of ordinary potatoes, split open and buttered, or topped with grated Parmesan or mature Cheddar, or soured cream and chives. I love them with bacon, with tzatziki, Greek yoghurt, and even tapenade. You might like to run up a snappy chilli and coriander butter for them (blend butter, fresh red chilli, coriander leaves and a shot or two of lime juice) or a classic French beurre maître d'hôtel (butter, parsley, garlic and lemon juice).

Sweet potatoes make a stunning **mash** – run the American route with

92

this one, flavouring the mash with grated nutmeg and cinnamon, to highlight the warmth. Add a big knob of butter, plenty of salt and freshly squeezed orange juice which matches not only the colour but also the flavour. Don't use milk in sweet potato mash – it just feels plain wrong.

Americans consider sweet potatoes (which they often call yams to confuse everyone else) an essential part of the Thanksgiving meal, served with the turkey and all the trimmings. Candied yams is a dish of sweet potatoes cooked with sugar and other flavourings (often orange juice and spices) to accompany the main course. Adding sugar to sweet potatoes? Overkill, unless we're talking pudding. It's certainly not an idea that appeals to me.

I'd far rather **sauté** cubes of sweet potato, finishing them with salt and ground cumin and coriander just before they emerge from the pan, or perhaps grate them raw to make a sweet-salt version of rösti, so good with game or white fish. You can use all sweet potato, or mix it with equal quantities of ordinary potato, or grate in raw carrot, or beetroot for something altogether more fancy. How about sweet potato and beetroot rösti, topped with a little soured cream and herring roe caviar (or the real thing when you are feeling extravagant) to serve as a chic starter to a dinner party? Put me on the guest list right now.

Using vegetables in **puddings** is not a natural activity. We've all grown used to carrot cake, but that's cake, not dessert. Put aside any reservations you may have in the case of sweet potatoes. They mash down to such a moist smoothness that they work brilliantly in all kinds of recipes. Be bold and try the meringue-topped sweet potato pie below, and you'll see what I mean. You could also enrich the mashed sweet potato with cream, butter and a little extra sugar to use as the filling for a two-crust pie, or to make a fool. I don't see why you couldn't concoct a superb sweet potato ice-cream if you fancied – then keep all your guests guessing the nature of your mystery pudding.

SEE ALSO KUMARA (PAGE 46).

Stir-fried sweet potato with lamb and green beans

Baking and boiling are all very well, but if you want to retain a degree of firmness to your sweet potato, then stir-frying is the natural choice. Stir-fry it on its own to serve as a side dish, but better still stir-fry it with lamb and salty Chinese black bean sauce for a quick feast, guaranteed to rev up the spirits, as it works the tastebuds.

For stir-frying I use either lamb leg steaks or chump chops, cut into thin slivers. The number of chillies is entirely at your discretion. I use medium-sized, medium-heat chillies here, to maximise the flashes of red in amongst the vegetables and meat, without totally blowing the roof out of my mouth. Tiny bird chillies are so ferocious that it would be wise to restrict yourself to one, foregoing the visuals in order to survive the heat. Unless, that is, you are a chilli fiend.

Serves 2–3

2 tablespoons sunflower or vegetable oil
2 cm (³⁄₄ in) piece fresh root ginger, peeled and chopped
2 cloves garlic, finely chopped
1 or 2 red chillies, deseeded and cut into strips
1 sweet potato, weighing around 400 g (14 oz), peeled, thinly sliced and then quartered

125 g (4 ¹⁄₂ oz) green beans, topped and tailed and cut in half
225 g (8 oz) tender boneless lamb, cut into thin slivers
3 tablespoons black bean sauce
1 teaspoon toasted sesame oil

Get all the ingredients fully prepared and measured out, and set them out close to the hob. Put your wok (which should be a good roomy one) over a high heat. Once it starts to smoke, add the sunflower or vegetable oil, then add the ginger, garlic and chillies and stir-fry for 20 seconds or so.

Next add the sweet potato and stir-fry briskly for 3 minutes. Add the green beans and stir-fry for 4–5 minutes, until the sweet potato is tender and the beans are patched with brown. Tip all the vegetables out on to a plate and return the wok to the heat. When it is back up to prime heat, add the

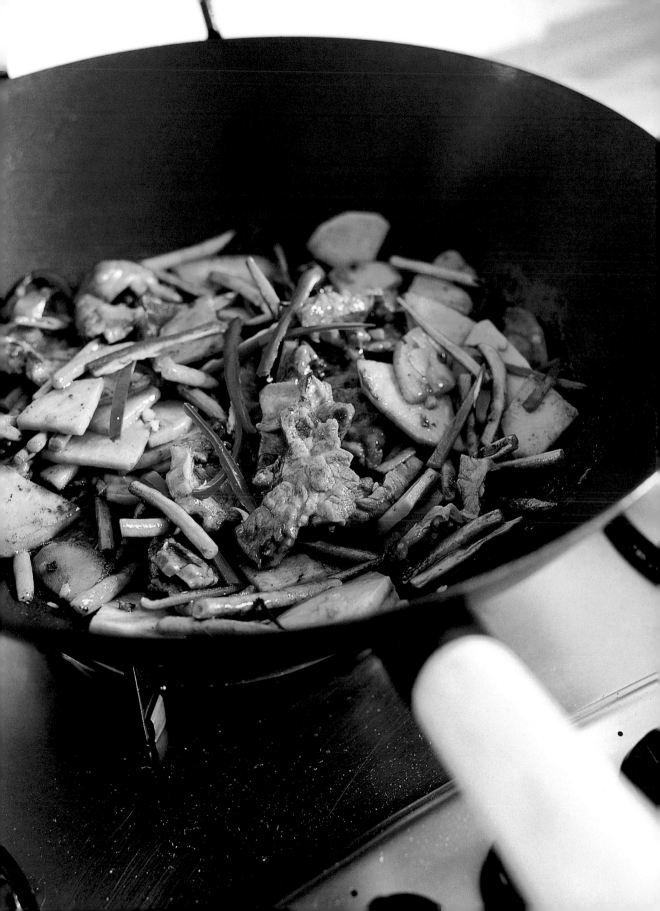

lamb and stir-fry for about 1 minute, until just barely cooked through. Return the vegetables to the wok and mix them well with the lamb. Add the black bean sauce and stir-fry for a final couple of minutes. Stir in the sesame oil. Taste and add a little more black bean sauce if you think it needs it.

* *

Sweet potato and red lentil soup with mint

What a splendid soup this is! Perfect stuff for a spot of cold weather (I'd be tempted to bring it out on Bonfire Night), with just enough lift from the lime and mint to stop it being dull. A whole star anise, by the way, has seven or eight 'petals' – useful to know if yours have collapsed in their jar.

Serves 6

1 onion, chopped
550g (1¼lb) sweet potato, peeled and cut
 into chunks
3 cloves garlic, chopped
4cm (1½ in) piece fresh root ginger, peeled
 and chopped
1 whole star anise
2 tablespoons sunflower oil

1 tablespoon tomato purée
1 heaped teaspoon ground cinnamon
150g (5oz) red lentils
1.5 litres (2¾ pints) water or
 vegetable stock
juice of 1–2 limes
150ml (5 floz) soured cream
leaves from a small bunch of mint
salt and pepper

Put the onion, sweet potato, ginger, garlic, star anise and sunflower oil into a roomy pan and stir around. Place over a low heat, cover tightly and leave to sweat for 10 minutes, then add the tomato purée, cinnamon, lentils and water. Bring up to the boil, then reduce the heat and leave to simmer until the lentils and sweet potato are very tender. Season with salt and pepper.

Remove the star anise, then liquidise the soup or pass through a mouli-légumes. Stir in as much lime juice as you like. Taste and adjust seasoning.

Reheat when needed, and spoon into bowls. Finish each one with a little soured cream and a small handful of mint leaves on top.

Southern sweet potato pie

This is far better than pumpkin pie. Don't be scared to line the pastry case with clingfilm – it's a pastry chef's trick and it works brilliantly, lifting out perfectly every time. And no, it won't melt either.

Serves 8

3 large sweet potatoes, about 1.5 kg (3¼ lb) in total
300 g (11 oz) sweet shortcrust pastry
30 g (1 oz) softened butter
100 g (3½ oz) caster sugar
1 teaspoon vanilla extract
½ teaspoon ground cinnamon
a generous grating of nutmeg

4 tablespoons double cream
1 egg
3 egg yolks

Meringue topping
3 egg whites
150 g (5 oz) caster sugar

Preheat the oven to 190°C/375°F/Gas 5. Put the sweet potatoes in to bake.

Meanwhile, line a 23–25 cm (9–10 in) tart tin with the pastry, prick the base with a fork, and chill in the fridge for half an hour. Line the pastry case with clingfilm and fill with baking beans. Bake blind for 10 minutes, then take out of the oven and remove the beans and clingfilm. Return the pastry case to the oven and bake for a final 5 minutes. Leave to cool.

Once the potatoes are done, scoop out the flesh and weigh out 950 g (2 lb 2 oz). Beat in the butter, sugar, vanilla extract and spices while still hot. Next beat in the cream, then the egg and yolks. Scrape the mixture into the awaiting pastry case, smooth down and return it to the oven. Once the door is closed, turn the heat down to 180°C/350°F/Gas 4 and leave to bake for around 20 minutes, until almost set.

As it cooks, whisk up the egg whites for the meringue topping until they stand in firm peaks. Sprinkle over half the sugar and whisk again until the meringue is light and glossy and billowing, then fold in the remaining sugar. Spoon the meringue on to the hot baked pie, spreading out right to the edge and completely covering the filling. Make swirls and peaks in the meringue, then return the pie to the oven (last time) and bake for 15 minutes, until the meringue is browned nicely. Serve warm or cold, with plenty of cream.

* *

Turnips

* * *

I got off to a good start with turnips, thanks to an alcoholic chef called Monsieur Bastard. He owned the restaurant at the end of the French village my family decamped to every spring and autumn. The evening we arrived we invariably ate at The Ariana. The first spoonful of M. Bastard's vegetable soup signalled the proper start of the holiday, and we cheered whenever jambon aux navets appeared on the menu. I still salivate at the thought of that thick slice of fine French ham and tender, glazed turnips that surrounded it.

Not everyone is so lucky. Bad turnips are enough to dismay the most ardent of vegetable eaters, let alone youngsters who are just embarking, often against their will, on the road to vegetable-appreciation. Or not. Which is a shame, because at their best turnips are downright sexy. Not the hefty, awkward lumps shrouded in tough green and grey skin fit only to be fed to cattle, not humans. No, I'm talking about the cute sorts of turnip: smaller than a tennis ball, with a handsome flush of pink or purple, waxy, tender skin and crisp white flesh.

The trouble is that the ideal turnip, sold marble-sized in fetching bunches, is horribly expensive and far too rare – good arguments for growing your own, so that you can enjoy them as fresh as can be. Failing that, you must regard turnips as a rare indulgence, especially if you have children. Never force-feed them rank monster turnip in the hopes that they will eventually grow to enjoy it. They won't. They'll probably never eat turnip again. Instead, restrain your turnip intake to once or twice a year, only when you can buy and cook small, sexy turnips that will tempt one and all.

Practicalities

BUYING Turnips must, must, must be eaten young and impeccably fresh. Over-large or stale turnips are a penance we could all do without. Beauty is for once a reliable guide. Look for pert small turnips, prettily blushed with pale purple or pink, over pearly white skin. Medium-sized green and white turnips are just about acceptable, but big bruisers are to be avoided unless you are a masochist. Only buy turnips, even the most perfect little darlings, when you are sure that you will be eating them within the next 48 hours.

Extra small turnips (think quail's egg or walnut-sized), bunched together fetchingly, are the ne plus ultra, the apex of deliciousness. Don't muck around with them – just trim the stems off a centimetre from the base, rinse well, nip off thready rootlets, then **steam** or **blanch whole** in lightly salted water for a few minutes until tender-crisp. Well drained and served immediately, they need no embellishment at all. If you want a dab of butter, fine, but it really isn't necessary. There's only one more complex dish that I'd recommend using them for, and that's a navarin printanier, the remarkable French stew of spring lamb and baby vegetables in a creamy sauce. Otherwise, leave them alone.

As they mature, the turnip flavour matures too and the outer skin toughens. As they approach tennis-ball size, they will probably need to be peeled. Before that it isn't necessary unless the skin is discoloured. Raw turnip is rarely used in salads, which is a shame, as it has a pleasing crisp juiciness – try it thinly sliced in the Malaysian rujak on page 121, for instance, or tossed with crisp sweet lettuce leaves, thinly sliced eating apple and walnuts in a lemony dressing.

Medium turnips are open to more adventurous approaches, as long as they do not include a crude white sauce, which does nothing for them. I often **roast** them with a little olive oil, or serve steamed or boiled turnip quarters sprinkled with a gremolata (a very finely chopped blend of lemon zest, parsley and garlic), or drizzled with bright green parsley and basil oil (literally a little olive, sunflower or avocado oil liquidised with a handful of tender herb leaves).

As they swell up, you: a) will have to peel off the tough skin, and b) would be well advised to blanch the turnips before finishing the cooking. In other words, cut the turnip into cubes or slices and drop into boiling water for 3 minutes or so, before draining thoroughly. This softens the less appealing aromas, without destroying the flavour or texture completely. Finish off the cooking when needed by sautéing them in butter or, better still, glazing them, for which I give a recipe overleaf.

Glazed turnips with orange and honey

There are many ways to glaze a turnip. The simplest is to finish the cooked turnips in butter and sugar, stirring them over a moderate heat until the sugar dissolves, and the turnips begin to colour. This recipe brings orange juice and honey into play as well.

Serves 4

500g (1lb 2oz) medium turnips
finely grated zest of ½ orange
juice of 1 large orange
30g (1oz) butter
1 tablespoon light runny honey
salt and pepper

Peel the turnips and cut into 2cm (¾in) cubes. Blanch in boiling water for 3 minutes, then drain thoroughly. Wipe out the saucepan and return the turnips to it, adding all the remaining ingredients together with a splash of water. Return to a moderate heat and stir until the butter has melted. Simmer, stirring frequently, until the liquid has all evaporated, leaving the turnips glossy with their buttery, orange glaze. Serve swiftly.

* *

Torshi lift
Turnip and beetroot pickles

I love the habit, at some North African restaurants, of bringing a plate of raw vegetables, olives and pickles to nibble on while you wait for the food. Very civilised, and naturally far better for you than stuffing in slices of bread and butter. I grab the startlingly pink crescents of pickled turnip – torshi lift – first. This pickle is crisp and juicy and very more-ish (as well as being Moorish). The colour comes from the inclusion of a few slices of beetroot, but the base flavour is the sweet, juicy, raw turnip. It doesn't take long to make, and is a good addition to a plate of charcuterie, or served with cheese at the end of a meal.

Fills a 1 litre (1¾ pint) jar

1 kg (2¼ lb) small/medium
  turnips
1 large raw beetroot
4 cloves garlic, thinly sliced

a small bunch of celery leaves
4 tablespoons sea salt
350 ml (12 fl oz) white wine vinegar

Peel the turnips and cut them in halves or quarters, depending on their size. Peel the beetroot, cut it in half and slice. Pack into sterilised preserving jars (see page 215), alternating layers of turnip and beetroot and interspersing with garlic slices and celery leaves.

Mix the salt with 1 litre (1¾ pints) water in a saucepan and bring up to the boil, stirring until the salt has dissolved. Add the vinegar, stir and then pour over the vegetables, making sure that they are completely submerged. Seal with non-corrosive lids.

Store in a warm (not hot) place – say a shelf in the kitchen. Leave them alone for 10–12 days. Once they are slightly softened and suffused with pink, move the jars to a cool place, where they will keep happily for a month or so.

* *

Crisp slow-roast duck with turnips

The discreet hint of bitterness in turnips is an excellent foil for the richness of duck – especially when they are semi-roasted in the duck's own fat. I adore this recipe, and make it time and again, relishing the moist tenderness of the slow-cooked flesh, the crisp skin and the juiciness of the turnips. I don't always bother with the sauce, good though it is, but the turnips are essential.

Serves 4

1 duckling, weighing around 2.3–2.7 kg
  (5–6 lb)
500 g (1 lb 2 oz) turnips
salt and pepper

Sauce
1 large carrot, diced
1 onion, chopped
2 sticks celery, diced

750 ml (1¼ pints) fruity red wine (1 bottle)
1 bouquet garni (a few stalks parsley, 2
  good sprigs thyme, 2 bay leaves, 1 small
  sprig sage, tied together with string)
750 ml (1¼ pints) duck stock or chicken
  stock
2 tablespoons redcurrant jelly

Preheat the oven to 220°C/425°F/Gas 7. Wipe the duck dry with kitchen paper. Prick the skin all over with a skewer, or a fork if the tines are sharp, so that the fat can run out more easily as it cooks. Season generously with salt and pepper. Sit the duck on a rack over a roasting tin and slide it into the oven. Turn the heat down to 180°C/350°F/Gas 4, and leave it to cook for 2½ hours.

During that time, all you need do, whenever you've a mind to – perhaps just before setting off for a walk, or the church, and again when you return – is drain off the fat that has gathered in the roasting tin (it's brilliant stuff for sautéing potatoes).

Once you've harvested your first crop of fat, take 1 tablespoon of it and heat it up in a frying pan. Add the carrot, onion and celery and sauté until the vegetables are tender and lightly browned. Now add the wine and the bouquet garni. Bring up to the boil, stirring thoroughly, then boil hard until reduced by half. Add the stock and boil again until reduced by about a third to a half, giving a syrupy sauce. Now stir in the redcurrant jelly until it has melted, then strain into a small pan. Add a little salt and pepper, and simmer

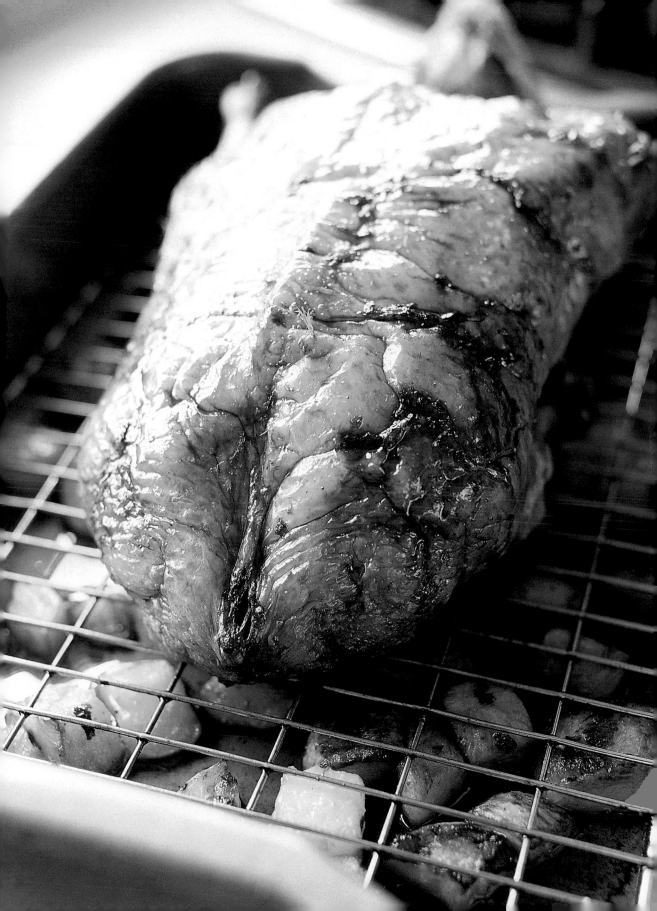

for about 2 minutes. Taste and adjust seasoning. Reheat when needed.

Peel the turnips, cut into 2 cm (¾ in) cubes and blanch in boiling water for 3 minutes. Drain and run under the cold tap. Leave to drain thoroughly. About 40 minutes before the duck is done, drain off most of the fat, leaving just a little in the roasting tin. Add the turnips and turn them in the fat, then leave to roast with the duck.

When the duck and turnips are cooked, turn off the oven and leave the door ajar. Let them rest like this (or in another suitably warm place, supposing you need the oven for something else) for about 15 minutes.

Using a sharp knife or poultry shears, cut the duck into four pieces – cutting first from head to tail end, along the breast bone and through the back bone to give two halves, then simply dividing each half in two. Serve quickly, while still warm, with the roast turnips and reheated sauce.

* *

Yams

* * *

They're big, they're ugly and they weigh a ton. So why are yams so widely grown all around the warmer regions of the world? Because they grow vigorously and plentifully in the moist heat, because they keep brilliantly despite it, because they fill up the stomachs of large hungry families at little cost, and above all because they taste great. I'm a recent convert to the yam and now I'm keen to sing its praises. I just adore the taste, something akin to that of a potato but a touch sweeter and nuttier, and the floury texture that soaks up juices and butter so deliciously.

The yam works as a perfect carrier of other flavours, ready to fall in with spicy foods, or big meaty stews in a companionable way. Even though they have to be imported, they remain cheap when bought in small Caribbean or

Asian food stores, the only catch being that they can be hard to identify amongst other big brown tubers.

It won't help to be told that although the yam you are most likely to come across is the greater yam, identified more precisely as *Dioscorea alata*, at least nine other related edible members of the genus *Dioscorea* are in cultivation around the world. And then there are dozens of cultivars of the Greater Yam itself. The good news is that they can all be cooked and eaten in much the same way.

The word 'yam' is used in the Southern states of America to mean the sweet potato (see page 91), as in candied yams, a staple of the Thanksgiving dinner. Ersatz yam crops up again in the Antipodes, where a New Zealand yam is actually an oca (see page 52), native to the high Andes not the tropics. And the last time I bought taro in a Chinese supermarket, I was told firmly that it was a yam. Whilst they have similarities, the slippery texture of taro is not at all the same as the dry, floury fluff of genuine yam.

Moral of story so far, if you are not familiar with yams, treat the whole business of buying and cooking them as something of an adventure. Chances are that a friendly shopkeeper or his or her customers will be keen to help you with identifying the right big brown long lump, and suggesting ways to cook it at its best. If you are a keen yam eater, can I beg you to offer help to anyone staring perplexedly at the display of yams and the like in your local foodstore. Encourage them to try yam as an occasional, pleasing but not too wayward alternative to potatoes.

Practicalities

BUYING Whilst you are unlikely to come across yams in your average supermarket or farm shop, any city dweller with a yen for a yam will find them in most West Indian or Asian food stores. Look for large, weighty, dull dark brown, cylindrical vegetables, which aren't banded with rings (that's probably a taro). They aren't smooth, either, but the skin is pretty much uniformly uneven all over.

I've read that yam tastes best when it is slightly matured. In other words, not freshly picked, nor as old as the hills. Since my trips to yam-growing countries have been all too few and all too short, I have no idea how much difference 'ageing' makes. Still, at least I can deduce that freshness is not critical. Yams keep well, for several weeks if necessary, in any cool, dark spot. The fridge is too cold, and besides a whole yam would take up an absurd amount of shelf space.

Preparation is much as you would imagine: wash, cut up into large chunks, peel if you want or need to (or leave it until after cooking, when the skins pull away easily), cut into smaller pieces as required. Left hanging around for hours, a cut yam eventually discolours, but half an hour of exposure to the air is not a problem. Next the cooking – and here you can do practically anything you would with a potato. **Boil** – of course; **steam** – fine; **sauté** – why not?; **roast** – yes, please. Yams are often added to **stews** for the last half hour or so of cooking time – a particularly good place for them. As they soften they draw in the grace notes of the other ingredients, adding their own substance to complete a big, filling meal-in-a-pot with no extra washing up on the side. If you wish, crush some of the yam with a wooden spoon to thicken the juices.

In parts of Africa boiled yam is pounded with a touch of its cooking water, to form a thick, all but solid, smooth 'mash' known as fufu. Bland in taste, it is absolutely designed as an accompaniment to spicier, richer dishes. Pounding is hard work, though, and being a lazy so-and-so, I just make a buttery mash out of them, which is absolutely gorgeous. In fact, yams and butter might have been made for each other. Just try roasting yam, then splitting open and slathering on the butter. Fantastic. To roast, either wrap large hunks of yam in oiled foil, or simply rub the pieces with oil and leave it at that. Roast in a hot oven (around 200°C/400°F/Gas 6) until tender – allow marginally less time than you would for a potato of roughly the same girth. Foiled roast yam is tender right the way through, whilst the open-roast yam develops a chewy, golden skin which is really rather good.

Yams can also be sautéed, just as if they were potatoes. In theory they should make good chips, but in practice I've found that they have a tendency to collapse if not handled with care.

Yam balls

These extremely good little morsels hail from West Africa, where they are a favourite item in celebratory buffets. They are at their best, however, hot from the frying pan, so I keep them to serve as a first course, perhaps with a light salad of watercress, or even as the main part of a more homely supper. Don't be put off by the bizarre coating mixture. It works and works very well indeed. If the idea of dipping them into corned beef purée is just too much for you, or if you don't eat meat, then simply coat them in beaten egg – they will still taste fine, though lacking that subtle edge of piquancy.

Makes 24

500 g (1 lb 2 oz) yam
3 eggs
1 tomato, deseeded and diced
1/3 red pepper, deseeded and cut into
　small dice

1/2–1 red chilli (depending on strength),
　deseeded and finely chopped
50 g (scant 2 oz) tinned corned beef
sunflower or vegetable oil for frying
salt and pepper

Cut the yam into big chunks then boil in salted water until tender. Drain, peel, then mash well. When it has cooled slightly beat in an egg, then mix in the tomato, red pepper, chilli, salt and pepper. Roll dessertspoonfuls of the yam mixture into balls and flatten to about 1 cm (1/2 in) thick.

Crush the corned beef to a pulp with a fork then beat in the remaining eggs, one at a time. Sounds weird, looks revolting, but don't let such trivialities put you off.

Pour enough oil into a frying pan to cover the base generously. Heat over a moderate heat. One by one coat the balls in the egg and corned beef mixture, and lay in the frying pan. Don't overcrowd (if they touch they'll stick together). Fry, not too fast, in the hot oil until golden brown underneath. Turn over and brown the other side. Serve hot and steaming.

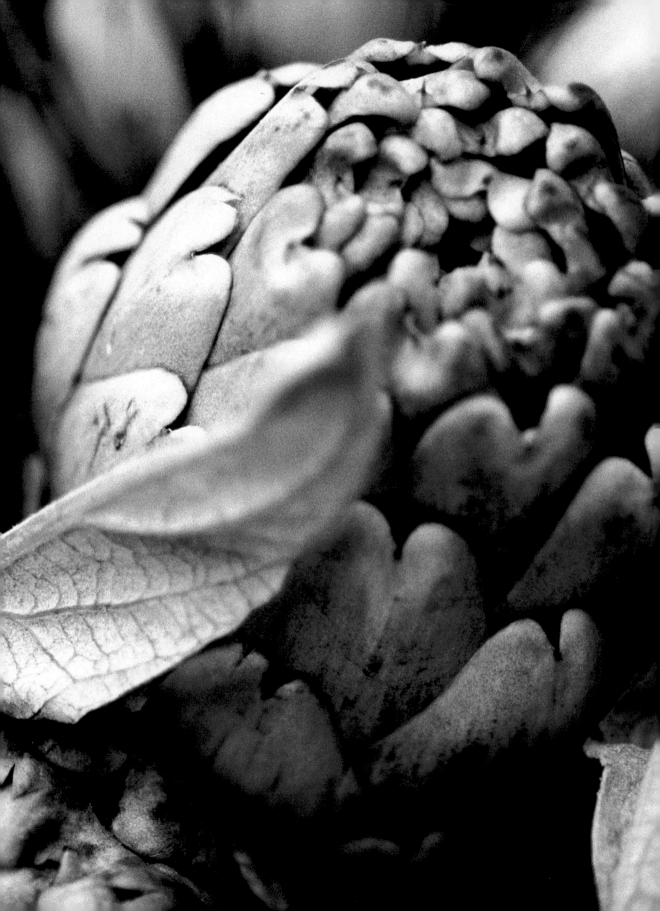

Shoots and stems

* *

Asparagus Beansprouts
Cardoons Celery **Fennel**
Globe artichokes **Kohlrabi**
Samphire **Wild asparagus**

* *

Asparagus

* * *

Asparagus are really something special amongst vegetables. Partly, of course, this is to do with their taste, but it comes almost as much from their immaculate sense of timing. The first asparagus of the year (exclude imports, for the moment) is a keenly anticipated pleasure, a harbinger of warmth, of light, of summer, of an easier life for a few months at least. Yes, even today, even in this modern world of high-flying internationally jet-setting vegetables, the opening of the asparagus season is cause for a humble domestic celebration. Here is a gorgeous treat – expensive by vegetable standards, but cheap by any other – that marks the end of the cold, the return of Persephone with the prospect of all that is good about summer ahead.

If you have your own asparagus bed or live in the countryside or a small town, you can hardly fail to notice the arrival, in early May, of the first choice asparagus. City-dwellers may have to search it out deliberately. Whatever. The point is to make the most of one of our most delightful seasonal offerings while it is around. At first, when prices are highest, treat your asparagus with due reverence. The initial reacquaintance should be a straightforward one, where the asparagus itself is allowed to take every single last drop of the limelight. In other words, steam or boil it until just perfectly cooked, no more, no less, then serve it warm with lemon-sharpened melted butter, or a hollandaise sauce. Savour every mouthful. Then after that, let rip while the going is good, watching hopefully for prices to plummet as the season gets into full swing. Throw asparagus into everything imaginable – stir-fries, medleys of roast vegetables, chicken stews, pies, omelettes, salads and anything else that appeals.

Do you consider this approach over the top? If you nod, if you mutter that you can buy imported asparagus at any time of the year, then it is you who

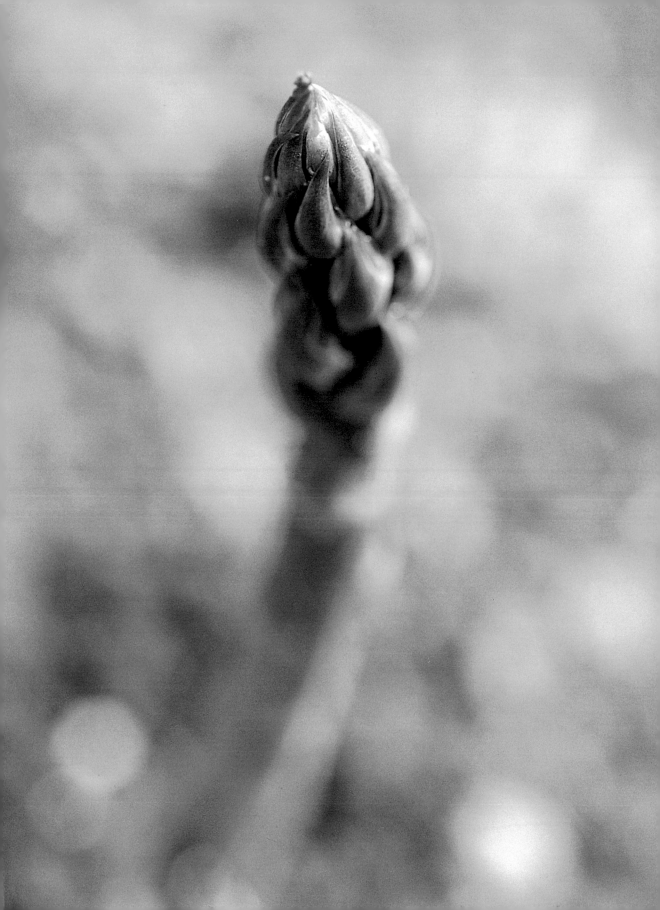

are losing out. I'm not for a minute suggesting that imported asparagus isn't worth eating. It is. Occasionally. But our own home-grown asparagus is far better, and part of the pleasure is that we can't have it any time we want. There's no gainsaying the fact that asparagus loses flavour once it has been cut. The most wonderful and amazing asparagus I have ever eaten was the one and only spear that we grew ourselves (subsequently moving house before the bed matured). It was rushed straight from the earth to the kitchen, rinsed and slipped into a pan of water all within the space of 20 minutes. 10 minutes later we ate it ceremoniously, with a little melted butter. The taste was breathtakingly exquisite and clear.

Only those with an asparagus bed of their own will be able to experience this perfection. As the hours pass, flavour dampens and diminishes. Eat asparagus within 24 hours of picking and it is still damn fine. 48 hours ain't bad at all. This is a possibility when asparagus is grown in our own country. When it has to cross half the world, hanging out at airport storage, then in some gigantic central warehouse, before even getting to a supermarket shelf… well, the loss of flavour is going to be clearly evident. It'll taste okay, but it will no longer be special.

The logical outcome of this is that anyone with a wee taste for asparagus is well advised to revel in it throughout the months of May and June. Eat it when you can, and try it in myriad different dishes. Learn, too, to respect that rather odd side-effect – smelly wee. Go to the loo within minutes of consuming asparagus, even in small quantity, and you can hardly fail to notice it. It's not exactly offensive but it is curious.

In this country we prefer the **green asparagus** that pops its stems up through the earth to the light, reaching upwards in long slender spears. Extra slender ones, by the way, are known as **'sprue'** and are considered inferior, rightly, to fatter stems which pack a richer tasting, more satisfying mouthful. Sprue should be cheaper than grade 1 asparagus, though I suspect the price is occasionally hiked up for the unsuspecting, on the grounds that small is cute and high-maintenance. A load of tosh, so don't be taken in.

On the Continent, the fashion is for the even sturdier bulging **white or purple asparagus**, that spend their entire growing-life shrouded in damp, moist soil to blanch them into pallor. The taste is perhaps nuttier, but often comes with a hint of bitterness which I find less pleasing. Talking of the

Continent, next time you happen to be perusing a classic French menu, bear in mind that anything 'Argenteuil' means it comes with asparagus. Potage Argenteuil, for instance, is a romantic name for asparagus soup. Argenteuil was once considered France's premier asparagus-growing region, just as the Vale of Evesham is ours. Continental asparagus is making its way across the Channel, and is definitely worth trying, though I doubt it will ever replace our much-cherished green asparagus.

Practicalities

BUYING   For a start, check that the asparagus you are buying in May and June is actually British. Complain when, as happens far too frequently, air-imported 'grass' from South America and other far-flung shores appears on our shelves in high asparagus season. Buy, if you can, from local growers to guarantee freshness. Before you stump up, cast an eye over your handsomely bunched asparagus. First, the cut ends of the stems (especially if they are covered up – call me suspicious, but...) which will be green or straw-coloured when the stems are recently cut, not brown and dry as a bone which suggests an over-extended parting from the earth. Now to the tips, which need to be tightly closed into neat points. This tells you something about the youth of the asparagus when they were cut. If the bracts are loose and opening the asparagus was too mature and long in the tooth. Too much of the stem will be tough and stringy – acceptable only towards the end of the season when you have decided to simmer up a big bowl of asparagus soup.

COOKING   Asparagus steamers are useful for precious little but steaming asparagus, and take up a good deal of room in the kitchen cupboards. It might be worth investing in one if you grow your own, but otherwise forget it. I find that asparagus cook beautifully on their sides, tip to base lying in **simmering** water. My favourite asparagus-cooking vessel is a deep frying pan, which is wide enough to take the whole length without compromise. For this most straightforward cooking method and for most others, too, I indulge in only minimal preparation, trimming off the lower inch or two of stem, before submerging the asparagus in their bath of salted simmering water. I don't spend ages peeling off the tougher skin of the lower half of each sphere, largely because I am too time-challenged/lazy (take your pick). I don't mind biting off the tender upper reaches of the cooked spears, then dragging out the remaining tenderness from the fibres of the base with my teeth. Only when the asparagus is going to take its place as a component in a more complex dish (e.g. a quiche or light stew) do I make the effort to remove the tougher outside layer of the lower regions.

Simmered asparagus will be cooked in some 5–10 minutes, depending on thickness. Keep an eye on it, and whip the pan off the heat as soon as the asparagus is tender, but before the tips turn to a mush. Even if you are serving them hot, drain quickly then run under the cold tap for a few seconds to put a stop to the ravaging effects of heat. Gobble up straightaway, or leave to cool for later on.

It's now well established that there is more than one way to cook asparagus. My favourite, both for taste and ease, is **roasting**, which keeps all the juices miraculously locked up inside the spears. Trim off the bottom inch or two (that's 2.5–5 cm for more youthful readers), then lay the asparagus out in a single layer in a roasting tin, or shallow ovenproof dish. Drizzle over a few tablespoonfuls of crackingly good olive oil and season with coarse salt. Roll the asparagus around a little until evenly sheened with oil, then slide, uncovered, into a hot oven – around 200°C/400°F/Gas 6. Roast for some 15–20 minutes until just tender, then serve up swiftly, perhaps with shavings of Parmesan strewn over them. Hard to beat.

More slender stems of asparagus are also good **stir-fried** – fatter ones may need to be slit in half, unless you really like them on the crunchy side. If the barbecue is lit, you might also have a go at grilling them, though you will need to pay them plenty of attention, turning vigilantly to prevent burning.

Asparagus go with so many other foods that it's hard to know where to begin. When asparagus is to be the star, the classic partners are melted butter or a plain hollandaise. A hollandaise flavoured with orange or mint works spectacularly well, too. I also love warm asparagus with a soft-boiled egg – the combination of that green spring scent with runny egg yolk is bliss. The Italian style is to serve them with a fried egg and Parmesan, which is almost as scrummy. Cold asparagus demand a light vinaigrette, which may be made up of little more than wine vinegar, olive oil, salt and pepper. Or some variation on the theme. In other words, try balsamic or sherry vinegar, or a nut oil, add a little mustard, or a touch of horseradish. Or you could stir in masses of chopped fresh herbs – tender spring chervil is brilliant, or chives, or parsley perhaps. The addition of a sprinkling of chopped hard-boiled egg is fabulous (charmingly known as 'mimosa'), or some crisply fried breadcrumbs, or a 'wrap' of tender Parma or Serrano ham.

Once you move away from straight asparagus on their own, the possibilities are curtailed only by imagination. Asparagus and eggs are notably good together (think omelettes, scrambled, quiches), but then so too are asparagus and chicken, or asparagus and pasta, or asparagus and tender new potatoes, or asparagus and shellfish or salmon or white fish. Darker meats and fish (e.g. beef, tuna) are perhaps too domineering, but to ban them from taking to the plate together would be too pernickety. Spices do wonders for asparagus, too, so don't exclude them from gorgeous Asian dishes either. Asparagus sing loud and clear in an aromatic Thai green curry, for instance.

SEE ALSO WILD ASPARAGUS (PAGE 151).

* *

Asparagus mimosa

In the culinary sense, 'mimosa' is the charming term for a scattering of finely chopped hard-boiled egg – those little flashes of yellow should remind you of the boughs of scented mimosa that hang down over the hills of the French Riviera. Or something like that.

Serves 6

1 kg (2¼ lb) asparagus, trimmed
2 hard-boiled eggs, shelled and finely
  chopped
40 g (1½ oz) shelled pistachios, chopped

Dressing
1 tablespoon rice wine or tarragon vinegar
½ teaspoon Dijon mustard
4 tablespoons extra virgin olive oil
salt and pepper

Cook the asparagus in gently simmering water until almost but not quite tender (they will carry on cooking a little as they cool), then drain and run under the cold tap. Drain again and leave to finish cooling. Cover until needed.

To make the dressing whisk the vinegar with the mustard, salt and pepper, then whisk in the oil a tablespoon at a time. Taste and adjust seasoning.

Make sure that the asparagus is at room temperature, then divide between six individual plates, or arrange on one large plate. Spoon the dressing over them, then scatter with chopped egg and pistachios. Serve at once.

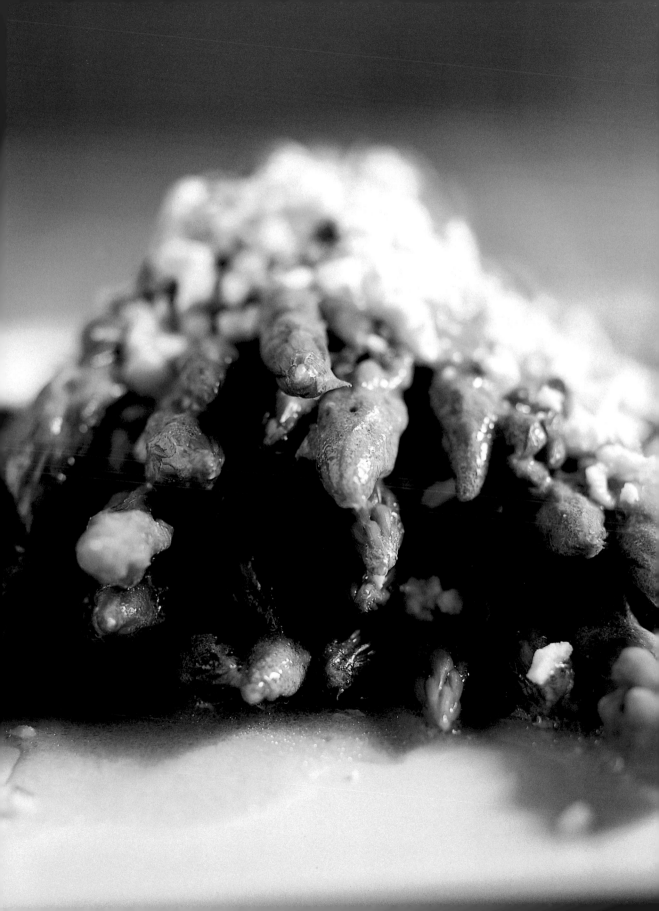

Asparagus and salmon lasagne

Lasagne, marvellous dish that it is, does not fall into the speedy cook's repertoire. Take some time to make this version – it's worth it – but be thankful that you can get away without pre-cooking either the salmon or the lasagne, both of which will soften happily in the heat of the oven.

Serves 6–8

500g (1lb 2oz) green asparagus
500g (1lb 2oz) salmon fillet
200–250g (7–9oz) dried green (spinach)
 lasagne sheets

Béchamel sauce
6 cloves
1 onion, halved
2 bay leaves
1.5 litres (2¾ pints) milk

2 pinches saffron strands, or 2–3
 tablespoons chopped dill
90g (generous 3oz) butter
90g (generous 3oz) plain flour
good grating of nutmeg
salt and pepper

To finish
30g (1oz) Parmesan, freshly grated

First start the béchamel. Push the cloves into the onion halves. Put them into a pan with the bay leaves and milk. Heat until hot, but not boiling. Turn the heat right down to the merest trace of warmth, and leave to infuse for 10–20 minutes. Discard the onion with its cloves, and bay leaf. Put the saffron, if using, into a small bowl and moisten with 1 tablespoon hot water. Set aside until needed.

Melt the butter in a saucepan large enough to take all the milk, then stir in the flour. Stir for about a minute, then draw off the heat and gradually whisk in the hot milk. Once it is all incorporated, return to the heat, add the dill, if using, and let the sauce simmer, stirring frequently, for 10 minutes. The sauce should have the consistency of runny, but fairly thick double cream. Now season with salt, pepper and nutmeg and stir in the saffron, if using.

While the sauce is simmering, trim the asparagus and blanch in lightly salted boiling water for 4 minutes – it should be slightly undercooked. Drain. Run under a cold tap to halt the cooking process then leave to cool. Slice the salmon moderately thinly, at a 45° angle (roughly speaking – no need to drag out the protractor).

Preheat the oven to 200°C/400°F/Gas 6. Grease a 25 x 20cm(10 x 8in) oven-proof dish with a little butter. Spread a thin layer of béchamel over the base. Now cover with sheets of lasagne, making sure that they don't overlap. Cover these with another thin layer of béchamel, and strew the asparagus pieces over that in a single layer. Now more béchamel to cover the asparagus, another layer of lasagne, still not overlapping, more béchamel. Now arrange the slices of salmon on the sauce and spoon over the next layer of béchamel. How are we doing? Pretty well, I imagine. Now time for the last layer of lasagne, and the rest of the béchamel goes over the top of that, making sure that the lasagne is evenly covered.

Finally, finally, finally, scatter the Parmesan over the top and get that lasagne into the oven. Bake for some 40–45 minutes until the top is nicely browned and the sauce is bubbling. Eat.

* *

Beansprouts

* * *

The purpose of every seed is to sprout. Some fail, some need precise and unusual circumstance, some do it at the sight of a single drop of moisture. Beans are merely seeds that began life protected by a pod. Therefore any bean will sprout, given half a chance. It just so happens, however, that one particular bean dominates the beansprout market. This is the **mung bean**, and from it we get those lovely little translucent white and yellow shoots that are so good in stir-fries or tossed into salads.

Other types of beansprout can be good too – **aduki beans** produce a decent sprout, and in China **soy beansprouts** are popular, though they have to be properly cooked before eating. Any bean with a high level of toxic haemaglutins (such as kidney beans or haricot beans) should not be eaten raw and neither should their sprouts. The latest addition to the world of edible sprouts-that-are-not-from-Brussels is the delectable **peanut sprout**. Obviously, this is a nut sprout rather than a beansprout, but it bears enough similarities to steal into this section. With the remains of the split peanut still clamped around the nascent leaves, it has a distinct nuttiness in the literal sense of the word.

Sprouting beans at home is easy and amazing. Children should enjoy the process as much as adults will (though that's not guaranteed). Try it with aduki beans, mung beans, **chickpeas** or **lentils** or even **peas** (though not frozen ones). Soak a handful of beans in lukewarm water overnight, then drain but don't allow them to dry. Tip them into a jam jar to form a layer no more than 1 cm (½ in) deep. Cover the jar with a double layer of muslin, held in place with a rubber band, and put it in a warm dark place (an airing cupboard is ideal). Every morning and every evening, and once or twice in between if possible, fill the jar with water (through the muslin), roll it around gently, then drain. Within 3–5 days the jar should be jam-packed full to the brim with the freshest possible beansprouts. They taste best when they are between 5 and 7.5 cm (2–3 in) long. Over-grown sprouts can sometimes taste bitter.

Tip the sprouts into a bowl of water and swish around gently to loosen the bean husks and little roots. Leave to settle, then skim off the husks that have floated to the surface. Drain well and eat as soon as possible.

Practicalities

BUYING The thing to remember about beansprouts is that they don't last. Beansprouts have a short lifespan so you just can't get away with buying them on Saturday to eat on Thursday. The chances are that by then they will have begun to go slimy and brown at the ends. Home-sprouted sprouts might keep more than a few days (in an airtight container or plastic bag in the vegetable drawer of the fridge), but I wouldn't leave them hanging around for much longer than that.

Old-school cooks advise one to nip off tiny roots still hanging on to the end of any of the beansprouts. This seems utterly mad advice to me, and I have consistently ignored it, with no ill effect or negative comment. I check over the beansprouts swiftly just in case the odd rogue sprout has started to deteriorate, I rinse them and shake dry, and that is the sum total of preparation necessary.

COOKING **Raw** beansprouts add a brilliant shot of healthy freshness to salads of all sorts, though they do take particularly well to the raunchier Asian dressings with big doses of chilli, garlic and ginger. They are best mixed in with other vegetables and ingredients – on their own the lingering bean-flavour is a touch overbearing – especially when added as a final flourish.

Beansprouts need only a minute or two in the wok when **stir-fried**. Just enough time to soften but not so long that they lose all their crispness and freshness. Stir-frying softens the flavour, transforming them into a vegetable which can be served on its own as a side dish, as well as an excellent element in a mixed stir-fry of vegetables and pork or chicken.

* *

Rujak
South-East Asian spicy vegetable and fruit salad

Rujak is a salad that came originally from Java but has been enthusiastically adopted in Singapore and Malaysia, where over time distinct Chinese and Indian versions have developed as well as regional versions. Common to all of them is a collection of the freshest crisp fruit and vegetables, brought together with a highly pungent sauce. Every time I've eaten it, it has included plenty of cucumber and beansprouts, but as for the rest – well, it's a veritable cornucopia. The important elements are a mix of crisp vegetables and sweet, firm fruit. Try it with the mixture I've suggested below first, then vary it to your heart's content.

Tamarind, that lovely bringer of fruity sourness, is fairly easily available these days, but if you have trouble locating the blachan or shrimp paste, replace it with old-fashioned anchovy sauce or purée or even that classic of the gentlemen's clubs, Patum Peperium, better known as Gentleman's Relish.

Serves 6

½ cucumber, cut into sticks
85 g (3 oz) beansprouts
10 pink summer radishes, trimmed and
   quartered
½ jicama or mooli, peeled and sliced
½ pomelo or ugli or red grapefruit,
   segmented
1 under-ripe mango, peeled and sliced, or 1
   scented apple (e.g. Cox or Kidd's Orange
   Red), cored and sliced, then tossed in
   a little lemon juice

60 g (2 oz) shelled roasted peanuts, chopped
a small handful of coriander leaves

Dressing
3 fresh bird's eye chillies, chopped
1 clove garlic, roughly chopped
3 tablespoons palm sugar or dark
   muscovado sugar
½ teaspoon blachan or 1 teaspoon anchovy
   purée or sauce
2 tablespoons tamarind paste

Work the chillies, garlic and sugar to a paste in a mortar, then work in the blachan or anchovy purée, the tamarind paste, and enough water to make a thick cream. Spoon into a bowl.

Prepare all the vegetables and fruit, arrange on a large serving plate and then scatter the coriander leaves and chopped peanuts over them. Serve the pungent dressing alongside, so that each person can take as much as they like.

* *

Cardoons

* * *

As vegetable plants go, this one is a humdinger. Left to its own devices a cardoon will shoot upwards, upwards, and outwards in a thrust of majestic proportions. It is what is often and in this case quite justifiably known as an architectural plant. Like the artichoke (to which it is closely related), it is an edible thistle, but unlike the artichoke, it is the stems, not the flowering heads, that are eaten. Sadly this means the demise of the entire, architectural mass of silvery foliage.

It is rare that one finds cardoons for sale in this country. They are not exactly commonplace elsewhere, though you may come across them in markets in the south of France (**'cardons'**) or in northern Italy (**'cardi'**), where their unique flavour with its hint of bitterness is much appreciated. These rare stems are not simply lopped from the plant – growing cardoons requires more than a plain cut-and-come-again technique. A natural stem of cardoon would shock the palate of even the most dedicated devotee of bitterness in food. So, cardoon gardeners will swaddle the stems of each massive plant in a jacket of cardboard or some other suitable, light-excluding medium for several weeks prior to harvesting to blanch the bitterness out. Actually, this happens before the plants have reached their full stature. By then, I imagine, it is too late to try to eradicate either the bitterness or the tough fibres that run the length of the stalks.

Practicalities

BUYING
If you don't grow your own cardoons, then you will just have to wait until you stumble across them somewhere, perhaps in a farmers' market or a very upscale greengrocery here, or somewhere on the Continent or possibly in Morocco, where they are also eaten. Since light encourages bitterness to reappear, common sense dictates that you should only buy stems that are firm and obviously freshly cut. And then you should keep them in the dark until you eat them within the next day or so.

To prepare, rinse then lop off any leaves including the little ones that run down the length of the edges. Trim top and bottom and pull away as many of the strong fibres running from top to bottom as possible. Cut the stems into manageable lengths.

COOKING
Simmer them in acidulated salted water (i.e. water with the juice of a lemon squeezed into it) until crisp-tender. Halfway through the cooking time (i.e. after around 4 minutes) nibble a small corner to gauge the residual bitterness. Once or twice (but not always) I've discovered too late that this is stronger than I find palatable. If so, drain the cardoon, rinse under the cold tap, then finish simmering in a pan of fresh water – with any luck that will do the trick. Once cooked, serve the steaming hot cardoons with a slick of melted butter and lemon juice.

I've also enjoyed them in a **gratin**, mixed with a creamy béchamel, salted with finely chopped anchovies and dotted with black olives, finished with a generous dredging of Parmesan, or with a tomato sauce spiked with capers and mint, again with that veil of golden-brown Parmesan over the top. Moroccan cookbooks may also contain recipes for spiced cardoon tagines. Lightly cooked in small strips, then dipped in egg and flour before deep-frying, they make delicious **fritters**. The most famous cardoon dish, however, is the Italian 'bagna cauda', a forceful blend of anchovy, garlic, olive oil and butter, into which cardoons and other vegetables are dipped.

* *

Celery

* * *

I wonder whether we should be demanding the return of old-fashioned **green celery**, its stems caringly protected from the light to mute the strong celery buzz? With rare exceptions, it is a thing of the past. Modern varieties of celery have been bred to grow slender, **pale celadon stems** with only the gentlest tinge of green to them, and a correspondingly mild taste. No need for the growers to blanch; no need for retailers to keep them from the light until they are sold. You get a hint of what true green celery might have tasted like from the few loitering leaves left on each head of celery – far punchier and more demanding on the palate.

Economics have had a hand in the demise of true green celery. Banking up the earth around the stems was something that was done by hand, and meant that harvesting was a longer job too. More labour, higher prices, lower sales. Where once celery was something of a speciality, it now sits alongside other salad vegetables, loved and loathed in equal measure. I doubt that it ever makes it on to anyone's favourite vegetables list. And that may just be because it has lost its vital character over the years. Sad.

One of the chief virtues of celery is its crunch and juiciness. So darn juicy is it, that we're often told you use up more calories eating it, than you get from it. Perfect dieters' snack food, in other words. In an attempt to prove this, I conducted a small experiment. The calorie content of celery is 15 per 100 g (3½ oz). I weighed one stem. 42 g, approximately 6 calories. It took me 1 minute and 45 seconds to consume it. In my subsequent search for the energy expenditure of chewing, I discovered that the process is all but irrelevant. You would use virtually the same amount of energy if you merely sat and contemplated all 6 calories laid flat on the plate. The critical figure, apparently, is the TEE of digestion. That's Thermic Energy Expenditure. And no-one, but no-one, would let me in on how to work that one out in relation to my very own stick of celery. The only way I can see to prove conclusively that the TEE is indeed greater than CPS (that's Calories Per Stick) is to eat nothing but crates of celery for a week without moving a muscle. Damn. My thirst for knowledge doesn't stretch that far. I'm pretty certain, though, that the CETFO must have exceeded the CCIC. Oh come on… Calories Expended Trying to Find Out, and Calories Consumed Ingesting Celery. Don't you know anything?

Practicalities

BUYING This one is easy. Only buy celery when the stems are stiff as a ramrod, and leaves (if there are any left) are not wilting. Look at the base too. If it looks slimy, soft or too brown, then the celery is old and not worth having. Once purchased, celery should be kept in the vegetable drawer of the fridge, and used up before it starts to wilt, 4 or 5 days at the outside. Once it has started to droop, the only place for it is the stockpot or the compost heap.

Preparation is also pretty obvious. Separate the stems (unless you want to cook whole celery hearts – skip to next paragraph), rinse away dirt, dry. Trim off leaves (they have an intense flavour, so treat them as a herb, for flavouring rather than as a salad green) or the drying tips of the stems. If you are leaving stems whole, pull away some of the tough strings that run the length of the outer curve. If you are the thoughtful, caring, patient type you will also do this when you are about to slice the stems. Most of us, most of the time, will not bother. To slice, nestle two or three stems together, then cut across all of them at one go.

Celery hearts are just what they say they are – the inner clump of the head of celery, where the stems have not yet had time to form strings and retain a youthful sweetness. In the past these were sometimes braised whole or halved lengthways, in stock, to serve as a side dish. You need a good deal of excellent stock to make this worthwhile. It's far more sensible to slice celery before braising. When celery hearts are sold ready trimmed for the pot (you see them every now and then in supermarkets) they come with a comparatively chunky price tag attached. Unless you genuinely won't make use of the outer stems (which are fine for salads, stocks, stews and soups) they are an unwarranted extravagance.

Celery plays three important roles within the culinary theatre. **Raw**, role one, it brings its exemplary crispness and juiciness as well as its unique flavour. **Cooked**, the quietest, now much diminished part – almost a one-liner these days – it can be surprisingly good, as long as it is handled considerately and coaxed to give of its best. Role three, **background** part, but absolute linch-pin of the plot, it is an essential member of the chorus of vegetables that gather to give stocks and sauces and stews of one kind and another, their depth of flavour, their complexity and backbone.

Let's begin with role three. It is no mere whim that celery appears in the ingredients list for every **classic stock**. It adds a kind of savouriness, to support the sweetness of carrot and the boldness of onion and leek. It doesn't stand out, but it does make a considerable difference. For the same kind of reasons it appears as a flavouring vegetable in many other dishes. I love to add a few stems, diced small, to a vegetable soup, for instance. Not enough to turn it into celery soup, but sufficient to lift the whole that little bit higher. In Louisiana, celery comprises a third of the 'holy trinity' together with onion and green pepper, the diced vegetables that are sweated in oil or butter as the foundation for the more obvious layers of flavour to follow.

Few people cook celery these days. If you've ever had to eat plain boiled celery, you'll understand this. Cooked in water, it is as dull and lifeless as a limp rag. It doesn't have to be like that. Celery hearts **simmered** in stock (real stuff only, not cube) until tender, then drained and finished with a gloss of butter are as good as any other vegetable. Or try slicing the celery, **braising** in stock or sweet wine and water, then draining and reheating with cream, chopped herbs and a final squeeze of lemon juice. Then you'll get a measure of how good cooked celery can be.

It takes an age to **shallow-fry** celery – all that water must sizzle off before it can begin to brown – but what you are left with is packed with flavour. Similarly, and rather less bother, you can concentrate all that is worthwhile, by **roasting** sliced celery in a hot oven. Treat it like any other vegetable, in other words toss with a little olive oil, add a few whole cloves of garlic in their skins, a few sprigs of herbs, salt and pepper and then leave it to swelter in a hot oven for some 50–60 minutes until all the liquid has evaporated, and the celery has shrunk and begun to brown. The taste is astonishing.

I was introduced to **deep-fried** celery by the chef, John Tovey. He suggests dipping batons of celery into flour that has been seasoned plentifully with curry powder, shaking off the excess then deep-frying until lightly browned. This is, I think, the best of all ways of cooking celery.

Role one is the big one. This is how most celery is consumed. In **salads** or perhaps with cheese. A mouthful of real, traditional Cheddar or creamy Stilton is undoubtedly enhanced by the crisp counterpoint of celery. Celery might have been designed to romance any number of our fantastic British farmhouse cheeses.

The most famous of celery salads is the Waldorf and there's a recipe for that below. Don't leave it at that, though. Add sliced celery to a crisp mixed green salad – with lettuce leaves, rocket, watercress, fresh raw peas and handfuls of tender-leaved herbs, or toss with cubes of watermelon and roughly chopped hazelnuts, or mix thin batons of celery with similarly sized lengths of carrot, beansprouts, shredded lettuce and spring onions, then add an Asian style dressing (see page 381), and finish with a scattering of finely chopped roasted peanuts. Or almost any salad needing crispness.

And of course, few vegetables are better kitted out to serve **raw** with dips of whatever sort. As I get older, I find that I am less and less inclined to serve a proper starter every time I invite people round to supper. Instead, there is a plate of cured meats on the table – salamis and Serrano ham, say – a few bowls of good olives, and bowls of hummus or htipiti (Greek red pepper and feta dip, see page 176), or taramasalata and sticks of celery to scoop it out. If that's not a good way to get the gastric juices flowing, then what is?

SEE ALSO CELERIAC (PAGE 29).

Roast celery and flageolet soup with coriander and lime pesto

Roasting celery draws out the best of its flavour which, as it happens, blends delightfully with that of flageolet beans. The basic soup is good all on its own, but the lively blend of coriander, lime and creamed coconut (that's the solid stuff, not the liquid coconut cream) gives it a final lift out of the ordinary. You'll end up with more of the pesto than you need, but the remainder can be stirred into a mayonnaise or vinaigrette, spooned on to baked potatoes with some soured cream, or spread under the skin of a chicken before roasting to scent it as it cooks.

The soup is good, too, finished with a spoonful of black olive purée, and a few pieces of diced, deseeded tomato.

Serves 4–6

1 head celery, cleaned and sliced
1 onion, cut into wedges
1 head garlic, cut in half horizontally
1½ tablespoons vegetable or olive oil
2 sprigs thyme
1 x 400g can flageolet beans, drained and rinsed, or 140g dried flageolets, soaked overnight and cooked until tender
500ml (18floz) chicken or vegetable stock
salt and pepper

Coriander and lime pesto
a big handful of fresh coriander (around 30g/1oz)
1 large clove garlic, quartered
50g (1²⁄₃oz) creamed coconut
1 green Thai chilli, deseeded and roughly chopped
juice of 1 lime

Preheat the oven to 220°C/425°F/Gas 7.

Put the celery, onion, garlic and oil into an ovenproof dish with the thyme, salt and pepper. Turn so that all the veg are coated lightly with oil, then roast for 40–50 minutes until very tender and browned here and there. Stir the vegetables around every 15 minutes or so. At first the celery will throw out a fair amount of water, but this will eventually evaporate.

While they cook, make the pesto. Put all the ingredients except the lime juice into the bowl of a processor and process to a paste. Keep the blades whirring as you trickle in the juice. Scrape the pesto out into a bowl.

Once the vegetables are done, remove and discard the thyme stems. Tip the vegetables into the liquidiser or processor, scraping in all the brown bits stuck around the edges. Add the drained flageolet beans and the stock and liquidise – you may have to do this in two batches. Rub through a sieve – a fairly wide-meshed sieve makes this a pretty straightforward, speedy job.

Just before serving, reheat the soup and adjust seasonings. Ladle into bowls and serve with a spoonful of coriander pesto stirred into each one.

* *

Waldorf salad, with a hint of horseradish and tarragon

The original Waldorf salad was simply a mix of equal parts of celery and apple, dressed with mayonnaise. It's good, but it gets even better when you add a scattering of toasted walnuts, and even better than that, I think, when it takes on a gentle twist of tarragon and horseradish.

If you make the salad in advance, the mayonnaise has a tendency to turn claggy, so either leave mixing until the last moment, or stir in one last tablespoon of mayonnaise just before putting the salad on to the table.

Serves 6

2 crisp, first-rate eating apples
juice of 1/2 lemon
4 sticks celery, sliced
60 g (2 oz) shelled walnuts, lightly toasted
4–5 tablespoons home-made mayonnaise
  (see page 35)

leaves of 1 big sprig tarragon, chopped
1 tablespoon creamed horseradish
salt and pepper

Quarter, core and dice the apple small (we're thinking 1 cm/1/2 in cubes, give or take). Toss with the lemon juice. Mix with all the remaining ingredients adding just enough mayonnaise to coat lightly. All done. Now it's ready to serve.

* *

Tonno alla stemperata
Tuna marinated with celery, olives and sultanas

This old Sicilian dish of marinated tuna is marvellous for a hot summer's day, as it positively benefits from being made a day in advance. The collection of ingredients is unusual, but be bold enough to give it a try. Somehow the sweetness of the sultanas, with the softened, caramelised strips of celery make a perfect foil for the tuna itself.

Serves 4

75 g (2½ oz) sultanas
6 tablespoons extra virgin olive oil
4 tuna steaks, cut about 2 cm (¾ in) thick,
  each weighing around 200 g (7 oz)
4 sticks celery, thinly sliced
3 cloves garlic, chopped

45 g (1½ oz) capers
125 g (4½ oz) green olives, stoned and sliced
  (approx. 75 g/2½ oz after stoning)
5 tablespoons white wine vinegar
a little chopped parsley
salt and pepper

Pour warm water over the sultanas and soak for 10 minutes, then drain.

Warm 4 tablespoons olive oil in a wide frying pan until good and hot. Lay the tuna steaks in the oil and fry until browned on each side – allow 1½–2 minutes on each side, depending on how well cooked you like it. Take the steaks out of the pan and arrange them side by side in a shallow dish.

Add the celery to the oil in the pan and sauté until it begins to brown (this takes far longer than you would imagine because of all the water trapped in celery – 10 minutes or more is not unusual). Now add the garlic and capers and cook for a further 30 seconds or so. Tip in the olives and drained sultanas and stir for another minute until everything is piping hot. Finally tip in the vinegar – it will sizzle and steam and quickly evaporate leaving just a damp mush. Season with salt and pepper.

Pour the contents of the pan over the fish, then drizzle over the remaining 2 tablespoons oil. Leave to cool, turning the tuna steaks once in a while. Serve at room temperature, sprinkled with a little parsley.

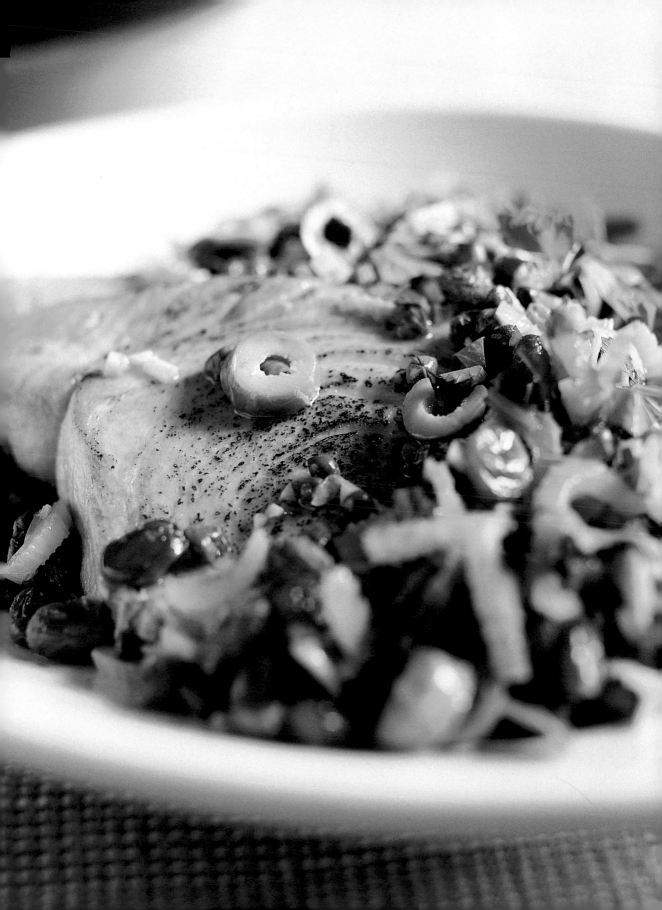

Fennel

* * *

Here is a vegetable that sits on a throne all of its own. There is nothing else quite like it. It's that aniseed taste that does it, a taste you will find amongst spices and herbs, but rarely amongst elemental foodstuffs of substance. Liquorice is about as close as it gets, but that's hardly substantial. Oddly, though I have never liked liquorice, I do have an enormous fondness for fennel. Does this mark me out as contrary? No, for fennel is blessed with a crisp, juicy firmness that balances and transforms the aniseed taste.

Florence fennel, to give it its full name, is a specialised form of *Foeniculum vulgare*. If you grow herbs, then you will probably be familiar with the high, swaying, feathery fronds of fennel, particularly the beautiful bronzed variety. You will not unearth a bulb of **Florence fennel** at the base of the plant. Vegetable fennel is a different play on the plant, with deliberately swollen succulent stem bases that curve around each other tightly to create its characteristic form.

There has been a vogue, now dampened I'm rather pleased to say, for slender, **miniature 'bulbs' of fennel**. They can be good, but far too often they turn out to be laced with tough fibrous strings running down their length. This does not make for happy eating. They are also inordinately expensive. This strikes me as an unsatisfactory brace of characteristics, and I have now learnt to ignore them. Fully formed fennel is a much better prospect.

Practicalities

BUYING Examine each bulb of fennel before you slip it into the bag. What you are after is a plump firm, tight white bulb, with stubs of green stems and frondy leaves poking out of it. Do not buy fennel that is a) dry looking or wizened, b) distinctly bruised or damaged. Minor blemishes mean that you may have to discard the outer layer, but no more than that.

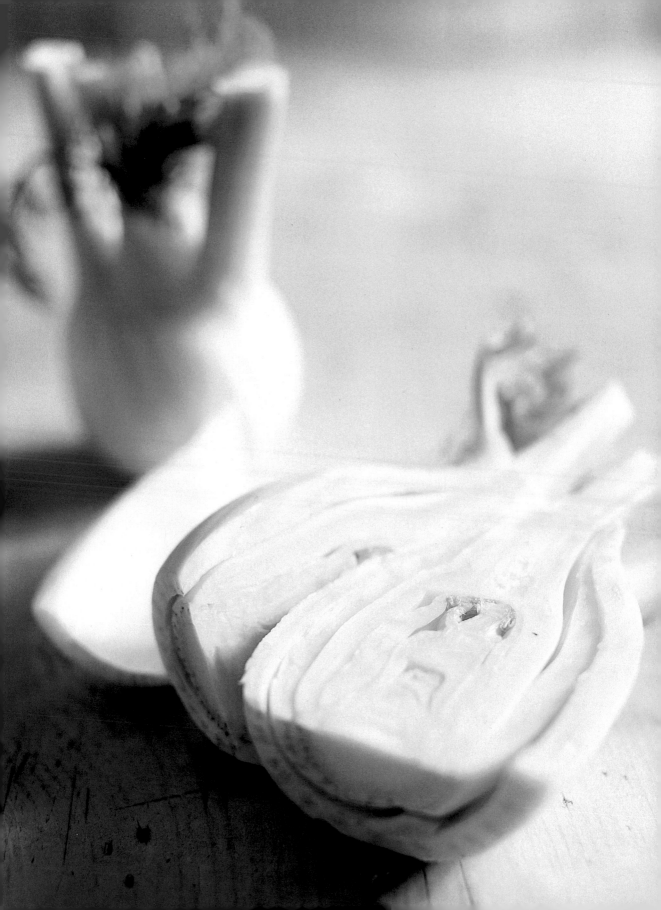

Fennel holds its form reasonably well for several days in the vegetable drawer of the fridge, and may last as long as a week. There will be some loss of flavour, but since it has so much in the first place it can cope.

Basic preparation is straightforward. Lop off the green stems – they are too stringy to eat, though good for flavouring a stock. Likewise, cut off the leafy bit, but save it to use as a garnish. Trim a very thin disc off the base and if badly damaged or discoloured, remove the outer layer. In most instances, you will now cut the bulb into quarters, from stem-end to base.

COOKING For **salads**, the quartered fennel then needs to be sliced very, very thinly. Too thick and it becomes unwieldy and overbearing. The best of all fennel salads in my opinion is the simplest – nothing more than paper-thin slices of fennel dressed with lemon juice, great olive oil, salt and pepper. So good with fish or white meats, but possibly only for those who adore fennel. Less pure, less intense, are salads of fennel and orange (see recipes), but in fact thinly sliced fennel makes a welcome addition to green salads, tomato salads, or even in a Waldorf salad (see page 129) in place of the celery. In fact, any time you want a crunch and a touch of aniseed in a salad, fennel's your man. If you are a fennel fan, then eat it Italian style, with cheese, particularly Gorgonzola or goat's cheese – the point here, as with pairing celery and cheese, is the contrast of fresh juicy texture with the richness of the cheese, as well as the mutually enhancing tastes.

Heat works a major transformation on fennel. Not only does it soften, but the aniseed flavour quietens down and the natural sweetness comes to the fore. Many people who don't appreciate raw fennel love the taste when cooked. The most obvious cooking method is straightforward **blanching**, in other words simmering quartered fennel in salted boiling water until tender – time will vary from one batch to another, but think in terms of 6–7 minutes. Be sure to take extra care over draining, pressing down gently on each piece to expel all the water trapped between the layers of fennel. Then serve it just as it is, dressed perhaps with a spot of butter and a sprinkle of chopped parsley.

Fennel is also extremely good **braised** in a tomato sauce, flavoured with a touch of oregano or chilli if you wish. Give it plenty of time to cook down to a melting tenderness, then serve hot, warm or at room temperature.

Alternative cooking methods include **grilling** (or griddling or barbecuing) and for more on that look at the recipe for griddled fennel with tomato and anchovy dressing on page 138. **Griddled or barbecued**, it gains an extra good smudge of smokiness, whilst retaining more of the raw aniseed scent, a combination that goes extra well with a good steak.

I have mixed feelings about **frying** fennel. It works, of course, in as much as the fennel softens in the fat, but for some unknown reason the taste becomes rather dull. Why, I have no idea. Theoretically it should taste delightful, but unless it is mixed with other vegetables it just comes over as insipid. **Deep-frying**, on the other hand, is a better bet even if you only undertake it once in a blue moon. Coat strips of fennel in flour that has been seasoned with a touch of curry powder, shake off the excess and deep-fry until browned. Now that's really tasty.

Last but by no means least interesting, is a rather curious way of using fennel that I came across a few years ago in a modern Provençal cookery book: candied fennel. No, I'm not joking. Fennel cooked in a thick sugar syrup until very tender is extraordinarily good served for pudding – mix it with toasted flaked almonds or pecans, and top with a swirl of whipped cream. Go on, I dare you.

* *

An unimprovable fennel gratin

This is nothing new, but then it doesn't need to be. Fennel baked with sizzling butter and lots of Parmesan is just perfect and I can't honestly think of any fennel dish that gets better than this. You could serve it with any number of things (chicken or fish in particular) but why? Just savour it on its own, with decent bread to wipe round the plate when the last morsel of fennel has gone.

Serves 4

3–4 bulbs fennel, depending on size
a generous 30g (1oz) butter
plenty of freshly grated Parmesan
salt and pepper

Preheat the oven to 200°C/400°F/Gas 6.

Trim the fennel bulbs, removing outer layers if damaged. Quarter lengthways, then blanch in boiling salted water until just tender. Drain extremely well, pressing out any excess water. Use a little of the butter to grease a gratin dish just big enough to take all the quarters in one tight single layer. Pack in the fennel, then season with plenty of pepper, dot with the remaining butter and dredge generously with Parmesan. Bake until the Parmesan is browned and the butter is sizzling. Serve hot or warm.

* *

Fennel, orange (or pink grapefruit) and olive salad

This is a salad where every component falls perfectly into place with no glitches. It's fresh, refreshing, lively and looks a picture. I couldn't tell you which is better, orange (as long as it is sweet) or pink grapefruit, as I love both.

Serves 4

1 large bulb fennel, trimmed, quartered and very thinly sliced
2 oranges or 1 pink grapefruit, peeled to the quick and sliced or segmented
12 black olives, stoned and roughly sliced

a small handful of fresh mint, shredded
juice of ½ lemon
4 tablespoons extra virgin olive oil
salt and pepper

Mix the fennel, oranges or grapefruit, olives and mint in a shallow serving bowl. Whisk the lemon juice with the olive oil, salt and pepper and drizzle over. Serve.

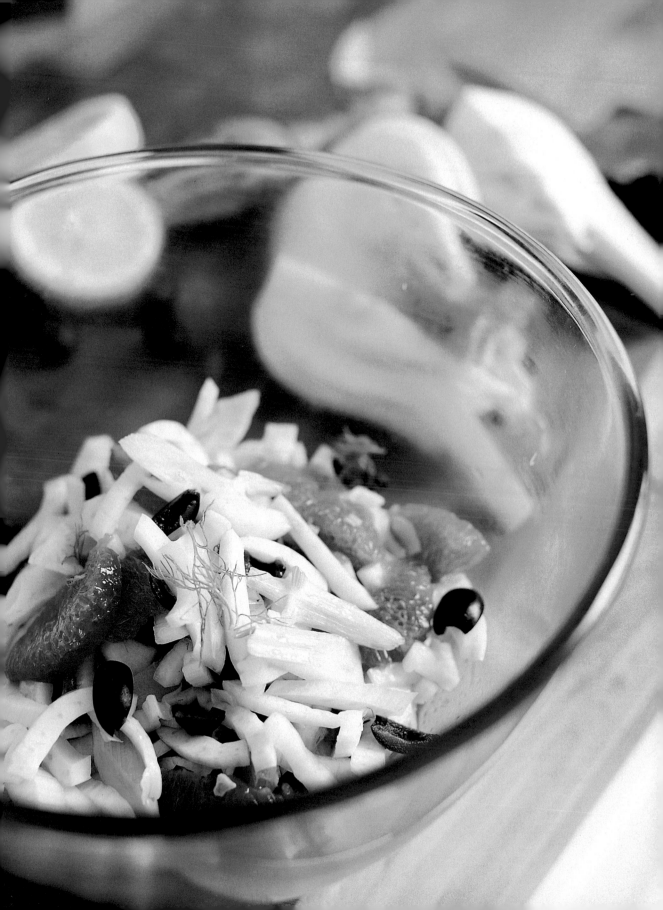

* *

Barbecued or griddled fennel with tomato, garlic and anchovy dressing

Fennel revels in the heat of the griddle or barbecue. That full-on pelt of heat swelters it up gleefully, yielding semi-soft slightly smoky flesh, that delivers sweetness and a touch of aniseed in perfect harmony. It's fantastic warm from the fire, and as good as a dressed salad at room temperature. This fried garlic and fresh tomato dressing, salted with anchovy, highlights all that is best about grilled fennel. It takes just a few minutes to make, but be careful not to burn the garlic.

Serves 4–6

2 bulbs fennel, trimmed
1½ tablespoons extra virgin olive oil

Sauce
2 tablespoons extra virgin olive oil
2 cloves garlic, finely chopped

4 canned anchovy fillets, chopped
2 tablespoons chopped parsley
2 tomatoes, deseeded and finely diced
1 tablespoon balsamic vinegar
salt and pepper

Preheat the barbecue or a griddle pan over a fairly high heat.

Cut the fennel into wedges from stem to stalk. Aim for wedges that are roughly 1.5 cm (just over ½ in) thick – quite how many you get from each head of fennel depends on their size. Toss with olive oil, so that each wedge is lightly coated. Grill, griddle or barbecue, turning the pieces once streaked with brown – this should take around 4–5 minutes per side.

Meanwhile, rustle up the dressing. Heat the oil in a small saucepan, then add the garlic and anchovies. Fry gently, mashing the anchovies down into the oil so that they dissolve a little. As soon as the garlic is beginning to brown whip the pan off the heat. Stir in the parsley, then the tomato followed by the balsamic vinegar and plenty of pepper.

Pile the fennel into a bowl and spoon over the dressing. Nibble a little corner and see if it needs salt – it probably won't as the anchovy is pretty salty. Serve immediately while still hot, or cool to room temperature.

Globe artichokes

* * *

Here's an odd thing about globe artichokes. They love salty, sea winds. The most beautiful artichoke field I've ever seen was on the west coast of Ireland, set amongst the rocky hills that tumbled down into the crashing waves at the rim of the Atlantic. Cold day, leaves and flower heads swaying with each gust. I could taste the salt on the air, and so obviously could those strong stately plants with their silver foliage.

Brittany, so famous for its globe artichokes, bears this out. Salty sea winds blow in from the long coastline to season the fields planted with globe artichokes. There they have become a major crop, and in early summer lorries piled high with densely packed artichokes are a common sight, as they trundle their load to market. Though these cultivated thistles grow peaceably and handsomely inland, they never seem quite as magnificently at home.

The part that we eat, the actual globe artichoke itself, is the hefty flower bud of the plant, secreting at its core, a hairy hoard which forms the eponymous choke. When the artichoke is left unpicked (or picked and left in a warm airing cupboard) the tough 'leaves' (technically not leaves at all but bracts) open out allowing the now purple choke to show through. What's been lost to the dining table is gained as a startling spot of beauty in the vegetable garden.

In France, globe artichokes are considered a regular summer treat for the family. Everyone loves the slow, satisfying performance of stripping off the leaves until the hidden heart is revealed as final pay-off. This is a habit I would love to see building here. It's the total antithesis of the fast-food culture and a perfect way to encourage children to enjoy the shared table.

While the French favour the **bigger, rounded artichokes,** Italians have a penchant for other, smaller varieties, often bearing sharp, aggressive spines. **Small spring artichokes,** too young to have developed the usual hairy choke, are cooked whole, or preserved in oil. More developed artichokes are stewed with wine and garlic, or fried and tossed with pasta, or puréed (heart only) to form a rich and all-but-addictive creamy dressing.

Practicalities

BUYING Most of what follows will concern the larger, French-style globe artichoke. This does not reflect a preference, just the fact that the smaller Italian artichokes are rarely sold in the UK, and when and if they make it to our greengroceries, are often rather tired and dried out. My advice on these is to snap up mini-chokes should you be lucky enough to find them in gloriously healthy and sprightly condition, then turn rapidly to Italian cookbooks to find suitable recipes for deep-frying whole, in the Roman Jewish style (utterly gorgeous), or pickling ('sott'olio') in oil to serve eventually with an antipasto of Parma ham, salami, and tomato and mozzarella salad.

Large globe artichokes occasionally suffer, like their wee relatives, from dismal, dry desperation. Don't waste money on artichokes with that pinched desiccated look. Even at rock-bottom move-'em-fast prices, they are not going to deliver. Brown-tipped, crisp-edged leaves are beacons that signal avoidance. What you want is a curvaceous, plump, well-fed sort of a look. Think Rubens, not El Greco. Bought in fine fettle, you can afford to let artichokes wait for up to two or three days (in the vegetable drawer of the fridge) before cooking, but don't tarry too long.

Preparation begins with a soak in a cold salt bath – upside down, stems waving, heads plunged into the salted water. Not 100 per cent essential, but it loosens and flushes out hidden insects. Leave them bobbing for half an hour or so, then shake off water (and insects), and dry roughly.

At the chopping board, begin by snapping the stems (which can sometimes be used, read on) off close to the base of the artichoke head. This will pull some of the tough fibres out of the base. Rub the exposed flesh with a little lemon juice to diminish browning. If you want to serve them whole that's really all you need to do. Unless, that is, you have bought a variety with extraordinarily hard and sharp needle-like tips to the leaves (more common in mini-chokes), in which case you will be thoughtful enough to snip these off with scissors.

Bring a large pan of salted, acidulated water, to the boil. To acidulate the water, simply squeeze in the juice of ½–1 lemon, depending on the quantity of water, or add a few splashes of white wine vinegar. Cram the artichokes in, stalk-end downwards in the water, bring back to the boil and leave to simmer until the outer leaves can be pulled away easily with a small nugget of tender artichoke at their base, around 30–40 minutes. Drain the artichokes thoroughly. Serve at once, while still hot, with jugs of melted butter sharpened with a touch of lemon juice, or leave to cool and serve with a lively vinaigrette. More on the eating etiquette below.

To make **artichoke bowls**, prepare and cook as before. Once they are well drained, take the first artichoke and carefully ease open the leaves until you detect the inner purple-white cone of soft leaves in the centre. Grasp this firmly and twist until it comes away. Now use a teaspoon and/or hands to pull out the soft hairy choke underneath, taking care to extricate every last tuft. Voilà, first bowl done. Now on to the next. It's pretty obvious that it is not practical to serve artichoke bowls hot for more than two at a time, unless you have a kitchen team on the case. In my house, I always leave them to cool before filling.

All kinds of delicious things can then be inserted into the bowl – lemony scrambled eggs perhaps, or a thick dressing of soured cream mixed with chopped fresh chives and dill, or a fabulous crab, mayonnaise and tarragon concoction, or a purée of broad beans (my mother's favourite), a pretty little salad of diced tomatoes, olives, basil and sautéed courgettes, and so on and so forth. The idea is to pull the leaves off and dip into the dressing one by one.

Still on preparation, it's time to progress on to trimming **artichoke hearts or bottoms**. To many this seems like wanton wastefulness – all those leaves that are heading straight for the compost heap. However, in the summer you do, just once in a while, get blessed by finding some market-trader selling off heaps of artichokes at comparatively rock-bottom prices, a chance not to be missed. So, arm yourself with a sharp knife, a bowl of acidulated water and a washing-up basin to hold all the rejected leaves. Begin by snapping off the stem close to the base. Slice the top portions of the leaves off. Now begin to whittle leaves off the sides of the base of the artichoke, working your way around and around again, until the flesh proper is exposed. Dip in that acidulated water. Using the tip of your knife, ease the cone of immature leaves (which is all you should have left by now) away from the base and discard. Next, carefully cut and scrape the exposed choke away from the top of the base, revealing the petite naked base in full glory. Drop immediately into acidulated water.

The base can be cooked in any number of ways. The most obvious is to simmer in salted acidulated water until just tender, then you could slice and dress in a vinaigrette to incorporate in a mixed salad, or with prawns, which have an affinity with artichokes, and rocket to make a pretty summer starter. Or you could serve them hot, using them as an edible saucer, which you might fill with a mess of peperonata, topped with basil, or sautéed spinach with pine nuts and feta or those lemony scrambled eggs again, with smoked salmon folded through. Clever clogs could even make a cheese soufflé mixture, spoon it into the artichoke saucers and whip them into a hot oven until puffed and golden – very impressive.

Slices of raw base make good **fritters**, and are even nicer sautéed in olive oil until tender – more of that in the pasta recipe.

Most people throw out the artichoke stems along with the leaves, but not Cypriots. Or at least not the Cypriot greengrocer I used to go to when I lived in London. When the artichokes are good and fresh and tender, the stems can be peeled to remove the long, chewy fibres, then what is left can be sliced thinly, dressed with lemon and olive oil, salt and pepper to make an unusually good, raw salad. Try it.

Do not, in a thrifty manner, throw a handful of artichoke trimmings into the stockpot – they will make the stock bitter.

How to eat an artichoke
Despite all that stuff I've penned about how to do this and that to artichokes, the very best way to eat them remains the most obvious – boiled whole and served either hot, warm, or at room temperature. The paced, timely process of sitting down with friends or family and an artichoke apiece, and pulling them apart, is culinary theatre at its most appealing and relaxed. Not

something to be rushed. If this has not been part of your life up until now, this is how to do it:

Prop your plate up by sliding your fork underneath it at the opposite edge to you. Now take a few spoonfuls of the dressing (hot butter, touched with lemon juice or a tart hollandaise to go with hot artichokes, vinaigrette to go with cold ones) and put it on your plate so that it puddles in the lower part. The artichoke sits, when you are not pulling leaves off, in the upper centre of the plate. One by one, pull off leaves, starting at the outside, and dip the base of each one into the dressing. Now suck and nibble off that little plumpness of sweet artichoke flesh and then discard the leaf. Continue in this way until you work your way down to the cone of soft, baby leaves in the centre.

Grasp the cone in one hand, the base in the other and twist it off. Scrape away any hairs caught on the inside of the cone, then nibble off the rim of flesh, before discarding. Scrape and tug the choke off the artichoke heart. Take the fork out from underneath your plate so that it sits flat, with the heart on it. Take your final helping of dressing and spoon it over, then devour the heart.

Note to the cook – always make about twice as much dressing as you think you'll need.

SEE ALSO JERUSALEM ARTICHOKES (PAGE 39).

* *

Penne with fresh artichokes and saffron

Sautéed, sliced globe artichoke hearts are just heavenly, on their own or like this, finished with cream and saffron and tossed with pasta.

Once you've prepared the artichokes, the actual cooking of the sauce is a swift process – it shouldn't take any longer than the pasta itself.

Serves 4

4–6 medium globe artichokes
finely grated zest of ½ lemon, the juice
    of 1½
400g (14oz) penne pasta
30g (1oz) butter
1 tablespoon extra virgin olive oil

300ml (10floz) double cream
a generous pinch of saffron threads
2 tablespoons finely chopped parsley
freshly grated Parmesan
salt and pepper

Prepare the artichokes as for hearts (see above). Cut into 5mm (¼in) thick slices, and keep in water acidulated with the juice of 1 lemon until ready to cook.

Put a large pan of salted water on to boil. As soon as it reaches a rolling boil, tip in the penne. Bring back to the boil and cook until tender (around 10 minutes, but check packet instructions).

Melt the butter and oil in a frying pan over a medium heat. Drain and dry the artichoke slices then add to the pan when it is hot. Sauté for about 5 minutes until browned and tender. Now add the cream, saffron, lemon zest and two-thirds of the parsley. Season, stir and simmer for about 2 minutes until the sauce is slightly thickened. Draw off the heat and stir in the remaining lemon juice. Taste and adjust the seasoning. Keep warm.

Drain the pasta, then return to the pan and toss with the artichoke and saffron sauce. Sprinkle with the last of the parsley, then serve immediately, making sure everyone gets their share of artichoke pieces. Pass the Parmesan around to scatter over the pasta.

* *

Kohlrabi

* * *

What sounds, at first, an exotic and strange vegetable loses much of its romantic gloss with translation from the German. 'Kohlrabi' – glamorous; 'cabbage-turnip' – dull as ditchwater. No wonder those who have tried to promote it in this country have stuck with the untranslated name. I can't think offhand of any other vegetable beginning with a 'k' except kale and kidney beans. That in itself lends it a curious cachet. Even so, kohlrabi has remained marginalised amongst the bevy of vegetables that crowd the shelves of supermarkets and greengrocers. Odd, I think, because at their best they can be extremely appetising, even if they don't blow your socks off.

The turnip part of the uninspired name refers purely to the shape of the kohlrabi, not to the taste. The vegetable is actually the swollen stem of a cabbage, an edible corm in other words. It has a pleasingly barmy look to it, with the stems growing out of the corm here and there at quirky angles – and if you are lucky enough to get kohlrabi complete with a handsome complement of leaves at the end of the barmy stems, you'll discover that the leaves, too, are good to eat. Most of the kohlrabi sold here is pale green, but you may also come across a fetching purple variety, which tastes exactly the same.

Back to that corm. When fresh and not over-swollen the taste is sweetish, somewhat reminiscent of immature green coconut flesh (not the desiccated stuff, which is quite different), with a crisp, juicy texture that holds from raw through a fair amount of cooking. This crispness is something that both children and adults appreciate, so make the most of it.

Practicalities

BUYING In practice you may not have a great deal of choice, but if you can pick out small- to medium-sized kohlrabi, then they will taste all the better for their lack of size. They should be firm, pale green or purple, and still complete with the stubs of stalks sticking out. The leaves, which shamefully are usually shorn off, should be treated like spring greens when the opportunity arises.

COOKING With their crisp texture, kohlrabi are excellent **raw** – in salads maybe or cut into fingers to dip into hummus or some other pungent dip. I love thin slices of kohlrabi, mixed with paper-thin slices of fennel and tossed with a perky Asian dressing rich in chilli, lime, ginger and fish sauce.

Before you start making your salad, though, you will need to assess whether the skin should stay or go. As the kohlrabi grows, the skin toughens. In smaller corms the skin will be tender enough to eat with pleasure, whereas with larger ones you would be well advised to trim it off. Those funky stalks will have to go too, I'm afraid.

To cook, you can opt for the obvious – just dunk it in **simmering salted water** for 4–5 minutes depending on thickness, until softened enough to develop the flavour, or you may prefer to **braise** it (cut into 5 mm/¼ in thick slices) with a knob of butter over a low heat, with a sprig or two of tarragon if you have any around, for around 6–7 minutes, in a covered pan. Check to make sure that it doesn't burn, and if necessary, add a small splash of water.

Hot kohlrabi needs little more than a knob of butter to set it off, though you can take matters further than that. In Germany, Austria and eastern Europe, it is often cooked then **baked** in a white sauce (a Hungarian acquaintance enriches his with a generous helping of soured cream), perhaps with a little cheese scattered on top. I like to add a spot of mustard to the sauce, or fresh dill or fennel, or some chopped ham, to liven matters up. It is good, too, napped in a rich tomato sauce, with a few chopped green olives thrown in for good measure.

* *

Antonio Carluccio's braised kohlrabi

This most unusual way of cooking kohlrabi is a total winner with its sweet and sour overtones. It comes from the excellent *Antonio Carluccio's Vegetables* (Headline, 2000), and makes a pleasing contrast to the many eastern European kohlrabi recipes that nap the vegetable with a white sauce.

Antonio recommends serving it with pork or lamb dishes, though we found it excellent alongside a golden roast chicken.

Serves 4–5

40 g (1½ oz) unsalted butter
30 g (1 oz) caster sugar
800 g (1¾ lb) kohlrabi, peeled, sliced and
  then cut into fingers

2 tbsp white wine vinegar
1 tbsp plain flour
½ tsp cumin seeds
250 ml (9 fl oz) vegetable stock
salt and pepper

Gently melt the butter in a saucepan and add the sugar. Cook until the butter starts to turn golden brown. Add the kohlrabi and the vinegar and simmer for about 10 minutes. Add the flour and cumin seeds and gradually stir in the stock. Continue cooking until the kohlrabi is cooked. Season.

* *

Smothered leeks and kohlrabi

Smothering is not as violent as it sounds, at least not here. It's simply a way of cooking vegetables with a little fat and the least possible amount of water, in a covered pan (I guess that's the smothering bit) until very, very tender. You can smother one vegetable on its own, or a collection, which gives the tiny amount of liquid left at the end of the cooking time a particularly good flavour. Kohlrabi holds together well, adding its own natural sweetness.

Serves 6

3 leeks, trimmed and cut into 2 cm (³/₄ in) lengths
2 kohlrabi (around 650 g/1 lb 7 oz), trimmed, peeled and cut into 2 cm (³/₄ in) cubes
3 large carrots (around 550 g/1¹/₄ lb), peeled and cut into 2 cm (³/₄ in) pieces
6 cloves garlic

1 bay leaf
2 sprigs thyme
40 g (1¹/₂ oz) butter
salt and pepper

Put the leeks, kohlrabi, carrots and garlic into a wide shallow pan which will take them in a single layer. Tuck the herbs down among them. Pour in enough water to come about 1.5 cm (¹/₂ in) up the sides of the pan. Season with salt and pepper and dot with butter. Bring up to the boil, then reduce the heat right down to the lowest thread of warmth. Cover the pan with a lid or foil, and leave to cook very gently for about 1 hour, stirring occasionally to make sure that it doesn't catch. If necessary add a splash or two of water. Alternatively, if you're left with a swilling pond, uncover and boil it off.

Either way, you are aiming to end up with meltingly tender vegetables, perhaps slightly patched with brown towards the end of cooking, with little more than a few tablespoonfuls of syrupy liquid left in the pan.

* *

Samphire

* * *

Marsh samphire is a seashore vegetable, not a seaweed. Resembling small forked shoots of green coral, it grows wild around our coasts but is not unique to our shores. Not only does it dot the coasts of Europe, but it even grows as far afield as Mexico. Or at least that's where my fishmonger assured me the unseasonably early samphire he was selling had been flown in from. Now there's unnecessary food miles for you. In the UK Norfolk is its most famous home, and it has been gathered here for centuries, not only for eating but also for use in the making of glass, hence one of its alternative names, glasswort. A friend of mine remembers the samphire seller's cart doing the rounds of the Norfolk back streets when he was a child in the 1960s.

Samphire tastes like nothing else. It tastes of the pure salt sea, of winds whipping through your hair, of waves crashing on to the shore. It is juicy, crisp and salty and in a class of its own. Almost. Because there are two samphires. As well as plump, succulent marsh samphire, there is flat-lobed ozone-scented rock samphire. They are not related, they don't grow in the same terrain, they don't even look that similar. However, they are of much the same size and they both love the sea air. This rarer second samphire is one that you must learn to recognise in the wild if you want to taste it, for it never sees the inside of a shop. It carries in it a whiff of iodine which some love and others loathe.

Marsh samphire is easier to get acquainted with, and its sea-salt savour makes it a natural companion on the plate with fish. The season begins in late April or early May, and continues right through the summer. It is at its best in May and the first weeks of June. By mid-July the maturing plants develop a tough, stringy core, and the price drops precipitously.

If you go gathering samphire yourself, remember Edgar's words in *King*

Lear: '...halfway down, Hangs one that gathers samphire, dreadful trade!'
He's really talking about **rock samphire** which grows on cliffs, but the advice
holds for harvesting **marsh samphire** in salty seaside marshes. In other
words, be careful for it often grows in perilous places. Next, of course, must
come the modern words of warning – don't eat it unless you are one
hundred per cent sure that you have picked the correct plant.

Practicalities

BUYING Go to the fishmonger's for samphire, not the greengrocer. The flavour is
intense, so you won't want huge amounts. A big handful of samphire is
enough for three to four people. The succulent green stems should be firm,
olive green, slightly translucent and dry. Slimy samphire is rotting
samphire.

Store your samphire, wrapped in a paper bag, in the vegetable drawer of
the fridge for a day or two. It will dry out and wrinkle like old skin if you
keep it much longer. Before using, rinse it well, then pick out any stray bits of
root, the odd twig, or brown pieces.

Samphire is nearly always cooked, though I rather like it **raw**, a few sprigs
tossed into a salad to add unusual crispness. **Steaming or blanching** in
boiling water are the best ways to cook samphire as they will soften the
saltiness a little. About 2–3 minutes in boiling water is all that it needs,
3–4 minutes if steaming. Drain it well, then dot with butter and serve.
Frying or roasting is disastrous, making samphire unbearably salty and
quite inedible.

The fact that samphire is sold alongside fish confirms that this is a
vegetable that works best with seafood. It enhances any fish you care to
mention, and counterpoints the sweetness of shellfish neatly. The best-
known samphire dish is a simple one – steam salmon fillet on a bed of
samphire until just cooked through but with a thread of translucence
lingering in the centre (around 5 minutes), and serve with a lemony beurre
blanc (see page 338). Perfect, especially if the salmon is wild.

I don't think you should get too carried away with fancy recipes for
samphire, but if you only have a small amount, you could eke it out by
mixing warm cooked samphire with potato and mayonnaise to go with
grilled halibut, perhaps, or toss with cool cucumber, flaked hot-smoked

salmon, and a tarragon vinaigrette.

When you have lots and lots of samphire to use up, the most obvious and I think most delicious recipe to turn to is old-fashioned **pickled** samphire. This is how I like samphire best of all, preserved in a sweet, sharp, spicy liquid, always at the ready to serve with fresh or smoked fish, or even with a fine piece of cheese or a pâté.

* *

Pickled samphire

The essential thing to remember is that the samphire must be completely covered by the spiced vinegar. As long as you've got that right, the exact weight of samphire is neither here nor there. If you have more than you can cram comfortably into one jar, then pack the rest into a second jar, and make up a little extra vinegar if necessary.

Fills a 1–1.5 litre (1⅓–2¾ pint) preserving jar
500 g (1 lb 2 oz) samphire

Spiced vinegar
1.2 litres (2 pints) white wine vinegar
600 g (1 lb 5 oz) caster sugar
24 allspice berries
12 cloves

2 cinnamon sticks
2 tablespoons coriander seeds
20 black peppercorns
2 star anise

Put all the ingredients for the spiced vinegar into a saucepan and bring gently up to the boil, stirring until the sugar has dissolved. Draw off the heat, pour into a bowl, then cover and leave to cool and settle for 2–3 hours. Strain out the spices.

Meanwhile, pick over the samphire, removing roots and damaged parts. Rinse thoroughly and dry. Pack into cold sterilised jar(s)(see page 215), then pour in enough vinegar to cover completely (you probably won't need it all, but the remainder will keep in the fridge until your next batch of pickling). Seal tightly, label and store in a cool dark place for at least 2 weeks, preferably 4, before delving into the jars.

* *

Wild asparagus

* * *

My father had a bit of a thing for wild asparagus. Looking back, it seems as if he always knew where to find it, every spring, wherever we were. I was not overjoyed as he marched us onwards to gather his harvest. I never much cared for it back then – it has a bitterness that did not appeal – and when we found some, it invariably dominated that evening's supper. I'm sorry to admit that I have never quite suppressed the dislike.

As it happens, it is unlikely that I will be faced with many more plates of wild asparagus, as it is now considered an endangered species in the UK and is on the decline in continental Europe, too. I don't think my father was entirely to blame for this state of affairs – erosion, lack of managed grazing and other less controllable forces have played a greater part in the plant's demise than foraging by those in the know.

The odd thing is that you may still find wild asparagus from time to time on restaurant menus and even at posh greengroceries. Despite the name this is no more 'wild' or 'asparagus' than the so-called wild rocket that abounds in supermarkets. It is, for a start, far nicer than real wild asparagus, in my opinion. And it looks quite different – short fine stems topped with a bulging green head. This is the young shoots of cultivated *Ornithagalum pyrenaicum*, **'aspergette'** in French, and **'Bath asparagus'** in English. It grows wild in the Pyrenees as its Latin name suggests.

Should you come across real wild asparagus, leave it alone. Don't go hunting for wild Bath asparagus, either. Cultivated Bath asparagus is another matter. Try it when you come across it, which won't be often unless you frequent very high-class veg stores. I would suggest that you simply blanch Bath asparagus in lightly salted water for 2 minutes, then drain and eat with melted butter, or use as a garnish, perhaps on a dish of scrambled eggs.

SEE ALSO ASPARAGUS (PAGE 110).

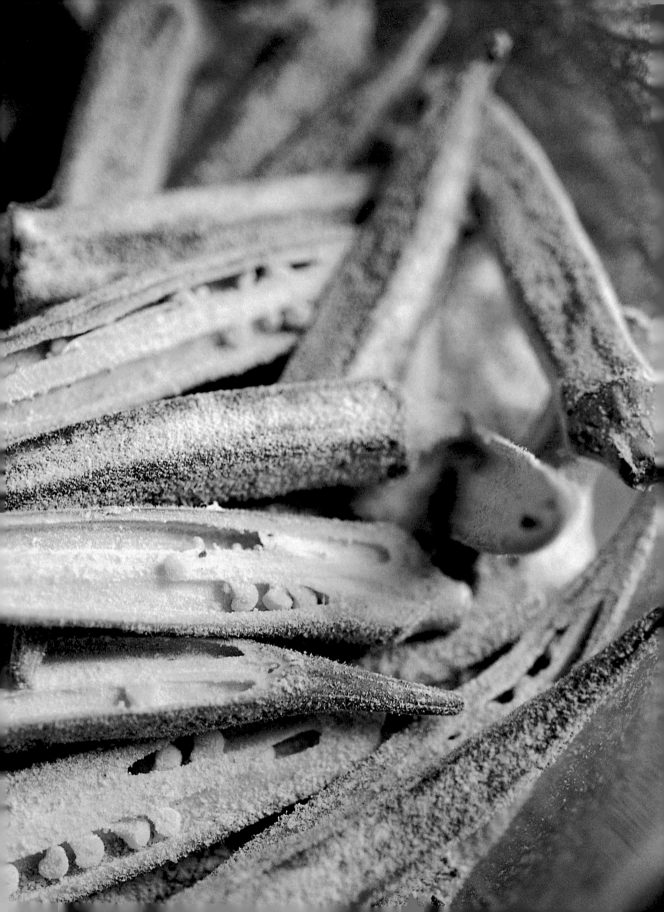

Fruits

****

Aubergine Avocado
Bell peppers Okra
Tomatoes

* *

Aubergine

* * *

Aubergines like to play tricks on people. You may think that an aubergine is a large, dark purple-black vegetable, and some of the time you would be quite correct. Then off you go to the local Thai restaurant and swimming around in your green curry are some oversized peas. Gotcha! They're not peas at all. They're aubergines in their most inspired disguise. Bite into these cleverly camouflaged 'peas' and your error is revealed. Though you may not be able to place it instantly, there's a touch of bitterness, a familiar hint of texture, all concentrated essence of pure aubergine, encapsulated in one mini sphere. **Pea aubergines** grow in clusters and bear no visual resemblance whatsoever to what we think of as an aubergine.

Aubergines have also been known to dress up as eggs. Pure and white and oval, the one give-away is the grey-green stem tacked on to one end like an absurd hat. If it weren't for this, you might find yourself trying to crack one open some bleary, hungover morning. The **egg-sized aubergine** also comes in a fetching bright yellow and that more familiar polished purple. You would have to have had a seriously heavy night to mistake either of these for your breakfast egg, but they can still cause confusion. Incidentally, it may well be this type of aubergine that gave rise to the American name for the vegetable, 'eggplant'.

Some aubergines look as if they've had a session on the rack to stretch them out to an unexpected slenderness. Often streaked with white, perhaps because of the stress of all that stretching, they're bereft of the pleasing plumpness of most full-sized aubergines. Some of the most handsome aubergines are the **violet Mediterranean aubergines**; less sleek than classic aubergines, their curves have an unruly swell to them, clad in glowing violet and white skin. In the south of Italy they are known as **'nostrano' aubergines,** which translates simply as 'our very own' aubergines, but always

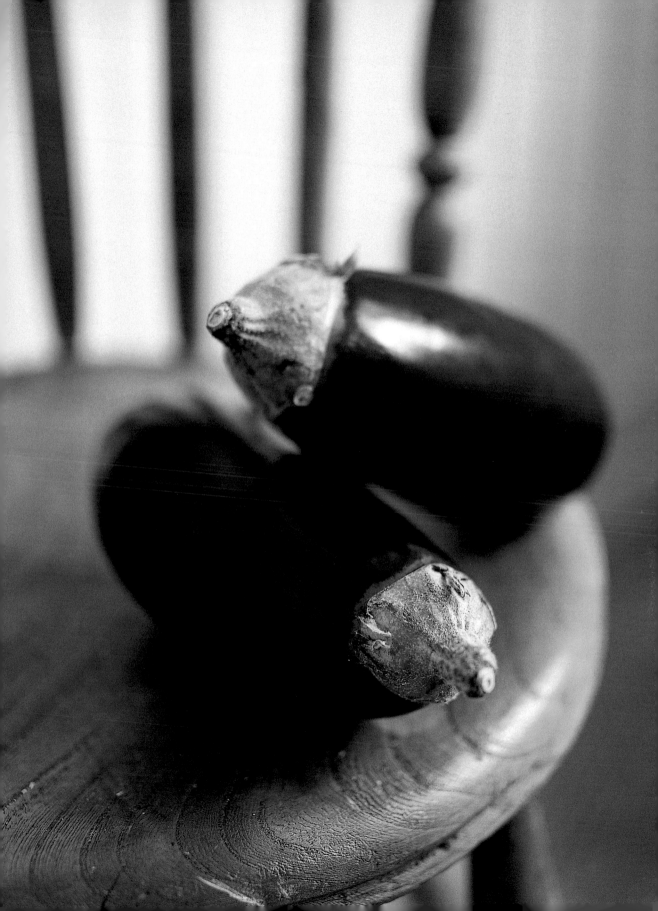

makes me think of the Neapolitan Mafia, the Cosa Nostra – our thing. All that sunshine breeds possessiveness, violence and the most sublime, barely disguised aubergines.

Practicalities

Let's assume that you are purchasing larger classical black-purple skinned aubergines, or if you are lucky the paler, streaky violet aubergines. It's the skin you should be looking at above all. It must be taut, with the healthiest of sheens. A high gloss may just mean someone's given them a polish, but polishing can only be effective on a firm aubergine. Firmness will come with the taut glowing skin. Wrinkles, soft patches, brown bruising (not always easy to detect) and/or dull lifeless skin (this is beginning to sound like an ad for an anti-aging cream) are bad signs.

The same principles go for the purple-skinned egg-sized aubergines, but white and yellow-skinned varieties usually have a matt skin, as do pea aubergines.

Aubergines need to be kept in the vegetable drawer of the fridge, where they can hang out for 4 or 5 days as long as they are used before they begin to sag.

When making **purées** there is absolutely no preparation involved. The whole aubergine is either **grilled or barbecued** (to give a smoky flavour) until the skin is charred and the flesh is soft. Alternatively, **roast** them in a hot, hot oven for 20–30 minutes until soft. Then cut them in half or quarters lengthways and leave to drain in a colander until cool enough to handle, before discarding the skin and whizzing the flesh with olive oil, yoghurt, garlic, lemon, cumin, and/or herbs. 'Hunkar begendi', sultan's pleasure, is a fabulous hot dish of aubergine puréed with a béchamel sauce and flavoured with Parmesan, an unexpectedly good alternative to mash.

For most other dishes you need do no more than cut the stalk end off, and then slice or dice the aubergine as required. The flesh will discolour on exposure to the air but since you are likely to go on to **fry or bake** the aubergine, this doesn't matter. Older recipes for aubergines will always instruct you to salt the cut aubergine 'to remove the bitter juices'. Modern varieties of aubergine are virtually never bitter, but that doesn't mean salting is entirely redundant, merely no longer a necessity. Salting still improves the flavour, reducing that hint of tinniness, but perhaps more relevant is that a salted aubergine will absorb less oil as it fries. What this means in practice is that if you have the time, it's still a good idea to salt, but you can get away without it. To salt sliced aubergines, lay the slices out on baking trays and sprinkle lightly with salt. Diced aubergine is better salted in a colander, set over a bowl to catch the drips. Either way, leave the aubergine for 30–60 minutes to disgorge its juices, then dry before cooking. Most of the salt will have been lost with the liquid, but go easy on the seasoning at first, just in case.

You don't need to peel aubergines – the skin holds the flesh together and has a brooding drama to it that is rare in most vegetables. Some Middle Eastern recipes will tell you to peel off strips of skin, leaving half in place. This is both decorative and practical, allowing oil or other flavourings to seep in where the flesh is exposed, but leaving enough skin to hold the softening aubergine together.

Aubergines are popular through a broad swathe of countries – from the south of France through to China – because their oddly spongy flesh is extremely absorbent and the flavour mild enough to support an extraordinary range of flavourings. Wherever they are used, they fit effortlessly into the local style of cooking as long as the seasonings are bold and enthusiastic. Aubergine fares less well in northerly muted cuisines.

Aubergines need oil. No getting around it. One rare successful oil-free aubergine dish is a purée of grilled aubergine blended with yoghurt (see above) but otherwise it's essential. Straight boiled aubergine is foul. Woe betide anyone who chucks a handful of aubergine cubes into a pan of water, or even tomato sauce. There is no point in massacring aubergine in this way. It won't make anyone happy.

The way to an aubergine's heart is to **fry it**. Cubed or in slices, there is nothing aubergine likes better than to dive into a frying pan holding a slick of fragrant, sizzling hot oil, especially olive oil. Turn the heat up high and sauté cubes, or fry slices flat, marvelling at the greedy way they guzzle up that oil. Once they are browned nicely they will release some of it back into the pan, but not as much as the calorie conscious would like. Too low a heat, or an overcrowded pan makes for greasy aubergine. For some dishes (I'm thinking in particular of moussaka) I find it easier, and more economical, to brush the aubergine slices with oil, then roast them on a baking tray in a hot oven (220°C/425°F/Gas 7) for 10–15 minutes until browned.

Grilling, griddling or barbecuing sliced aubergine is a winning option, imbuing it to varying degrees with a pleasing smokiness. As with baking, the aubergine must be brushed or tossed with oil, preferably olive, before it meets the heat, then cooked until tender and striped or patched with brown.

Stuffed aubergines come in several guises. The easiest way is to halve the aubergine lengthways, scoop out a little of the flesh to form a cavity and pile the stuffing straight in. In the Levant the prepared aubergine may be deep-fried before stuffing, but this is not enormously practical, and since it will subsequently be baked with its stuffing in anyway, it's a step that can be ignored. The aubergine will not turn out as creamy, but it will still absorb juices from the stuffing to give it richness. If halving your aubergine seems far too simplistic, you can go for more complicated excavation methods. With medium-sized squat aubergines, you could slice off the stalk end to form a lid, then tunnel in from here to create a well for the stuffing. With smaller, more slender aubergines, or little egg aubergines, leave the stalk in place, but instead cut a slit from just below the stalk, right down almost, but not quite, to the opposite end. The idea is to form a pocket, so don't plunge the knife right through to the opposite side of the aubergine. Pull the slit open so that you can force as much stuffing as possible inside. The disadvantage of both of these methods, it seems to me, is that you can't get as much stuffing into the aubergine. In some cases this may not matter, but it is worth considering before you take action.

About the simplest aubergine recipe worth its salt is the Italian melanzane al funghetto, aubergines cooked like little mushrooms. Cubes of aubergine are **sautéed** in olive oil with chopped garlic and parsley added towards the end of the cooking time. Another, more substantial Italian aubergine classic is melanzane alla parmigiana, a **gratin** of fried or grilled or baked aubergine slices, layered with plenty of thick, home-made tomato sauce and mozzarella, the top dredged with Parmesan and an extra drizzle of oil before baking in the oven until hot and sizzling. You might guess from the name that this dish is a speciality of the area around Parma in the north of the country, but interestingly the Sicilians also claim it as their own. Just too good to give up, I guess.

Sicily is also the home to my favourite aubergine dish, caponata, for which I give a recipe below. This is a sort of **aubergine stew**, one of the many that abound around the shores of the Mediterranean. The most famous and most maligned is the French ratatouille. At its best this is a fabulous dish that reeks of summer sunshine. At its worst it is a miserable penance forced on people in the name of health. Essentially a mix of aubergine, courgette and peppers captured in a tomato sauce usually flavoured with coriander seed, the individual vegetables need to be sautéed separately, then cooked gently together in a rich, thick tomato sauce for long enough for flavours to meld, but not so long that they collapse to mushiness. Made well, this is a dish that is as good served at room temperature as hot, perhaps even better.

In summertime, I often make **grilled aubergine salads**. Sliced to a thickness of around 1 cm (½ in), I marinate the aubergines in olive oil with crushed garlic, a few crushed spices (such as cumin, coriander, chillies, fennel and so on) or herbs, salt and pepper, then brush off the bits and grill or barbecue. In theory they could also be griddled but they take up such a massive amount of space that they would have to be cooked in multiple batches, thus smoking out the kitchen royally. As soon as they are browned and tender, I toss them with a vinaigrette and lots of chopped herbs, then leave to cool. Excellent just as they are, they can also be expanded with the addition of diced tomato, skinned grilled peppers, blanched green or wax beans, mozzarella, and so on.

Slices of grilled aubergine, cut from top to toe for maximum size are ideal for rolling around a filling to make a more deconstructed version of stuffed aubergine. As with all stuffings for aubergine, it will need to be boldly flavoured, such as the one used for the involtini di peperoni on page 180. In fact, you could simply substitute grilled slices of aubergine for the grilled skinned pepper to produce a different, but equally delicious dish.

Much as I love the fragrant, often sweet and sour, tomatoey aubergine dishes of the Middle East, I occasionally make forays further east, to India in particular, where aubergine is combined with spices to form splendid curries. The best, I think, include chickpeas whose firm mealiness is a good foil for the smoothness of the aubergine pieces.

* *

Aubergine and pomegranate cream

Now that pomegranate molasses is becoming easier to find in this country (good delis, Middle Eastern food stores and even a few supermarkets stock it), this gorgeous aubergine dip is something we can all make at home. The fruity sourness of the molasses (made from a sour variety of pomegranate) gives it a unique flavour. Serve it with warm pitta bread and strips of raw vegetables (cucumber, peppers, fennel and so on), radishes and cherry tomatoes.

Once you've got a taste for the molasses, try using it in salad dressings, tomato sauces, stews and other dishes.

Serves 6

1 large aubergine
1–2 tablespoons pomegranate molasses
150g (5oz) Greek-style or natural yoghurt
2 tablespoons tahina
1 clove garlic, crushed
salt and pepper

To serve
the seeds of ½ pomegranate
a little chopped fresh coriander

Either grill the aubergine slowly, turning as the skin blackens and burns, or else preheat the oven to 220°C/425°F/Gas 7 and roast the aubergines in it until very tender. The flavour is not quite so good, but you don't have to hang around turning them all the time. Set the aubergine aside until cool enough to handle, then strip off the skin and chop the flesh roughly. Drain in a colander for half an hour, then squeeze out excess liquid.

For an unevenly textured purée, mash the flesh with a fork, then beat in the remaining ingredients, before tasting and adjusting seasoning.

For a smoother purée, just drop the aubergine into the bowl of the processor, add the remaining ingredients and process until smooth. Taste and adjust seasoning.

Spoon the resulting purée into a bowl and just before serving, scatter over the pomegranate seeds and coriander.

Caponata

Caponata is something between a relish and a side dish, the kind of thing that you might serve with hot grilled chicken or lamb chops, or as a first course or as part of a summer lunch along with, say, a green salad and slices of cured hams, salamis and so on. The making of it is not a task to be hurried – the loving browning of celery and aubergine and onion is essential to the complex, rounded flavour of the finished dish – but the caponata will taste all the better for being made 24 hours in advance, allowing plenty of time for the taste to mature.

Even those who profess to loathe celery will not mind it in this context, as it melts into the whole almost imperceptibly. Do not be alarmed by the raw vinegariness of the caponata when it is first cooked and still hot in the pan. By the time it has cooled to room temperature the jagged notes will have settled down into complete harmony.

Serves 4–6

1 large aubergine, diced
6 tablespoons olive oil
6 sticks celery, chopped
1 onion, chopped
1 x 400 g can chopped tomatoes or 450 g
  (1 lb) fresh tomatoes, skinned and chopped
2 tablespoons caster sugar
4 tablespoons red wine vinegar

1 teaspoon freshly grated nutmeg
1 heaped teaspoon capers
12 green or black olives, pitted and roughly
  chopped
2 tablespoons chopped fresh parsley
salt and pepper

Spread out the aubergine dice in a colander, sprinkle with salt and set aside for ½–1 hour. Press gently to extract as much water as possible. Dry on kitchen paper or a clean tea-towel.

Heat 4 tablespoons of the olive oil in a heavy-based frying-pan. Sauté the celery until browned. Scoop out and set aside. Fry the aubergine in the same oil until browned and tender, adding a little extra oil if necessary. Scoop out and leave to cool.

Add the remaining oil to the pan and sauté the onion until golden. Add the tomatoes and simmer for 15 minutes until thick. Next add the sugar, vinegar and nutmeg and cook for a further 10 minutes, until you have a rich sweet-and-sour sauce. Add a little salt and plenty of pepper. Stir in the capers, olives, parsley, aubergine and celery. Taste and adjust the seasoning – the flavours will soften as the caponata cools. Serve in a dish when cool.

* *

Sweet and sour stuffed aubergines

Many Middle Eastern recipes for stuffed aubergines begin with deep-frying the aubergines. This gives them a silky richness, but is a real faff in a domestic kitchen and, of course, loads on the calories. In fact, they don't need to be pre-cooked at all, still emerging tender from the oven, having absorbed the flavours of their filling. As long, that is, as there is enough moisture in the dish to soften them properly. In this lovely recipe for aubergines stuffed with a sweet and sour minced beef filling, the moisture is provided by a blend of water, tomato purée, lemon juice and sugar.

Serves 4

2 medium aubergines
4 tablespoons tomato purée
juice of 1 lemon
2 tablespoons caster sugar
extra virgin olive oil
salt and pepper

Filling
2 tablespoons extra virgin olive oil
1 onion, chopped
2 cloves garlic, chopped
300 g (11 oz) minced beef
1 heaped teaspoon ground cinnamon
1 heaped teaspoon ground cumin
2 tomatoes, deseeded and finely diced
3 tablespoons bulgur wheat
30 g (1 oz) pine nuts
30 g (1 oz) currants

Halve the aubergines lengthways and scoop out a little of the centre (add to a soup or a stew). Season the aubergines with salt and then turn upside down on a wire rack to drain.

To make the filling, heat the olive oil and fry the onion until tender then add the garlic and fry for a minute or so longer. Add the meat and fry until it

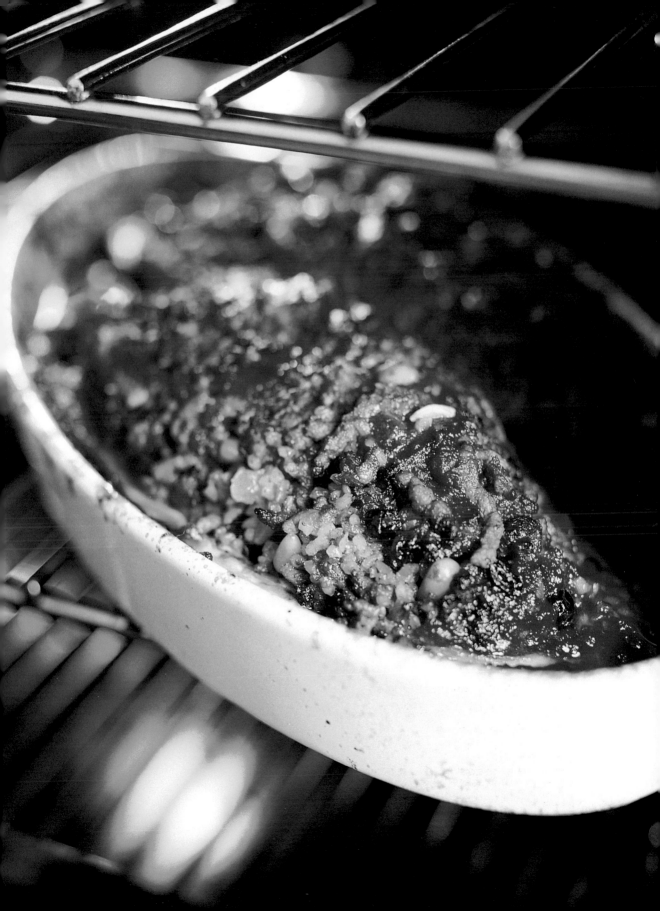

has changed colour, breaking up the lumps. Sprinkle over the spices, salt and pepper and fry for another minute. Stir in the tomatoes and just enough water to cover. Simmer gently for 30 minutes until tender. Taste and adjust the seasoning, then stir in the bulgur wheat, pine nuts and currants.

Preheat the oven to 170°C/325°F/Gas 3. Arrange the drained aubergines in an oiled ovenproof dish. Fill them with the spiced meat mixture. Mix the tomato purée with the lemon juice, sugar and 2 tablespoons olive oil, 150 ml (5 fl oz) water, salt and pepper and pour over the aubergines. Cover with foil and bake for 45 minutes.

Remove the foil, baste the aubergines in their own juice, and cook for a further 15–20 minutes. Serve hot or warm.

* *

Avocado

* * *

Size is not necessarily something to be proud of if you're an avocado. Not even when you know that the word derives from the Nahuatl for testicle, 'ahuacatl'. God's honest truth. What a thought – a tree laden with enormous green testicles. Scary, though that may just be a female perspective. For a bellicose Aztec warrior it could have been a source of inspiration, though even the smallest of avocadoes would seem a lot to live up to.

Anyway, size is not everything and the smaller avocadoes undoubtedly have the best flavour. This is because they are endowed with an extremely high concentration of oils. Juggernaut avocadoes, often from the Caribbean, are merely pumped up with water. Not in any sinister fashion; that's just how they grow. Higher water content means dilute flavour. Q.E.D.

There are two distinct types of avocado in production. The smaller varieties come from the **Mexican/Guatemalan** avocadoes, while the big bruisers have been developed from the **West Indian**. It is generally acknowledged that the finest of all avocado varieties is the dark-skinned knobbly **Hass**, discovered accidentally in the late 1920s by a Mr Rudolph Hass, postman of La Habra, California. They still thrive in California, but are also grown prolifically in Israel, which has provided a perfect home for avocado production. Twenty something years ago, I visited an Israeli avocado orchard and was shocked, in my youthful naivety, to be informed by the Jewish owner that his favourite ways to eat avocado were in a sandwich with bacon, or with shrimps. Bacon? Shrimps? Here was a direct introduction to the political divisions that dominate Israeli life. Kosher or not kosher? Liberal or orthodox? War and peace. All wrapped up in one avocado-grower's food choices.

Practicalities

BUYING The ideal avocado is firm but with a slight give to it. In this state they are ready to be eaten straightaway, or perhaps the next day, but you can't rely on them staying at this peak of perfection for too long. Squishy is hopelessly over-ripe – if the price has been sledge-hammered down to next-to-nothing, then it may be worth buying a few in the hopes that they are still good enough to make guacamole, but don't count on it.

There is hope for a rock-hard avocado – give it a few days and it should soften to edible creaminess, but there's no guarantee that it will slot into your timetable. Annoyingly, every batch of avocadoes will ripen at its own special pace. Speed up the ripening process by keeping it in the fruit bowl, or by putting it into a brown paper bag with a potato (or tomato or apple or banana or practically any fruit or vegetable). This neighbourly conjunction hastens ripening because both avocado and potato give off ethylene, a natural gas which encourages ripening. In the confined space of a paper bag, the effect is concentrated.

Unripe avocadoes are best stored at room temperature, whilst ripe ones can be held for as long as 5 days in the vegetable drawer of the fridge before they spiral into hopeless mushy over-ripeness.

To prepare an avocado, first cut in half, from stem end to base, swivelling your knife around the stone. Twist the halves apart. Put the side with the stone in on the work surface, then whack the knife into the stone and lift it out. If this dramatic method fails, opt for the sissy's method – ease the stone out with a spoon. To reduce browning (you can't halt it totally) wipe the exposed avocado flesh with a cut lemon. If you need to peel the avocado, turn each half skin-side up, and pull away the skin in thick strips.

Avocado is a remarkable fruit/vegetable, rich in nutrients, and at its best as smooth as butter. Although considered dated, I still think that avocado halves make a good first course, but instead of piling them high with dull prawns swimming in mayonnaise (as if you needed more oiliness) take a livelier, fresher approach. Get fine lightly cooked, fresh tasting prawns or fresh white crabmeat and toss them with diced tomato, chilli, chopped coriander and lime juice then pile high in the avocadoes. Or fill them with a properly herby tabbouleh (see page 195), or tzatziki (see page 208) or freshly grated carrot moistened with a lemony vinaigrette, sharpened with chopped spring onions and dill.

Diced or sliced avocado is a blessing for all manner of salads and cold dishes, adding healthy richness and substance, as well as its special texture and flavour. The best-known salad is probably the Italian 'tricolore' salad: slices of avocado, tomato and mozzarella, dressed with lemon, olive oil, salt and pepper and lots of basil leaves. This is a joy when made with the best ingredients, perhaps with a few crisp salad leaves thrown in for good measure, and a miserable whimpering disappointment when nothing is ripe, the mozzarella is cheap and the dressing factory-born.

Don't reserve avocado for the tricolore – sliced into a green salad it adds a new dimension of taste, or try alternating slices of avocado, ripe canteloupe or charentais melon and smoked chicken or Parma ham. For the most refreshing, invigorating salad, mix avocado with peeled and skinned pomelo or pink grapefruit, and then dress with dry-fried ground cumin and coriander, a little chilli and a few squirts of lime juice. No need for oil. Big on impact, fabulous with grilled squid, or tuna or practically any other simply cooked fish. Avocado goes well, too, with grilled, skinned peppers of any hue, and to flesh it out, add flaked smoked mackerel or crab for high days and holidays. Avocado, new potato, crisp bacon and watercress is another winner.

Diced small, it's a natural for the Latin American salsa – on its own seasoned with finely chopped shallot or spring onion, a little chopped chilli and garlic, lots of coriander and lots of lime juice, or mixed with diced tomato or mango or papaya or grilled skinned peppers, or even pear or apple. This goes down a treat with fish (again), grilled chicken, or in tortillas with slices of rare-grilled steak and a dab or two of soured cream. Alternatively include slices of avocado and add a straight tomato salsa. Diced avocado also adds life, particularly in winter, to thick warming bean and/or vegetable soups: sprinkle over the surface as a garnish, with coriander or chopped parsley.

A ripe or even marginally over-ripe avocado (as long as it is not turning brown and ugly) virtually demands to be mashed or puréed. Great all on its own for baby food, but even better for big boys and girls. Just because they sell tubs of guacamole in every supermarket the length of the land doesn't mean that you shouldn't make it at home. It is undoubtedly one of the most delicious things you can do with an avocado, but not the only way to enjoy a puréed avocado. 1970s cooks made an art of the swift avocado and yoghurt soup and in the summer it is a real treat – you'll find one version of it on page 170.

There was once a vogue for baked avocado, often smothered in cheese or cream. This is sooo not a good option. It's sickeningly greasy. I'm not totally against serving avocado hot, but there's only one dish I've come across where it makes sense, and that's avocado fritters. My mother, the food writer Jane Grigson, included a fabulous recipe for this in her *Vegetable Book* (Michael Joseph, 1978) laced with rum. The reason it works, I think, is that the batter takes the brunt of the heat, whilst the avocado itself is merely warmed through.

Puddings made with uncooked avocado can be extremely palatable, on the other hand. An avocado fool (avocado puréed with cream or yoghurt and sugar, scented with vanilla or rum) can be most enjoyable, but on the whole I think I'd rather have a savoury version, sugar and vanilla replaced with garlic and coriander. What I would urge you to try, on the other hand, is the utterly fabulous avocado smoothie. This is nothing more than ripe avocado liquidised with milk and honey to taste. It's rich and luscious and a beautiful pale, frothing green.

* *

Ceviche of gurnard or sea bass with avocado

Every good ceviche (marinated raw fish, thinly sliced) I've ever eaten has been served with a salad containing avocadoes. There's something about the pure, clear flavour of the fish that begs the richness of buttery avocado. Almost any fresh fish can be 'cooked' with acidic lime or lemon juice (it coagulates the proteins in much the same way as heat) but these days gurnard is an excellent buy, far cheaper than fashionable sea bass and less controversial than cod.

Serves 4

300 g (11 oz) gurnard or sea bass fillets
juice of 1½–2 limes
1 hot red chilli, deseeded and finely diced
salt

Salad
2 shallots, thinly sliced
juice of 1 lime
1 avocado, peeled, stoned and sliced
a handful of rocket leaves or 4 inner leaves
  of cos lettuce, sliced
12 cherry tomatoes, halved
a big handful of coriander leaves (optional)

Begin by chilling the fish fillets in the freezer for 20 minutes, or until firm but not rock hard. Using a sharp knife, cut into thin slices, at an angle of about 30°, towards the tail end. Mix with the lime juice, chilli and salt. Set aside for an hour, then drain off the liquid.

Mix the shallots with the juice of ½ lime and ½ teaspoon salt. Set aside for half an hour, or more. Drain. Peel and slice the avocado, then toss in the remaining lime juice.

Just before serving mix the shallots, avocado, rocket or cos, tomatoes and coriander leaves, if using. Arrange the fish in a single layer on a large serving dish, or 4 individual plates, then pile the salad on top. Serve immediately.

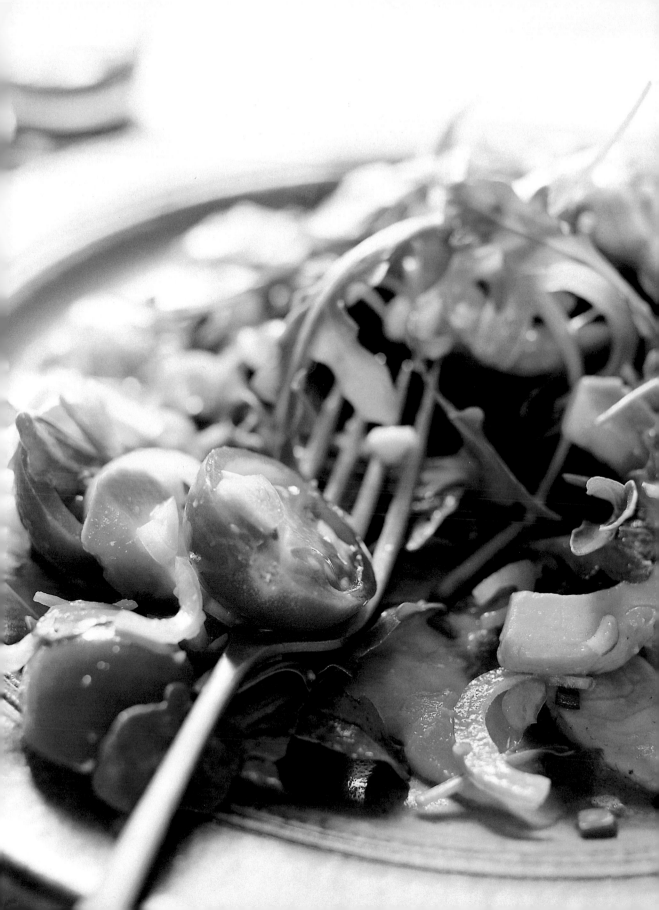

* *

Avocado, cucumber and sorrel soup

This is a cracking variation on an old standby. A cool summer soup that is made virtually instantly, at the flick of a switch. The only downside is that it doesn't like being kept hanging around, so just get everything ready and waiting and blitz the soup into being mere seconds before serving.

On a searingly hot day, cool the soup right down by floating a few ice cubes in each bowl.

Serves 6

1 ripe, buttery avocado
a generous handful of sorrel leaves (discard any tough stalks)
¼ large cucumber, roughly diced but not skinned

250g (9oz) Greek yoghurt
1–2 cloves garlic (fresh garlic is very good in this)
salt and pepper

To serve
avocado oil

Put all the main ingredients into the jug of your liquidiser. Add a good slurp of water and then flick that switch. As soon as it is all smoothly blended, taste and adjust seasoning, adding more sorrel, or salt or pepper, and thinning down with a little more water if needed.

Divide between six serving bowls or cups and drizzle a thin thread of avocado oil on the surface. Serve at once, or at least fairly soon.

* *

Guacamole

How purist do you want to be about this? Genuine Mexican guacamole is often no more than mashed avocado seasoned with lime juice, chilli and salt, perhaps with the addition of a little chopped coriander. Personally I like the full quota of ingredients, and each time I make it, I marvel at how extremely wonderful it is. Use it as a dip, in sandwiches, in wraps with feta and salad, as a sauce with grilled fish or chicken. There's plenty of room for improvisation.

Despite the lime juice, the guacamole will still brown if it has to hang around for a short while. It is not true that sitting the avocado stone in the centre of the bowl of guacamole will stop it browning. The part directly in contact with the stone will remain bright because the air has been excluded, that's all. Better to cover the surface with clingfilm, then stir the discoloured surface back into the guacamole seconds before serving.

Serves 4–6

2 ripe avocadoes
1 shallot or ½ onion, very finely chopped
juice of 1–2 limes
2 tomatoes, deseeded and finely diced

1–2 red or green chillies, deseeded and
 finely chopped
1 small clove garlic, crushed
a big handful of coriander leaves, chopped
salt

Peel the avocadoes and remove the stone. Mash the flesh with a fork then stir in all the remaining ingredients. Taste and adjust seasoning. Serve within half an hour while the colour is still bright, or cover with clingfilm and read the introduction to this recipe.

* *

Bell peppers

* * *

Peppers fall into two major categories: cooked and uncooked. Uncooked peppers are principally a northern seasonless foible. Cooked peppers are the stuff of warm summer days, of the Mediterranean, of long alfresco lunches with family and friends, of happiness. It's not that I don't like raw peppers, more that I can't get excited about them. Juicy, crisp, sweetish, burp-inducing ('they repeat on you,' my mother always said), colourful, all these qualities are fine, but they lack romance. More importantly, they mask an unremarkable mediocrity. Raw strips or rings of red pepper are what uninspired chefs throw into dull salads for the buffet table, in a sorry attempt to produce something more interesting. To be fair, I do occasionally include strips of raw peppers in a mix of crudités to go with something like hummus or the Greek htipiti (itself a blend of cooked peppers and feta) on page 176, but they sit there merely as a vehicle for greater things. For once, lack of distinction is useful.

All the more remarkable, then, the transformation that is wrought by the application of heat. Even the most standardised supermarket pepper becomes something special when it is cooked. Crispness and juiciness vanish, to be replaced, oh miracle of miracles, by a voluptuous, silken texture and a taste that sings of sunshine and mellowness.

There is, naturally, a sub-division to be made in the cooked category, separating unripened green peppers from the brighter coloured red, yellow and orange fully ripe peppers. Many people dislike the taste of cooked green peppers and I can see why, though I don't share their dislike. They have a splash of natural bitterness and a more savoury taste than riper peppers. This is something that can be harnessed to good effect, either by mixing them with red peppers to balance their sweetness, or to provide savoury depth to composite dishes, as in the excellent soup/stews or gumbos of Louisiana.

Most of the time, though, for most of us, it's the ripe and handsome **red and yellow peppers** that excel. But should it be? If you only ever shop in a supermarket, you might be forgiven for thinking that there was no other option. Heaps of almost identical peppers, bright as children's plastic toys, almost boxlike in shape are on offer. Here and there a few higher priced **speciality peppers, long and tapering, richly red or palest green,** make a token appearance. They are all perfectly pleasant, but if you want a truly sexy, fully flavoured pepper you will have to look elsewhere and be prepared to take, indeed be delighted by, a lack of uniformity.

For great peppers, look for a great market or a great greengrocer's. Then hunt out, in season, i.e. in the summer, peppers that twist and undulate with exuberant irregularity. Thrill to the sight of red peppers mottled with dark green, or green peppers randomly patched with splurges of orange and yellow. Peppers like this are rare in our over-organised and over-graded shops, but that makes them all the more precious.

Practicalities

Taut, glossy skin bursting with vigour is essential in a pepper. Any small suggestion of a wrinkle, any small suggestion of dullness, any small suggestion of weariness should be seen as a warning. 'Don't buy me; I am no longer worth your attention.' The corollary of this is that they should not be left sitting around in the vegetable drawer of the fridge for days on end. Up to 3 days may be okay, but more than that is asking for trouble. A less than vibrant pepper is at best sapped of taste and at worst tinged with mouldy overtones. Neither is worth the bother.

Preparation is elementary. For grilling or roasting (see below) you may want to leave them whole. For stuffing you will either cut them in half from stem to base to give two pepper 'bowls' to hold the stuffing. Alternatively, for whole stuffed peppers, slice off a 'lid' complete with stem-base handle. Whichever you go for, you will then have to cut out the plug of white flesh and seeds in the centre and scrape or shake out remaining seeds. If they are large and intrusive, you may want to remove the white inner ribs, too, but there's no absolute necessity to do this.

For any other use, begin by cutting out the stem and white seedy plug under it using a sharp small knife. Again shake out the seeds. Then just cut the pepper up however you want it.

I've not got a great deal to say about the use of raw peppers. If you like them in salads, put them in but if you really want to fathom out how extraordinarily good peppers can be you must cook them. Boiling or simmering or steaming, however, are not to be contemplated. Like all rules there is one exception: for stuffed peppers you can get away with blanching the peppers in boiling water for 5 minutes to speed up the time in the oven. I don't. Or at least not any more. Having tried them both ways, I've come to the conclusion that the peppers taste better after a longer spell in the oven. And that means less fiddling around with extra saucepans.

Grilling, roasting and frying are the methods that suit peppers. Of these three, grilling is the most important. Whenever you read in a list of ingredients '1 pepper, skinned' the implication is that you will have grilled it first in order to skin it. I have heard of people peeling the skin off a raw pepper with a vegetable peeler, but most cooks would consider this an abnormal and perverse thing to do. For more, see pages 175–6.

Grilled skinned peppers have many uses, but above all they make a divine salad. I usually include a green pepper in addition to a couple of red or red and yellow peppers, but they are not to everyone's taste. To make the simplest of grilled pepper salads, cut the skinned peppers into strips and place in a bowl together with any juices from grilling. Dress with a little red wine vinegar or balsamic vinegar, extra virgin olive oil, salt and pepper. Although delicious eaten as soon as it is made, this is a salad that improves from being left hanging around, covered, for an hour or so. It also keeps nicely in the fridge for a couple of days. Minor embellishments might be a little very finely chopped garlic, chopped parsley, torn-up basil, or fresh marjoram, dried wild oregano. Fresh herbs should be added only shortly before serving. Other things to add to a grilled pepper salad include ripe sliced tomatoes, strips of anchovy, black olives, capers, rings of shallot or red onion, chopped spring onion, blanched green beans, mozzarella, quartered hard-boiled eggs, cooked cannellini or flageolet beans, and so on.

Grilled (or **roasted**) and skinned peppers are also a good ingredient in themselves. I use them in stuffings, in sandwiches, on cheesy toast (under the cheese), in terrines, in flavoured butters, or as the basis for a sauce. To make a sauce of them, purée with a little stock or single cream, salt and pepper and reheat gently. Puréed red peppers also give a pretty finish to a soup – just swirl a spoonful into each bowl as you serve. For a red or yellow pepper mayonnaise, dice or process grilled skinned peppers and stir into the mayo along with a touch of crushed garlic and a slurp of sweet chilli sauce.

To distinguish them from chilli peppers, sweet or bell peppers are often called 'capsicums', a name derived from the Latin for a box. The connection is obvious, and their box-like shape makes them natural **containers for stuffing** (see above for preparation). My favourite stuffings are rice or grain based (couscous or burgul, for instance), but they need to be lifted out of the bland by emphatic seasoning and lively added ingredients. Under-seasoned stuffings taste very dull. You only need turn to the pages of any good Provençal, Greek, Turkish or North African cookbook to find inspired recipes for stuffed peppers, and remember that **baking** is the best way to cook them.

Sautéing or stir-frying is the third enhancing way to cook peppers. Make sure that the oil in the pan is extremely hot before adding the peppers – there's a good deal of water in them that will need to be sizzled off. Keep the heat fairly high as they cook. Inadequate heat allows liquid to gather in the pan and your peppers will stew rather than fry. For a straightforward, last-minute side dish, sauté strips of pepper in olive oil, adding finely chopped garlic towards the end of the cooking time, when they are beginning to soften and sport splashes of brown. I also like to toss in a handful or two of cherry tomatoes when the peppers are almost done, so that they have time to heat through but don't burst. For a more Asian feel, fragrance the hot oil in the wok with chopped garlic and ginger, add the peppers and stir-fry for 3–4 minutes. Throw in some mangetouts and stir-fry for a minute or two longer. Keep it simple by finishing with a shake of soy sauce and sesame oil.

To grill or roast peppers for skinning
With all of the following methods, the trick is to get the skin of the peppers burnt almost to a cinder, and at the same time to cook the flesh until soft, but not so soft that it collapses. To be frank, this is at first a matter of trial and error: get the peppers too close to a grill or flame that is too hot, and the skin will char before the flesh has cooked through. Grill them a mite too far from the heat, or under an inadequate heat and you will find, perversely, that by the time the skin is black enough to lift off, the flesh will be so soft that it disintegrates as you peel the peppers. If you don't get it quite right the first time, persevere, adjusting the distance between heat source and peppers or, if you can, the temperature itself.

Method 1 Appropriate when preparing 1–2 peppers only. You need a gas hob, or an open fire for this. Spear a pepper through the stem end on a fork. Hold it in the flame of a gas ring, turning frequently, until the skin is blackened and blistered all over.

Method 2 Appropriate for preparing a moderate number of peppers. Preheat the grill (or a barbecue). Cut each deseeded pepper into quarters or eighths and lay them on the rack, skin-side to heat. Slide them under the grill, or over the barbecue, getting them close to the heat source. Leave until the skin is completely blackened.

Method 3 Appropriate for a larger number of peppers. Preheat the grill (or barbecue) but leave the peppers whole, complete with stalks. Arrange the peppers on the rack and slide under the grill or over the barbecue. Leave until the side nearest the heat source is thoroughly blackened and blistered, then turn. Continue this way until the peppers are blackened all over.

Method 4 Appropriate for a moderate or large number of peppers, or if you happen to have the oven on at a belting heat for something else. Preheat your oven to 220–230°C/425–450°F/Gas 7–8. Arrange whole peppers in a roasting tin or baking dish in a single layer. Roast in the oven for 30–40 minutes until browned and sagging. The skin won't blacken this time.

Skinning grilled or roast peppers

As soon as the peppers are done, drop them into a hole-free, clean plastic bag and seal. Don't worry – the plastic won't melt. Leave until cool enough to handle. The trapped steam in the bag loosens the skin. By the time they are tepid, the skin will peel away easily, leaving luscious pieces of perfectly grilled pepper. Obviously, peppers that have been cooked whole will also need to have stalk and seeds removed. If there are a lot of black flakes left on the peppers, they can be rinsed off under the tap, but you lose some of the juice, and hence a little of their flavour.

* *

Htipiti
Greek red pepper and feta dip

From the north of Greece comes this blend of grilled peppers and salty feta cheese that you eat just as you would hummus. It is nicest made with freshly skinned peppers, but occasionally I cheat and use tinned or bottled grilled and skinned peppers instead.

Serves 5–6

125 g (4½ oz) grilled skinned red peppers, roughly chopped
1 medium-hot red chilli, deseeded and roughly chopped
175 g (6 oz) feta cheese, crumbled
1 clove garlic, roughly chopped

3–4 tablespoons extra virgin olive oil
paprika

To serve
crudités (e.g. strips of celery, green pepper, carrot, cucumber, fennel, etc.) and/or warm pitta bread, cut into fingers

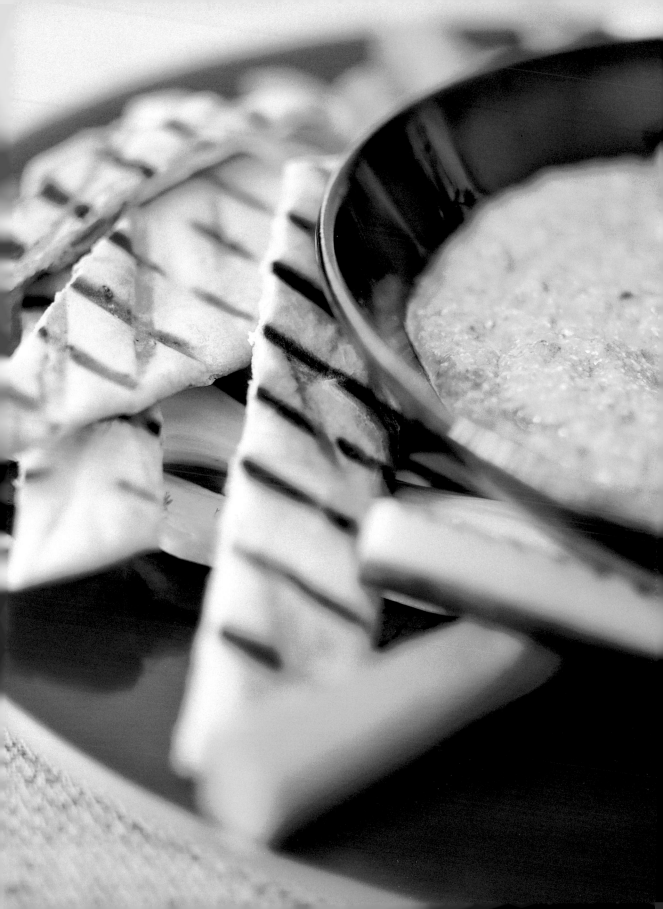

Process all the ingredients except the paprika together, adding enough olive oil to give a pleasing consistency. Spoon into a bowl and cover with clingfilm until ready to serve.

Just before serving, trickle a thread of olive oil over the htipiti and dust lightly with paprika. Serve with crudités and warm pitta bread to dip into it.

* *

Peperonata

This is Italy's most famous pepper stew. Cooked down to a thick, luscious tenderness, peppers and tomatoes come together in perfect harmony. Serve it warm, or at room temperature, as a side dish or as an hors d'oeuvre, or as part of a mix of antipasti, in other words alongside plates of sliced cured meats and cheeses. It also makes a fine topping for bruschetta: griddle or toast slices of good bread, rub with a halved garlic clove and top with peperonata and the halves of a mini ball of mozzarella or a curl of Parma ham.

Serves 4–6

1 onion, sliced
4 tablespoons olive oil
4 red peppers, deseeded, and cut into long
  strips
3 cloves garlic, crushed
½ teaspoon fennel seeds

450 g (1 lb) tomatoes, skinned and roughly
  chopped
1 tablespoon tomato purée
1 teaspoon caster sugar (unless your
  tomatoes are exceptionally good)
salt and pepper

Sauté the onion in the olive oil until lightly browned. Add the peppers, garlic and fennel seeds and cook for a further couple of minutes. Cover the pan and let them cook down gently in their own juices for 10 minutes.

Now add the remaining ingredients, bring up to the boil, then simmer gently for half an hour, uncovered, stirring occasionally.

Taste and adjust the seasoning. Reheat when needed or serve at room temperature.

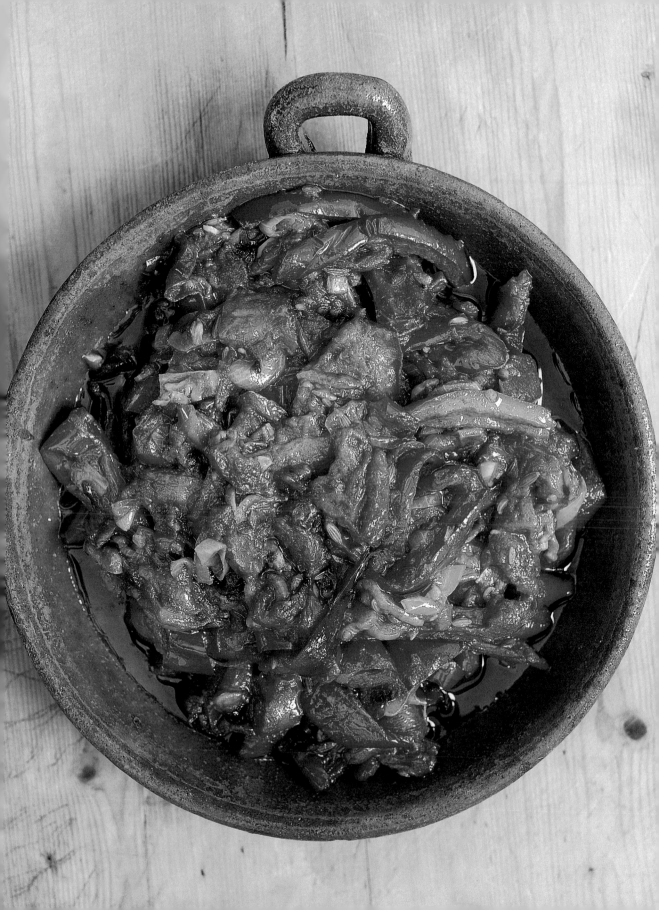

* *

Involtini di peperoni
Stuffed, rolled peppers

Another Italian recipe, this time from the south where they cook peppers so well. First grilled and skinned, the peppers are rolled up around a filling which sounds weird (anchovies and sultanas?) but turns out to be just piquant and sweet enough to set off the peppers perfectly. Serve the involtini hot, warm or cold.

Serves 8

2 red peppers, grilled and skinned
2 yellow peppers, grilled and skinned
2 tablespoons sultanas or currants
4 anchovy fillets
2 tablespoons capers, rinsed if salted

3 tablespoons chopped parsley
2 tablespoons pine nuts, toasted
4 tablespoons fresh breadcrumbs
extra virgin olive oil
salt and pepper

Preheat the oven to 180°C/350°F/Gas 4. Deseed each grilled pepper, and cut into quarters lengthways. Soak the sultanas or currants in warm water for 10 minutes, then pat dry.

Chop the anchovy fillets and capers finely, then mix with the parsley, pine nuts, sultanas or currants and breadcrumbs. Season with lots of pepper and a little salt (remember both anchovies and capers will have already contributed a modicum of salt). Add a few teaspoons of olive oil – just enough to moisten the filling, but not to leave it swilling and greasy.

Lay the pepper quarters out on the work surface and divide the filling between them. Roll up neatly and place in an oiled ovenproof dish. Drizzle a little oil over them, just enough to keep them moist, then slide into the oven for around 15–20 minutes. Serve warm or at room temperature.

* *

Okra

* * *

Okra is an elegant vegetable. When at their prime, the long tapering olive green pods, ridged right up to the cone that attaches them to the stem, are peerless. They came originally from Africa, then travelled with slaves in the hellholes of transport ships to the Caribbean and to the southern states of America. A taste of home that grew easily in these new lands, embedding themselves in the regional cuisines. They made their way from there to India, where again they thrived and were embraced with enthusiasm.

This extraordinary vegetable, imprinted with the weight of colonial history, has a unique characteristic which I imagine is why it was carried so far around the globe. It has the strangest, mucilaginous texture. This is not apparent when raw (and you can eat okra raw, sliced perhaps into salads), but as they cook they ooze a slippery glue. This can be used to advantage – Louisiana gumbos (rich soup stews) are traditionally cooked with okra to thicken and enrich the juices, whilst in parts of the Caribbean they are added to cornmeal mush to lubricate it – or just enjoyed for its own sake. There are techniques for reducing the slipperiness (salting or soaking in acidulated water) but unless force of circumstance means that okra must be a major part of your diet, this seems pointless. If you don't like the characteristic that singles okra out from other vegetables, then don't eat them. Problem solved.

There are two schools of thought about how long to cook okra. The first, and probably most prevalent, is that they should be cooked until very, very soft and tender, which releases more of that mucilaginous juice. The second is that they should be cooked fairly swiftly, so that they retain a slip of firmness at heart. This is the better method for those who are suspicious of the texture. I like both. When I want an appealing, comforting side dish, I'd stew them in tomato sauce until they almost melt. When I fancy something more invigorating, I'll deep-fry them swiftly to revel in the crunch.

Practicalities

The best places to buy okra are, without any doubt, West Indian or Asian food stores, where they are considered everyday vegetables and priced accordingly. On the rare occasions that they grace supermarket shelves they are considered exotica, and priced exorbitantly. Choose okra that are firm, olivey green and unblemished. Smaller ones are preferable.

At home, store okra in a paper bag in a cool place. Oddly, they don't like to be chilled, so only store them in the fridge if you have nowhere better. Don't leave them in a plastic bag or they will sweat and moulder within 24 hours.

Basic preparation is simple. Just trim off the stalk, leaving the cone of the okra in situ. Alternatively, you can travel the Greek route, which is to take the cone off completely, dip the cut end into salt, then leave them in a pan or baking tray in the sun (or a warm room) for a few hours so that some of their ooze is drawn out. Elsewhere, the prepared okra, cones removed, possibly sliced, are tossed with vinegar, then left lying around to the same ends.

COOKING Okra suit two cooking methods and two only: **stewing and frying**. Okra boiled in water are dull, dull, dull. Grilled or barbecued okra are not much better. The most obvious and enormously popular way to cook them, right around the known okra world, is in a thick tomato sauce, flavoured according to provenance. So, in Greece it will be made with olive oil, flavoured with dill or coriander seed and blessed with plenty of garlic. In northern Africa there will be cumin, coriander (seed or leaf or both), chilli and so on. In India, the spices are taken to greater heights, the tomatoes minimised, while in the Caribbean the sauce will be lifted with the violent heat of Scotch bonnet chillies, and flavoured with oodles of thyme. The okra are added to the sauce – whole or sliced – and simmered for as long as the cook likes. It's a formula that should be played with until you find a version (or two) that suits you.

Added to soups and stews for the last half hour of cooking, okra yields a wonderful smooth quality to the juices – again this is a favourite trick both in Louisiana and in the Caribbean, where okra is an important ingredient in many of the sustaining vegetable and meat stews.

I've got a bit of a soft spot for fried okra, too. Try sautéing okra, halved lengthways, with chopped onion in olive oil for some 10 minutes, adding chilli or crushed cumin and coriander halfway through. Finish with a few squirts of lemon or lime, some chopped coriander or parsley, and salt.

Sometimes I'll add a sliced red pepper, too, for colour and sweetness. Diced deseeded fresh tomato is good stirred in right at the end of the cooking so that it retains its substance.

* *

Pickled okra

A recipe from the southern states of America, where okra are big – not in size, but in status. The okra, stashed tail to nose (or rather stem to tip) in jars, are put away for safe keeping. After 3 weeks they mature and soften slightly, without losing their crunch. Eat them with a bowl of chilli con carne, Texas style, or serve as part of an antipasti with cured meats and cheeses.

Incidentally, don't be alarmed at the extraordinary colour of the cloves of garlic as they soak in the vinegar. Blue is an unusual colour in food, but in this case it doesn't indicate danger!

Makes 1 large jar or 4 jam jars' full

500g (1lb 2oz) okra
1 litre (1¾ pints) white wine vinegar
4 tablespoons salt
4 tablespoons caster or granulated sugar

4 cloves garlic, peeled
4 dried hot red chillies
4 sprigs dill
4 teaspoons mustard seeds, coarsely
  crushed

Trim the top of the stalk off the okra but don't cut right into them. Take one 500ml (18fl oz) sterilised (see page 215) Kilner jar or 4 sterilised jam jars (make sure that they are tall enough to take the entire length of the okra), and pack the okra really tightly into them, alternating tip to tail. Tuck cloves of garlic, chillies, sprigs of dill and mustard seeds down amongst them.

Bring the vinegar, salt and granulated sugar up to a boil, and then pour over the okra, making sure they are covered completely. Seal tightly.

Keep for at least 3 weeks, in the fridge, before eating.

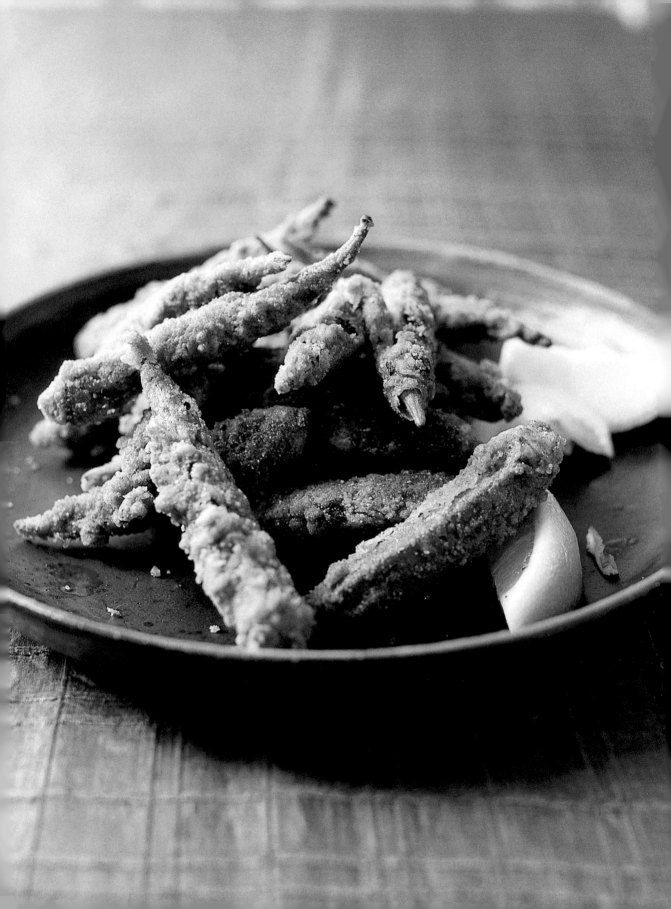

Fried okra with cornmeal

I love these okra fritters with the crunch of cornmeal in the outer coating (though not too much or it becomes overwhelming), and the inside cooked just enough to soften without losing a touch of firmness at the centre. Serve them as a first course or just a snack, with plenty of wedges of lemon to squeeze over them.

'Pimentón' is the Spanish word for paprika (and yes, also for bell peppers, which can cause confusion), smoked before grinding to a powder. You can now find it fairly readily outside Spain, and for this dish the hotter 'piccante' version is what gives the best flavour.

If you prefer a softer fritter, try tossing the okra, halved lengthways, in plain flour seasoned with pimentón, then dipping them into egg and dropping them straight into hot oil. The egg will puff up around each piece of okra like a golden cloud.

Serves 4

200 g (7 oz) okra
2 tablespoons cornmeal
4 tablespoons plain flour
1 teaspoon smoked paprika (pimentón piccante)

2 eggs
salt
sunflower oil or dripping for frying
wedges of lemon to serve

Trim the stalks off the okra, leaving the cap intact. Mix the cornmeal with the flour, paprika and salt. Beat the eggs together lightly in a shallow dish.

Heat a 5 mm (¼ in) depth of oil in a frying pan. Toss a handful of the okra first in the cornmeal mixture, shake off excess, then coat in egg. Lift out and return to the cornmeal mixture to coat again. Fry, turning once or twice, until lightly browned and crisp.

Drain briefly on kitchen paper, then serve swiftly, with wedges of lemon to squeeze over them.

* *

Bhindi sabji
Indian spiced okra

This is one of my favourite ways of cooking okra, softened with plenty of spices, a little tomato and the sharpness of lime.

Serves 4

2 tablespoons sunflower or vegetable oil
1 onion, chopped
4 cloves garlic, chopped
1 cm (½ in) piece fresh root ginger, grated
1 red chilli, deseeded and chopped
1 teaspoon turmeric

½ teaspoon ground cumin
1 teaspoon ground coriander
400 g (14 oz) okra, sliced into rings
2 tomatoes, skinned, deseeded and chopped
juice of ½ lime
salt

Heat the oil in a wide frying pan over a moderate heat. Fry the onion until tender, then add the garlic, ginger and chilli and fry for a minute or so longer. Sprinkle over the spices and stir again, then add both okra and tomatoes and 2 tablespoons water. Season with salt.

Fry until the tomatoes begin to soften and collapse, then cover and turn the heat right down low. Leave to cook for 10–15 minutes (check occasionally and add a little more water if really necessary, to prevent catching).

Stir in the lime juice, then taste and adjust seasoning. Serve hot or warm.

* *

Tomatoes

* * *

Controversial, variable, potentially sensational, often tedious, versatile, common, humble, cheap, expensive, irreplaceable, theoretically seasonal, international, local, where would we be without the tomato? Okay, much the same place, but undoubtedly much poorer foodwise. The tomato is a vegetable of so many facets and such vast importance the world over, that it is hard to imagine mealtimes without it. I know several people who don't like or, worse, are allergic to tomatoes. I feel sorry for them. What a huge gap that leaves – no pasta with tomato sauce, no pizza, no tomato soup (home-made or from a tin) or baked beans (ditto), no tomato salad. Tragic.

You don't need me to tell you that there are good tomatoes, great tomatoes and downright miserable tomatoes that taste of precious little, barely providing more than a smear of dampness. Nor do you need me to tell you that the best tomatoes are **summer tomatoes**, and high summer at that. Even in Italy, European cradle of tomatodom, they don't really rate tomatoes before late June or early July. On one early summer trip to the Amalfi coast, I was surprised to be served classics like bistecca alla pizzaiola (steak with a swiftly cooked tomato sauce perked up with capers, olives, anchovies and lots of garlic) with a dressing made up of briefly cooked cherry tomatoes. When quizzed the answer was always the same – it's too early for decent tomatoes, so these are the only option.

A lesson to us all, there. Out of season, in other words any time except for July, August and September, think twice before you cook with fresh tomatoes. If **cherry tomatoes** are viable, and they often do carry a sufficient quantity of essential sweetness, balanced with a shot of acidity and a distinct tomatoey zing, they're the better option. And better still in many recipes, is a **can of chopped tomatoes** or **whole plum tomatoes**, or a few slurps of **passata**.

The world of the tomato has changed a great deal over the past few decades. Where once travellers complained endlessly that it was impossible to buy a decent tomato anywhere but the Mediterranean and other hot, hot regions, now we are offered a wealth of new varieties (grown for flavour; ha ha, as if we didn't know that they are grown for profit). They cost more, unless you are growing them yourself, but they taste much better, full of individuality and energy. Usually. One shouldn't, however, assume that all is as it should be in the premium 'grown for flavour' market. Have you noticed that plum tomatoes, which we once praised to high heavens, are no longer the dead cert that they once were? Some are good (especially the ones I picked from my own plants); some are, at best, mediocre. Same goes for marmande and beef tomatoes. Still, I mustn't be too cynical and defeatist. There are some fantastic tomatoes around these days, tomatoes that make a plain tomato salad a sheer joy, which of course, it should be. Listing varieties is pointless – new ones appear all the time, and such a lot depends on growing conditions. Try new varieties when they appear, grow your own for maximum pleasure (and that heavenly smell of the foliage), and make the most of the summer tomatoes when they are at their zenith.

Practicalities

BUYING Colour is the first clue to a potentially fine tomato. A rich, deep, deep red is a good sign, but not conclusive. There are marvellous orange, yellow, pink, cream and even bruised purple tomatoes to be found from time to time. Firm, all but ripe green and red tomatoes can be excellent, too, as long as they are of good variety and have been grown in the sun. The one colour to avoid is a watery, pallid red which almost always suggests lack of flavour.

A good tomato should be firm with a taut burnished skin, but regularity of shape is of absolutely no consequence. Many of the most delicious tomatoes I've eaten have been lumpishly irregular, with the odd blemish here and there. Size is not an issue either, as long as it suits the dish you will be making with them. The one characteristic that is fairly reliable is the smell. A ripe tomato should smell fragrantly of ripe tomato. When they are wrapped in plastic there's no way to detect this, but at a market or in the greengrocer's it's worth having a sniff.

When you see tomatoes being sold 'for making sauces', make sure that you pick out the ones you want yourself. Sauce-tomatoes are über-ripe tomatoes and an unscrupulous vendor might slip a few over-ripe, mouldering tomatoes into the bag, and they are no use to anyone.

If you will be using them up within a couple of days, tomatoes are nicest kept in a bowl or a dish out on the kitchen table. Then you can throw together a **tomato salad** in minutes, and enjoy their true deep flavour. A salad made with tomatoes taken straight from the fridge will need time to lose the chill which mutes the taste.

During the summer months, my family and I eat tomato salad almost every day. Don't we get bored with it? No, never. There are infinite variations to be made on the basic salad, and we run our way through a fair number of them. Tomato salad was the first dish that my children learnt to make entirely by themselves, and they still love imprinting their own particular tastes on each new salad they make. Although we all love the most obvious combination of sliced tomatoes, dressed with balsamic or red wine vinegar, olive oil, salt, pepper and a handful of basil, it is only an occasional visitor. Other days we replace the basil with fresh mint, coriander, chives, tarragon, parsley, marjoram or Greek rigani, dried wild oregano. Sometimes we add capers or caperberries, olives, grilled and skinned peppers, chopped spring onion, sliced shallot, slices of orange or even slices of ripe peach or nectarine. The remains of a tin of tuna may be flaked over the tomatoes, or strips of tinned anchovy or silvery marinated anchovies; drained and rinsed canned flageolets or cannellini beans get a look in, and of course we love to add mozzarella, preferably buffalo mozzarella, or crumbled goat's cheese or feta, and sliced avocado. Toasted chopped nuts are an occasional addition, though nut oils are not great on tomato. Limpid green avocado oil is, on the other hand. See too the Chilean tomato salad on page 309.

Our other raw tomato favourite is the **salsa**, both South American and Italian style. The Italian salsa cruda, literally raw sauce, is simply a bowlful of finely diced, deseeded tomatoes (technically known as tomates concassées), mixed with finely chopped shallot or onion, finely chopped garlic, salt and pepper, a little olive oil and lots of roughly torn fresh basil. Left to stand for an hour or two to allow flavours to develop, it is sensational tossed into steaming hot pasta. South American salsas are made in much the same way – finely diced tomato, garlic, onion or spring onion, oodles of coriander, chilli and lime juice instead of oil. That's the basic salsa, but as with a salad it is a formula to play on. Some of the tomato may be replaced with finely diced avocado, or mango or papaya or other fruit. Sweetcorn, lightly cooked or freshly slashed from a raw or grilled cob, is good in with the tomato, as is diced grilled and skinned red, yellow or green pepper.

For these raw dishes, I never bother to skin tomatoes; I like the cheery red of the skins. I do deseed them, on the other hand (see opposite). Nor do they need to be skinned when they are to be stuffed or halved and grilled or seared or griddled. For many cooked tomato dishes, on the other hand, tomatoes do need to be skinned unless you are seriously pushed for time.

A **tomato sauce** is another preparation which can take on board any number of variations. The first thing to decide is whether you need a quick-cooked frisky sauce, or a slow-cooked mellow sauce. The two taste quite different. When your tomatoes are supremely good, go for the speedy version: fry chopped garlic (and chillies if you wish) in olive oil until beginning to colour then swiftly add diced, skinned and deseeded tomatoes. Fry for a few minutes longer, season, take off the heat, stir in basil or oregano, and use immediately, poured over pasta, on a rare or medium steak, with fish, or a frittata. For a more rounded sauce, look to the recipes at the end of this section. In either case, you might choose to add capers, olives, chopped tinned anchovies (fry them gently with the garlic, so that they dissolve into the mass), other herbs, ginger and so on. Slow-cooked sauces love a glass or two of wine.

For most purposes, I prefer to leave the sauce knobbly and textured, but if you want a smooth sauce, liquidise, adding a little extra water or stock if necessary to get the right consistency. For perfect smoothness rub the liquidised sauce through a sieve. Reheat when needed, and for something extra suave, stir in a few slurps of double cream.

Roasting is another exceptional way of cooking tomatoes, this time to serve as a side dish, rather than as a sauce. Again, open to variation, but the basic method goes like this: halve tomatoes around their equator (or stem to stalk for plum tomatoes) and arrange in a closely packed single layer, cut side up, in an ovenproof serving dish. Drizzle over a little oil, season with coarse salt, pepper and a pinch or two of sugar, tuck a few whole cloves of garlic down amongst them and sprigs of thyme or rosemary, then bake in a hot oven (220°C/425°F/Gas 7) for some 40–45 minutes, until patched with brown and very tender. Serve them hot, warm or at room temperature.

These are the most elementary ways to use tomatoes, essential preparations for every cook from novice to senior chef. From these spreads out a vast array of tomato-imbued dishes adored on every continent, except perhaps Antarctica, where I imagine tomatoes are rare and the penguins don't give a damn about them. Still, I'll bet that the explorers and scientists who camp out there take a stash of tinned tomatoes or tomato soup, or at least ketchup with them. Tomatoes know no bounds.

Deseeding/skinning tomatoes

A ripe tomato is easier to peel than an under-ripe one. For ripe tomatoes it is enough to boil up a kettle of water and pour it over the tomatoes to cover them completely. Leave them for about 40–60 seconds, then take out. Now the skin will pull away easily. With firmer, paler tomatoes, I suggest that you bring a saucepan of water up to the boil, then place the tomatoes in it. Simmer for 40–60 seconds, then take them out but leave the pan on the stove just in case. Try to skin the tomatoes – if the peel still clings tenaciously, return the tomatoes to the hot water and leave them to swelter for another 30 seconds. Try skinning again. If it still won't peel, then either give up and leave it in place, or take a blowtorch to them and singe the wretched stuff into oblivion. This more drastic approach will inevitably cook the tomato flesh a little (or even a lot if you get carried away). This doesn't matter too much when you are making a sauce, but if you want to keep them raw, it's better to give in to the skin after the first steaming dunk.

Deseeding can be tackled in several different ways depending on how you will be using the tomatoes. Where they are to be cooked to a sauce, the easiest way is to cut them in half around the equator (i.e. halfway between stem and base), then simply to squeeze the seeds out into a bowl or straight into the bin, but be careful not to drop the tomato into it too. If you don't want mangled tomato halves, scoop the seeds out with a teaspoon instead. For perfect tomato 'petals' (a fanciful term for deseeded quarters), cut the tomatoes into quarters from stem to base. Slide a small vegetable knife down the quarter, between the thick outside flesh and the seeds and sticky-up bits, which can then be discarded or added to a vegetable stock.

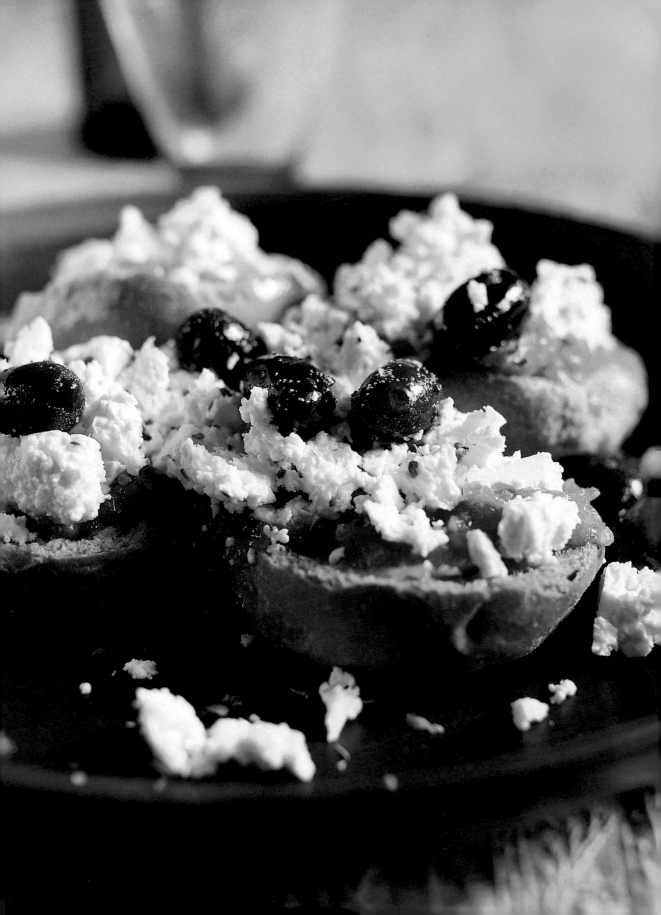

* *

Dakos
Greek tomato and feta rusks

Greek food is based on fabulous ingredients; think ripe, red, sweet tomatoes, salty, ivory feta, spicy fragrant dried wild oregano (rigani) from the hills, and of course, olives and green-gold olive oil. Five stars of the Greek table that come together in a Greek salad and in this simple first course or light lunch.

You must have the best summer tomatoes for this to sing and if you can lay your hands on barrel-aged feta it will taste even better. 'Dakos' are Cretan double-baked rings of bread some 15cm (6in) across which you may be able to find in Greek or Cypriot groceries. If you can't find the larger ones, smaller versions, say 10cm (4in) across will do just as well – use 2. Italian delis may also sell friselle which are the southern Italian equivalent and work just as well. If neither of these are forthcoming, don't give up! Most supermarkets sell double-baked Swedish-style rusks in packets.

The point is to end up with a mound of tomato and feta (be generous) piled high over a crisp base, which is softening here and there with the juice of the tomatoes and the oil. You can't eat it neatly, and that, really, is half the point.

Serves 2–4

2 large dakos, 3–4 smaller ones or 4–6 crisp
  rusks
extra virgin olive oil
2–3 gorgeously ripe but not squishy
  tomatoes, halved and deseeded

150 g (5 oz) feta cheese, crumbled
dried oregano
8–12 black olives (Kalamata olives are ideal)
pepper

Drizzle 1 tablespoon water over the dakos or rusks and place on a serving dish. Drizzle with a thin trickle of olive oil. Grate the tomatoes, pressing their fleshy cut side against the grater, and discarding the skin when you've grated off all the flesh. Spoon over the rusks, and then pile the feta over the top. Sprinkle with oregano, season with pepper and scatter the olives over the cheese and tomato. Let the mixture sit for 5–10 minutes, then drizzle with a final helping of olive oil, and serve.

* *

Tomato confit

Confit tomatoes are baked for several hours, surrounded by a lake of olive oil, until divinely tender. The result is not the same as roasted tomatoes, browned by a stabbing heat. Confit tomatoes are richer and more mellow, though equally good. Both standard-sized and cherry tomatoes respond well to the treatment. If using small cherry tomatoes, leave them whole, but cut a small cross through the skin of each one to prevent them bursting. You may also find that you need a little extra oil.

What to do with the tomatoes once cooked – serve them hot as a side dish, or make them part of a first-course salad, mixed, at room temperature, with rocket and salty feta, dressed with juices from the dish. Or you might like to toss them, again with some of the cooking juices, with pasta for a hasty supper.

Once cooked, the tomatoes will keep, covered, for 4 or 5 days in the fridge.

Serves 4–6

650 g (1 lb 7 oz) plum tomatoes, halved
1 teaspoon fennel seeds
6 sprigs lemon thyme
1 generous tablespoon coarse salt
2 teaspoons black peppercorns, coarsely
  crushed

cloves from 1 head garlic, peeled, and
  halved
1 or 2 dried chillies (optional)
100 ml (3 ½ floz) extra virgin olive oil

Preheat the oven to 140°C/275°F/Gas 1. Halve the plum tomatoes lengthways. Scatter the fennel, thyme, salt and pepper over the base of an ovenproof dish just large enough to take the tomatoes in a closely packed single layer. Arrange the tomatoes over the seasonings, tuck in the garlic and chillies, if using, then pour over the oil. Cook for 3 hours, basting every 40 minutes or so with their oil and its flavourings, but trying not to disturb the tomatoes too much.

Serve the tomatoes as they are, straight from the dish, or leave to cool down and serve at room temperature, or reheat in the oven when called for.

* *

Tabbouleh

This is not the tabbouleh of the 1970s health-food café, but one with a closer resemblance to the original North African tabbouleh which is really a herb salad, softened with tomato, cucumber and a speckling of cracked wheat or couscous.

Serves 8

60 g (2 oz) cracked wheat (bulgar or burgul) or couscous
1 big bunch flat-leaf parsley
1 small bunch mint
1 small bunch coriander
finely grated zest of 1 lemon and the juice of 2 lemons
250 g (9 oz) tomatoes, deseeded and finely diced

1 cucumber, finely diced
6 spring onions, thinly sliced
6 tablespoons extra virgin olive oil
salt and pepper

To serve (optional)
inner leaves of cos lettuce or little gem lettuce leaves
some fabulous bread

Put the cracked wheat into a bowl and pour over enough cold water to cover generously. Leave for 20–30 minutes to swell and soften. Drain thoroughly.

Chop the leaves of the parsley, mint and coriander roughly. Mix with the cracked wheat, and all the remaining ingredients, making sure that it is generously seasoned. Cover and leave for a few hours in the fridge, or better still overnight, to allow the flavours to mellow and blend, and the leaves to soften.

Stir again and taste and adjust seasoning, adding more lemon juice if necessary – it should taste distinctly lemony and sharp. Serve as a first course with leaves of cos lettuce or good bread to scoop it up, or as an accompaniment to other dishes.

* *

Tomato sauce

There is no single right way to make a tomato sauce. Variations in technique, length of cooking time, basic ingredients, essential additions, inventive additions, favoured additions are just endless. It would be perverse not to include at least one recipe for tomato sauce in this section and this is a good one for pasta, or for gratins (mix with lightly cooked vegetables, spread out in a dish, top with a mixture of cheese and breadcrumbs, drizzle with oil or dot with butter and bake until browned and sizzling) amongst so many other things.

Just touching the tip of the tomato sauce iceberg, here are four minimal ways to ring the changes. 1) Italian touch – add a big handful of shredded or torn-up fresh basil leaves when the sauce is cooked. 2) Maltese touch (excellent with fish) – add a couple of tablespoons of capers and the finely grated zest of a lemon with the tomatoes, then stir in a handful of shredded mint leaves when the sauce is cooked. 3) Greek touch – add 1–2 teaspoons dried wild oregano (Greek rigani is the best) with the tomatoes. 4) Moroccan touch – slip a cinnamon stick and a teaspoon of coarsely crushed cumin seeds in with the tomatoes.

Serves 6

2 tablespoons extra virgin olive oil
1 onion, chopped
3 cloves garlic, chopped
2 x 400 g cans chopped tomatoes in their
   juice, or 1 kg (2¼ lb) fresh tomatoes,
   skinned, deseeded and roughly chopped
1 tablespoon tomato purée

1 bay leaf
1 sprig thyme
1 teaspoon caster sugar
salt and pepper

Heat the oil in a wide frying pan over a gentle heat. Add the onion and fry gently, stirring frequently, until translucent. Do not rush this stage – it should take around 10 minutes. Now add the garlic and cook for a further 2 minutes or so to soften it.

Tip in the canned or fresh tomatoes, the tomato purée, the bay leaf and thyme, the sugar, and salt and pepper. Bring up to the boil, then reduce the heat and simmer very gently for some 20–30 minutes, stirring frequently, until the tomatoes have reduced down to a thick sauce. You may need to add a little water to prevent catching. Taste and adjust seasoning. Fish out and discard the thyme and bay leaf. Use straightaway or reheat when needed.

* *

Tomates à la Provençale

In this recipe the tomatoes are both fried (don't be scared by the smoke) and roasted, crisply topped with garlic and herb imbued breadcrumbs.

Serves 8

8 medium-large, well-flavoured tomatoes
3 tablespoons extra virgin olive oil, plus a
  little extra
a little caster sugar

3 tablespoons chopped mixed parsley,
  tarragon, basil or rosemary
2 cloves garlic, chopped
3 tablespoons fresh breadcrumbs
coarse salt and pepper

Preheat the oven to 200°C/400°F/Gas 6. Cut the tomatoes in half. Put the 3 tablespoons of oil into a heavy frying pan, and heat over a high heat. Place the tomato halves, cut-side down, in the oil, without overcrowding the pan (you will probably have to do this in two batches). Now don't touch them for at least 3–4 minutes, until the edges are just beginning to show a hint of dark brown – it may even take a few minutes longer, depending on the heat of the oil. Once the cut sides are browned, carefully lift the tomatoes out, and arrange snugly, cut-sides up this time, in an oiled heatproof, shallow dish.

Season with salt, pepper and a little sugar (unnecessary if your tomatoes are a perfect synthesis of sweet, acidic and fragrant). Chop the herbs finely with the garlic, then mix with the breadcrumbs. Scatter the mixture over the tomatoes, then drizzle over the cooking oil from the frying pan, and another tablespoon or so of olive oil. Transfer the dish to the preheated oven and cook for a further 20–30 minutes, until the breadcrumbs are crisp and the tomatoes gorgeously squishy and tender. Serve hot.

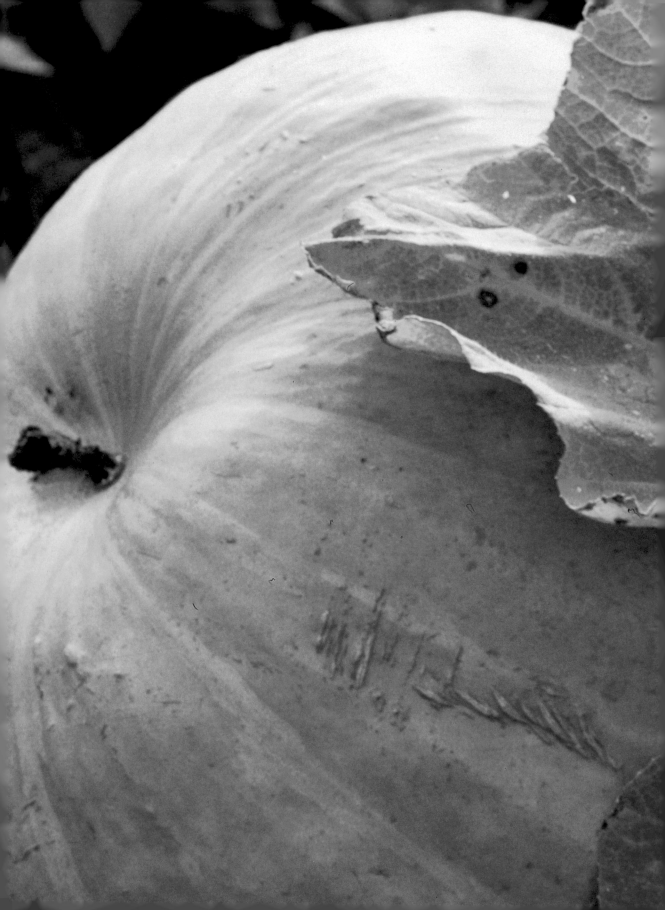

Squashes

* *

Courgettes Cucumbers
Marrows Summer squashes
Winter squashes

* *

Courgettes

* * *

Courgettes can take a certain pride in having conquered northern climes. Where once they were considered a foreign vegetable, an interloper from the warmer shores of the Mediterranean, now they are as common as older denizens of the summer, as common as, say, green beans and already poaching on the territory of the runner bean when it comes to allotment space. The origins are plain in the names we choose for them. Americans have whipped the name '**zucchini**' straight from the Italian, whilst we have swiped the word '**courgette**' straight from the French. Both are diminutives: the French '**courge**' is a marrow, while the Italian '**zucca**' is a form of pumpkin. The lesson to take from this, is that some of the best courgette recipes hail from the Continent, from France (particularly the south), from Italy and then, for the curious, on round to Greece, Turkey, and into the Middle East.

Courgettes are one of the only vegetables that I grow regularly in my garden, supplemented, in those years when I get it together in time, by tomatoes which partner them so well. The reason I grow courgettes, apart from the fact that they need so little attention, is that it gives me the opportunity to pick them at whatever size suits me and the plants. At the beginning of the season, we celebrate the first finger-sized courgettes, small and slender and delicate, their freshest flavour undiluted by the water that swells them out as the weeks progress. We treasure these babies, cooking them whole, sometimes swathed in a light tempura batter, accompanied with no more than a sprinkling of salt and a squeeze of lemon. They are fabulous steamed whole, sprinkled with a few drops of lemon oil, or a knob of sweet butter, though never so heavily dressed that their flavour is muddied by the onslaught. Once over the initial flush of tender delight, I let my courgettes swell a little more, so that I can enter in on the mainstream

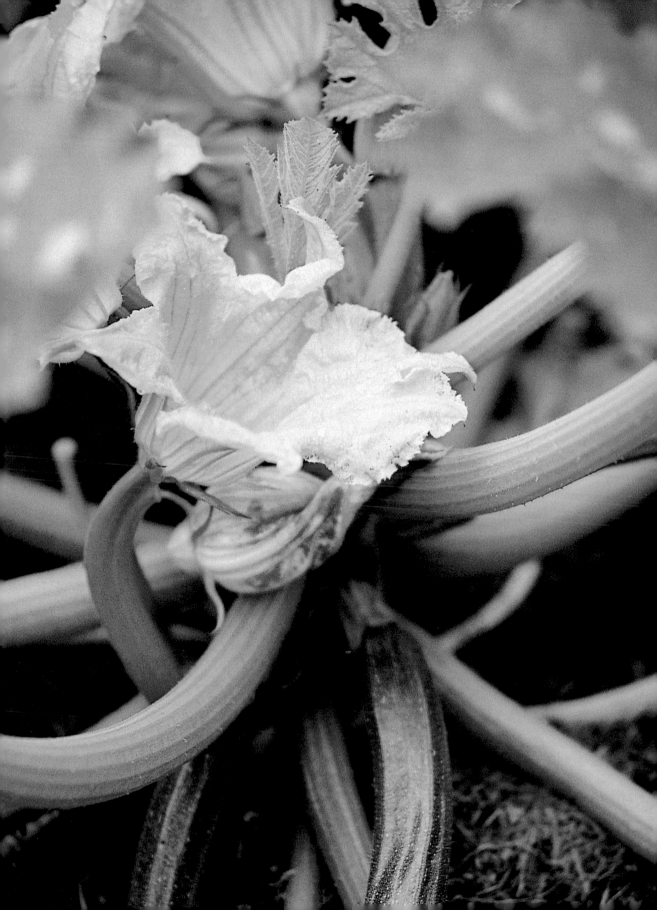

of courgette recipes, using them as hosts for myriad other ingredients, baking, frying, blanching, roasting and stewing as circumstance dictates. By the time late August and September arrives we have usually reduced our vigilance, and several courgettes will have blown themselves into giant proportion. They have turned into the dreaded 'courge', which is a nice way of saying marrow. For more on **marrows**, turn to page 218, where you will find what is, I admit, a less than enthusiastic attempt to come up with worthy ways of using a vegetable that does little for me.

The other marvellous advantage of growing one's own courgettes is the flowers. Now if you head off to a fancy greengrocer you may be able to purchase some at a vastly inflated price. The tips will inevitably have wilted and twisted together, but they will still be perfectly good to eat. Somehow, though, the whole point has been lost. If you are going to eat courgette flowers (or indeed the flowers of any other member of the squash family), then you should be aware that they are never going to be a substantial ingredient. It's the kind of thing that is a wonderful extra if you happen to have courgettes growing in your vegetable plot, so that you can snap the stems, and cook them instantly while at their peak of freshness, but a bit pretentious if you insist on buying them elsewhere.

Practicalities

BUYING Size matters. Very small courgettes will be better flavoured, but more expensive, cuter to look at, but less versatile. Medium-sized courgettes are what I pick out when I'm buying them. The price is reasonable, in season, the flavour still distinct, and you can cook them in all sorts of ways. Large courgettes, the ones that haven't quite made it to marrow status but are well on their way, may seem more economical, but bear in mind that most of what you are buying is water, delicately flavoured with a hint of courgette. Good for stuffing, perhaps, fine for soups, but less appealing in other dishes. Although, now that I think of it, they can be used in cake and bread doughs (like carrots) to bring extra moistness.

Whatever the size, it is imperative that you buy freshly picked courgettes, or as near as dammit, and store them in the vegetable drawer of the fridge. Fresh courgettes have firm, fresh stem-stubs (beware – they can be surprisingly prickly), and smooth, taut skins with an egg-shell finish. The odd brown blemish is nothing to be ashamed of. Wrinkles, soft spots, drying stem-stubs are no-nos.

Do not keep courgettes hanging round for more than 2–3 days. They may appear perfectly acceptable after that, but it doesn't take too long for courgettes to develop a nasty bitter taste which mars their light flavour.

Yellow-skinned courgettes, incidentally, taste much the same as **green**. Buy them because you love the colour, not for a radical new take on a familiar veg. They look pretty and inject a note of gaiety into a bowl of vegetables, which is an excellent thing in itself. Rarer, but not so unknown these days, are round courgettes. They can be cooked just in the same way as an ordinary courgette, though the skin may be a tad firmer. However, given their shape, the obvious use for them is as containers for a spicy stuffing – something Middle Eastern maybe, redolent of cumin and coriander, or spiked with chilli and garlic, or indeed just burnished with salty cheese and tomato. The meat stuffing on page 162 would be ideal.

Courgette flowers do not like being kept hanging around. It takes but a few short minutes – well, an hour or so, anyway – for them to begin wilting, their tips crinkling and softening and twisting together. A little bit of wilt doesn't matter – indeed it is hard to avoid – but too much is not appealing. In other words, courgette flowers should be cooked on the day they are picked, or bought. Keep them cool, wrapped in a damp layer of kitchen towel, in the vegetable drawer, until you can get them into a pan of some sort.

Preparation-wise there is only one thing worth debating when it comes to courgettes, and that is 'to salt or not to salt'. Before that point, all that needs to be done is to slice off the hard, prickly-haired stem-stub, wipe the courgettes clean, and then cut into whatever shapes your recipe suggests.

It's what happens next that matters. You can hardly have failed to notice that courgettes are full of water, water that oozes out damply as soon as you begin to cut them. You can ignore this and just carry right on. The downside of this is that if you fry your courgettes they will brown more slowly and any hint of over-crowding in the pan will produce a veritable lake of liquid, so that the courgettes stew in their own juices. No, if you want to fry unsalted courgettes, you must allow plenty of space and plenty of time. With other methods of cooking (e.g. roasting or stuffing) you will end up with a more watery vegetable.

The sensible alternative is to salt the courgettes for half to an hour before cooking them. This requires a degree of organisation and forethought, but not a great deal. Put the prepared (i.e. sliced or otherwise cut-up) courgettes into a colander or sieve set over a bowl. Sprinkle lightly with salt, turn the courgettes pieces to distribute it, then walk away. Return after 30–60 minutes and be amazed at the lakelet of salty liquid pooled in the bowl. Dry the courgettes on kitchen paper or a clean tea-towel before using.

The effect of **salting** is clearly noticeable – the flavour of the courgettes is more pronounced, the texture much improved and to cap it all, less oil will be absorbed when they are fried. Obviously, there is little point in salting courgettes if you are going to boil them afterwards. And almost as obviously, it is absolutely essential if you are thinking of deep-frying them in a batter.

On the subject of **boiling** or **steaming** courgettes, whilst I wouldn't suggest for a minute that this is a bad way to cook them, I should point out that far too often they are miserably over-boiled to a lacklustre slush. About 1–2 minutes of simmering (timed from the second the water comes back to a discreet simmer) is all that sliced courgettes require. Smaller whole courgettes may need all of 4–5 minutes, but no more. As soon as the timing is up, drain them, rinse in cool water, to knock the heat down a notch, then serve straightaway (perhaps with a knob of butter, some chopped chives or tarragon or mint, or a spritz of lemon oil) and get them on to the table pronto. When they are to be tossed in a dressing for a salad, err on the side of light cooking, and whip them into the dressing as fast as you can.

A spot of time on a violently hot **griddle** pan brings out the best in courgettes. Cut them into relatively large, long pieces (it makes turning a whole lot easier and less time-consuming), toss with some olive oil or sunflower oil, then arrange on the griddle pan. Leave until the underneath is striped with brown, then turn. Cook until just tender, and streaked with brown on all sides. Serve hot, warm, with added herbs, in a salad, or how you will.

One of my all-time favourite summer courgette dishes is a plain griddled courgette salad. Slice the courgettes lengthways into thin ribbons. Toss with peppery extra virgin olive oil, then cook on a griddle or barbecue (see above) until just tender. As soon as they are done, toss with lemon juice, a little extra olive oil, fresh mint, salt and pepper. That's all, and it is hard to get better than that.

Of course, if you want to, you can make griddled courgettes the basis of a more elaborate salad, adding tomatoes, green beans, broad beans, roasted peppers, prawns, chickpeas, goat's cheese and so on. The danger is that you lose sight, or rather taste, of the courgettes themselves, so don't get too carried away.

Number 2 on my list of top courgette salads, is the Italian 'zucchini al scapece'. For this the courgettes are **fried** in generous amounts of olive oil (having been salted first), with plenty of chopped garlic added towards the end of the cooking time. The whole lot is then tipped into a bowl, and dressed with red wine vinegar, salt, pepper and lots of fresh mint. Serve at room temperature.

PARTNERS When it comes to hot courgettes, I'd suggest first of all that if you want to tart them up, you whiz up some simple herb or anchovy butter, and dot it over the warm courgettes just before bearing them to the table. Most herbs, particularly those soft-leaved summer herbs, are good with courgettes. Mint is the one I go back to time and again, but parsley, chives, sage (in moderation), dill or fennel, lemon balm, marjoram, and so on are all fine friends. Alternatively, you will find that a judicious sprinkling of toasted flaked almonds or pine kernels has an enhancing effect.

I'm not big on raw courgettes, but many people adore them. A few slices or cubes can add appealing crunch and juiciness to a salad or a salsa, but they need plenty of animation and complementary flavours to play with.

Chefs, with their teams of minions, will make time to **stuff** courgette flowers. You may wish to do the same if you live a life of leisure. I, on the other hand, prefer to work with the less fiddly options – **deep-fried** in a light batter (best of all), or roughly chopped and stirred into something like a risotto, or even pasta.

For more exotic ways with courgettes (and there are plenty to be tracked down) look to the Middle East, where spices and succulent **stuffings** with nuts and dried fruit and meat and rice all abound. Italy and France, naturally, have a wealthy fund of courgette recipes to delve into, but that mild flavour makes them a good recipient for Asian spicings and gentle curries moistened with coconut milk. In short, courgettes are natural all-rounders limited only by their need for speedy cooking.

* *

Liliane's courgette gratin

Every summer we spend 4 weeks in a small village in France, along with
a brood of cousins. On high-days and holidays we head down to the islands
in the river at the bottom of the hill, where Liliane runs a small outdoor bar
and restaurant. Mostly it's sausages and steak and chips, moules frites, and
occasionally, when we're in luck, her fabulous gratin of courgettes.

The secret, she says, is to fry the courgettes and leave them to drain overnight, before mixing with eggs and cream. I've been trying to fathom why this
should be any better than salting them first to draw out water, and then frying.
I guess that one way or another, the 24 hours of hanging about improves the
flavour of the courgettes, rather in the way that a stew always tastes better
the day after it is made. Anyway, the point is that it makes a difference, and
the result is a minor snap of courgette heaven, good enough to merit the wait.

Serves 6

1 kg (2¼ lb) medium-sized courgettes, sliced
2 tablespoons extra virgin olive oil
200 ml (7 fl oz) crème fraîche

2 eggs
salt and pepper

Line a large sieve or colander with coffee filters, torn open, or with a double
layer of butter muslin, and set over a bowl. Fry the courgettes in batches,
in the oil over a medium heat, until tender and lightly browned. Tip into the
lined sieve, cover with a plate and weigh down with a tin of tomatoes or
beans. Once cool, leave to drain at least overnight or, better still, for 24–48
hours, in the fridge.

Next day preheat the oven to 170°C/325°F/Gas 3.

Beat the crème fraîche with the eggs and season with salt and pepper.
Uncover the courgettes and press down gently on them to expel the last
of the moisture. Fold into the egg and cream mixture. Transfer to an
ovenproof dish, just big enough to hold the mixture in a layer of around
2.5 cm (1 in) depth. Smooth down lightly and slide into the oven. Bake for
40–45 minutes until just set. Serve warm or at room temperature.

* *

Moroccan-style courgette salad

I will admit to having something of a passion for pairing fresh mint with vegetables. It brings an incomparable liveliness and almost never clashes. Here it is the finishing kick for a warmly spiced salad of courgettes.

Serves 4

1 teaspoon cumin seeds
1/2 teaspoon coriander seeds
juice of 1/2–1 lemon
3 tablespoons extra virgin olive oil
500 g (1 lb 2 oz) courgettes, sliced
leaves of 4 sprigs mint (or more),
  roughly chopped

30 g (1 oz) pine nuts
20 g (3/4 oz) currants
a handful of rocket or watercress leaves
salt and pepper

Dry-fry the cumin and coriander seeds in a small frying pan over a moderate heat until their miraculous spicy scent fills the room. Tip into a mortar or bowl and leave to cool, then crush to a coarse powder. Whisk the lemon juice with the olive oil, salt and pepper.

Bring a pan of salted water to the boil. Add the courgette slices, bring back to the boil and simmer for 1 minute and *no longer*. Drain, run under the cold tap, and then drain again.

Immediately toss the courgettes with about half the spices and dressing, half the mint leaves and all the pine nuts and currants. Leave to cool.

Just before serving toss the watercress with the remaining dressing and arrange on a plate with the courgettes. Scatter the last of the mint over the top and serve.

* *

Fried courgettes with tzatziki

I love fried courgettes, but they need something to bring out their flavour.
It could be no more than a squeeze of lemon juice, but next time you want
a quick and simple starter, try pairing them with tzatziki, that wonderful
cucumber, yoghurt and garlic sauce so popular in Greece and all around the
southern Mediterranean.

Incidentally, don't try to save time by skipping the salting of the
cucumbers. Unsalted cucumbers will leach torrents of water into the yoghurt,
creating a weak pale swamp instead of a beautiful white cream flecked with
green.

Serves 6

450g (1lb) very fresh courgettes, sliced
extra virgin olive oil for frying
salt and pepper

Tzatziki
½ cucumber, peeled and finely diced
1 tablespoon red or white wine vinegar
200g (7oz) thick Greek yoghurt
1–2 cloves garlic, crushed
2 tablespoons chopped mint leaves

To make the tzatziki, begin by spreading the diced cucumber out in a
colander. Drizzle over the vinegar and some salt. Stand over a plate and
leave to drain for 1 hour. Pat dry with kitchen paper or on a clean tea-towel.
Mix with the yoghurt, garlic, mint and some black pepper, then taste and
add more salt if it needs it. Chill until required.

Just as everyone is about to sit down to eat, fry the courgette slices
in a little oil over a brisk heat, until golden brown. Drain briefly on kitchen
paper, season with a little salt and serve at once, steaming hot, with the
cool tzatziki.

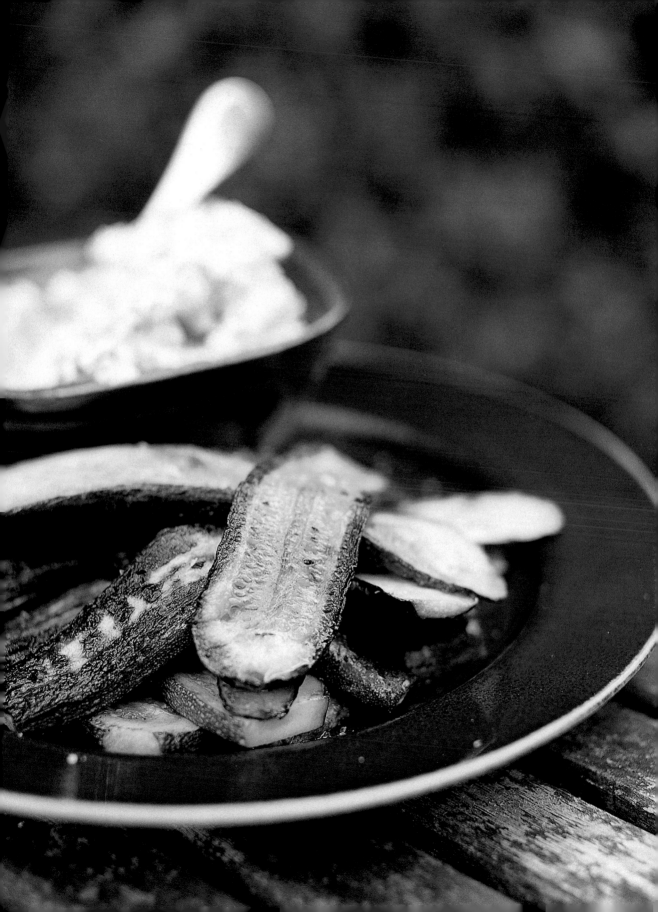

* *

Manuela's aunt's torta verde

My friend Manuela was born and brought up in Liguria and cooks like a dream. This is a recipe she makes often, varying it with the seasons, replacing courgettes with artichoke hearts and Swiss chard in spring (no rice needed for this version, she says), and pumpkin or butternut squash in the winter. The recipe came originally from her aunt.

Serves 6–8

500 g (1 lb 2 oz) small courgettes, trimmed and roughly chopped
1 medium onion, chopped
1 clove garlic, chopped
1 small bunch parsley, roughly torn up
60 g (2 oz) arborio or carnaroli rice
1 tablespoon extra virgin olive oil
2 eggs, beaten

75 g (2½ oz) Parmesan, freshly grated
salt

Pastry
400 g (14 oz) strong flour
6 tablespoons extra virgin olive oil
salt

First make the pastry. Sift the flour and make a well in the centre. Add the olive oil and some salt to it and then work to a dough, adding warm water a little at a time to form a soft, but not sticky, dough. You'll need around 120–150 ml (4–5 fl oz) water. Wrap in clingfilm and leave the dough to rest for 20 minutes.

Preheat the oven to 180°C/350°F/Gas 4 and oil a 23 cm (9 in) tart tin.

Whiz the courgettes, onion, garlic and parsley in the food processor and then pour the mixture into a bowl and add the rice and the olive oil. Do not add the salt, eggs and Parmesan until you are just about to fill the pie, otherwise the mixture becomes too watery.

Cut the dough in two, one part slightly bigger than the other. Roll the larger half of the pastry out thinly, and use it to line the tart tin, letting the edges overhang the sides.

Mix the Parmesan, eggs, and salt into the courgette mixture and pour into the lined tin. Roll out the second portion of pastry and lay over the pie. Using a sharp knife, cut excess pastry away, about 1 cm (½ in) away from the edges of the tin. Fold the pastry over on top of itself, sealing in the filling.

Crimp all around the edges with a fork, then brush the pastry all over with a little more oil. Make three holes in the top to let steam escape.

Bake the pie for 45–50 minutes. Probe discreetly with a skewer to make sure that the rice is cooked through. Let the pastry cool a little then turn the pie out of the tart tin and serve warm or cold.

* *

Cucumbers

* * *

We played hooky for a few hours. Escaping from the stuffy conference hall into the warm, polluted spring air of Athens, a colleague and I headed off in search of 'green pies' and returned eventually with a stash of cucumbers. Green pies, like spanakopitta (see page 388) and cheese pies, are the standard Greek snack, but it was the little cucumbers that stole our hearts. Half the length of British cucumbers, they tasted so sweet and fresh and so very, very cucumbery. Did the distinction of those ridgy cukes have anything to do with the shadow of the Parthenon, the thrumming traffic belting out fumes, the pleasure of being let loose for a moment or two? All I can say is that they still tasted good at breakfast the next morning and they reawakened my interest in this commonplace vegetable.

I'd forgotten how much I like cucumbers – easily done over the course of a long, dreary winter – but here suddenly, they made consummate sense, yet again. Cucumber is a sunshine vegetable, a vegetable that refreshes, and invigorates, or at least it should. All too often it gets lost on the plate, overlooked member of the general salad fraternity. I vowed, there in Athens, that I would not let that happen again in our house. From then on, I would make cucumber a focal point, give it status, let it shine. So far, so good.

If you doubt that cucumber can take too much limelight, then I urge you to re-evaluate the way you use it. A few slices in a sandwich? A couple more tucked in amongst the lettuce leaves and tomatoes? Two discs of cucumber reserved to refresh your tired eyes? If that's it, then believe me there's plenty of room for manoeuvre. Cucumber is largely made up of water (around 90%), but what lovely water it is, especially when given mild diuretic treatment to concentrate the flavour without destroying the texture. Salt, sugar and vinegar will all serve to draw out excess juice, whilst providing a base that supports and enhances the sheer cucumberiness. Far better cucumber enhancers, really, than grand Greek ruins or swathes of traffic smog,

Practicalities

BUYING Why should cucumbers be straight? My suspicion is that the only reason is that they pack better that way. In other words, it suits big commerce, and somehow they've persuaded the buying public that there is honour to be found in ram-rod conformity. I shall stick my neck out, then, and suggest that the very choicest cucumbers, those laced with a full-on cucumberiness, are the imperfect ones, with a bit of a curve here and there, with undulating swells, mildly or largely misshapen. So, even though much of the time you may be restricted to poker-straight duller supermarket cucumbers, make a beeline for summer farmers' markets where you may be blessed to find quirkier, tastier specimens.

Straight or curved, your cucumber should be firm to the touch, with a healthy mid-green skin. Bumps are fine, but yellowing and flabbiness are not. Size is neither here nor there. Small cucumbers, like our Athenian ones, can be extra good and when there is just a couple of you to feed, the perfect size.

That cool cucumber needs to keep its cool, in other words, make sure it stays in the vegetable drawer of the fridge to keep it crisp for as long as possible – up to 5 days if it was ultra fresh in the first place. The moment it starts turning flabby, donate it to the compost heap. Like most raw juicy vegetables, cucumber does not react well to excessive cold. Don't let it get pushed right up against the back wall of the fridge where it could freeze. All that water will expand as it freezes, bursting the inner cell walls. Restored to room temperature, it will be mushy and miserable.

The big cucumber question is 'to peel or not to peel?' Nutritionists tell us that the nutrients congregate just underneath the skin, so we should leave it right where it is. My mum, a die-hard peeler, said the skin 'repeated' on her, just like raw peppers, and indeed cucumbers are notorious for their burp-inducing quality. It's no coincidence that a whole slew of modern varieties are named Burpless This and Burpless That. One for; one against. Which kind of justifies my position as an occasional peeler. I don't mind the odd burp and I like the colour of the skin. I'm all for the extra nutrients and less work. However, peeling a cucumber takes seconds, and there is no doubt that my all-time favourite cucumber salad tastes far better minus skin. So, no definitive answer, other than doing what feels right at the time.

That all-time favourite salad is also one of the easiest to make, is oil-free, has the advantage of being made in advance, and will keep nicely in the fridge for several days. It's a Danish cucumber salad and this is how you make it: peel a whole cucumber, cut in half lengthways and scoop out the seeds, slice thinly and mix with 2 tablespoons white wine vinegar, 1 table-spoon caster sugar and 2 teaspoons salt. Cover loosely and ignore it for at least half an hour. Just before eating, drain off all the liquid, dress the salad with chopped dill or tarragon or parsley if you fancy it, though it's not strictly necessary, and serve. That easy, fabulously good. Be warned, however, that treated like this one cucumber will probably satisfy no more than four people. Danish cucumbers are brilliant with fish, with cheese, in sandwiches and so on. Despite releasing oodles of liquid, they retain a pleasing flexible crispness which is what makes them so utterly appealing.

Although cucumbers can be mixed into any summer salad you care to mention, the most famous, quite justifiably, has to be the wonderful Greek salad. Yes, back on Hellenic territory again, but they do have a way with cucumbers. Their other big cucumber gift to the world is tzatziki, cucumber in yoghurt, with garlic and mint (see page 208), another summer essential. Use it as a relish, a sauce, a starter.

On the whole, I think it advisable to hold back when it comes to mixing cucumber with other vegetables to form a salad, so that it isn't over-whelmed. Let it breathe – try cucumber and fennel, for instance, or cucum-ber, watermelon and feta, or cucumber, peach and rocket. Or even that old cutie, salad Elona, in other words cucumber and strawberry, which needs plenty of freshly ground pepper to bring out the best in it.

Raw cucumber is also a natural vehicle for dips of all sorts, a founder member of the 'crudités' club, along with carrots and peppers. For summer canapés, discs of cucumber can replace bread or pastry as long as the topping is piled on only just before serving (salty or vinegary toppings will soon draw out the water in the cucumber, leaving it flopping in your guests' hands). The enterprising will carve out cucumber boats and baskets, which though fun are not really the stuff of everyday meals.

Hot cucumber can be surprisingly good. It's not something one comes across a great deal, but it is worth trying once in a while. It's the kind of vegetable that goes well with white fish or salmon. Cucumber is usually cooked without skin, shaped into charming little rugby ball shapes, or more thriftily, into half moons (peel cucumber, halve lengthways, deseed, slice). Plunge it for 2–3 minutes in simmering water then drain and toss in a little melted butter, or with a spoonful of crème fraîche and some finely chopped dill, tarragon, basil or chervil. You could alternatively fry it in butter for a few minutes over a big heat, finishing it with cream and herbs if you wish. Or with a squeeze of lemon, lime or orange juice if that suits your mood better.

* *

Japanese cucumber salad

This is the Japanese equivalent of my beloved Danish cucumber salad (see introduction) and is just as good, retaining that cucumber purity, but adding a gentle waft of sesame and ginger that works brilliantly. The marinated cucumber can sit in the fridge for several days without spoiling – drain and dress with the sesame oil and chilli sauce when you are almost ready to sit down and eat, so that the cucumber is still lightly chilled.

Some like it hot, others don't – the chilli is entirely optional, a pleasing contrast with the cool cucumber, but not critical to the success of the salad.

Serves 3–4

1 cucumber
1 teaspoon salt
1 tablespoon caster sugar
1 tablespoon rice vinegar

1 teaspoon grated fresh root ginger
1/4 teaspoon hot chilli sauce (optional)
1 teaspoon sesame oil
1/4 teaspoon sesame seeds, lightly toasted

Peel the cucumber, halve lengthways and scoop out the seeds. Slice thinly. Mix with the salt, sugar, vinegar and ginger, and chill for at least an hour.

Drain the cucumber and place in a serving dish, drizzle over the chilli sauce if using, and the sesame oil, then sprinkle with sesame seeds. Serve.

* *

Bread and butter pickles

This American pickle is unexpectedly good, especially with cheese or in sandwiches. Make it when cucumbers are cheap in the summer and don't be tempted to replace the green pepper with a red one. I've tried and it isn't an improvement. The sweetness interferes with the cucumber, and the red stains.

To sterilise jam jars, wash with warm soapy water, rinse well and leave to dry, upside down, on a rack in the oven at 140°C/275°F/Gas 1 for half an hour. Remove from the oven when needed, but do not touch the inside with your hands or a cloth before filling.

Fills 2–3 x 450g (1 lb) jars

1 large cucumber, peeled and sliced
1 red or white onion, halved and very thinly sliced
1 green pepper, deseeded and cut into strips
1¾ tablespoons coarse sea salt
300 ml (10 fl oz) white wine or cider vinegar

280 g (10 oz) caster sugar
1 tablespoon mustard seeds
1 teaspoon celery seeds or dill seeds
1 cinnamon stick
6 allspice berries
2 dried red chillies

Mix the cucumber, onion and pepper with the salt in a large bowl. Sit a plate or saucer directly on top of the vegetables, weigh down with a tin or a bag of rice and then leave in the fridge for 8 hours or overnight.

Drain and rinse the vegetables under the cold tap. Nibble on a piece of the cucumber and if it still seems excessively salty, rinse it again. Drain well. Put all the remaining ingredients into a large saucepan over a moderate heat. Stir until the sugar has dissolved then bring up to the boil. Simmer for 1 minute. Stir in the vegetables and bring back to the boil. Immediately take the pan off the heat.

Spoon the vegetables and juice into hot sterilised jars (see above) and seal tightly with non-corrosive lids. Label and store in a cool dark place for at least 1 week, better still 3. Use up within 4 months.

* *

Greek salad

To me, this is one of the all-time great salads, up there with salade niçoise and Caesar salad. Made with good cucumbers and great tomatoes, it is a magic creation, so fresh and so full of life. The saltiness of the creamy feta and the olives bring out the full taste of the main ingredients. If you can get Greek 'rigani', dried wild oregano, then that gives the salad the ultimate finishing twist. Failing that, standard dried oregano will do, though it doesn't have quite the same power.

Serves 6

1 cucumber
4 very red, ripe tomatoes
6 leaves cos lettuce, thickly shredded
125 g (4½ oz) feta cheese, diced
12 good black olives, stoned
1 teaspoon rigani, or dried oregano

Dressing
juice of ½ lemon
4 tablespoons extra virgin olive oil
salt and pepper

Peel the cucumber, then cut roughly into cubes. Cut the tomatoes up roughly. Whisk the lemon juice with some salt and pepper, then whisk in the oil a tablespoon at a time.

Shortly before serving, pile the lettuce into a salad bowl, and scatter the cucumber and tomato on top. Spoon over the dressing, then finish with the feta, the olives and sprinkle with rigani. Serve.

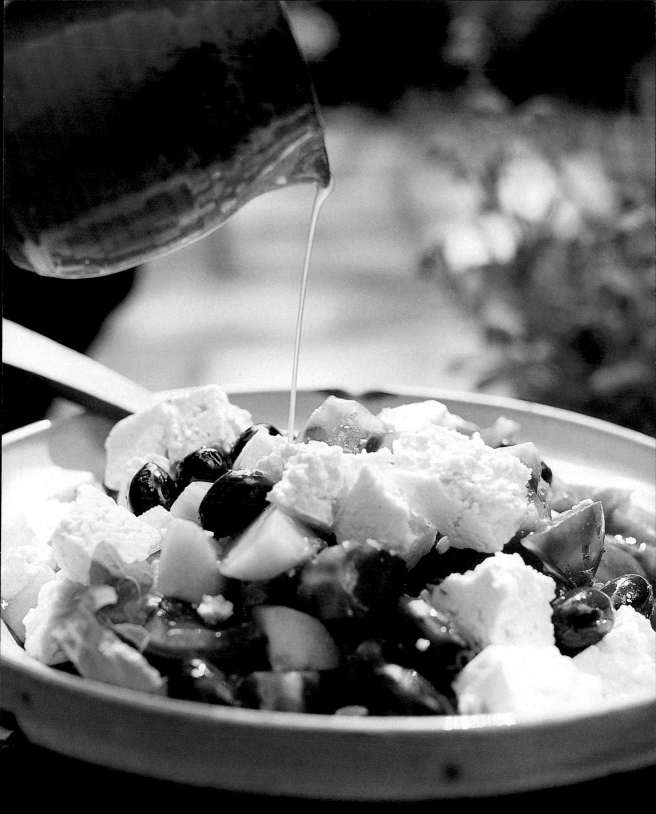

Marrows

* * *

Turn your back on a courgette plant in full swing for just a few days and what happens? A marrow happens, that's what. Admittedly your average marrow will feed a small army, whereas a lone courgette would barely satisfy a garden gnome, so you could argue that the marrow is a gift from heaven. Or Mother Nature. Then again there are some amongst us who heave a big sigh, and resign ourselves to the prospect of economical stuffed marrow. Unless we can palm it off on someone else, of course, but in the country and in city allotments there comes a time of year, late summer or early autumn, when everyone is trying to palm off their outsize courgettes. It can be an uphill task to find a willing taker.

It's not that I dislike marrow as a vegetable. There's really nothing there to dislike. That's the problem. Marrows don't taste of anything much. They're neutral hulks of watery flesh, not unpleasant but without distinction of any kind. Come to think of it, they can be unpleasant if pushed – have you ever been faced with a miserable helping of boiled pappy marrow embedded in undercooked floury white sauce? Now that's nasty.

It goes against the grain to be negative about any vegetable (which is why I won't consign my oversize marrows to the compost heap) so let me make amends. Marrows make sturdy containers for stuffings, and as long as the stuffing is big and brassy in flavour, the fresh, juicy texture of the marrow is a good foil. Marrows can be turned into a funky jam with a little help. A free marrow is better than no marrow at all. Just. I draw the line, however, at paying for one.

Practicalities

BUYING Assuming that you have grown your own marrow, accidentally or deliberately, or have charitably accepted one from a neighbourly gardener, you will just have to take what you get. To tell you that the skin should be firm and dry with no wrinkles, that the marrow should be heavy for its size, that the odd blemish or discoloration is irrelevant is neither here nor there. On the other hand, if you are fond enough of marrow to hand over your hard-won cash, then these pointers may be of some use.

Marrows are on the cusp between summer and winter squashes, and as such have a fairly good shelf-life. Keep them somewhere cool (but not as cold as the fridge) and dry, and they will hold out in a decent state for up to a month. Probably. Once cut, however, any unused marrow must go into the fridge, cut-side covered in clingfilm, and be used up within a couple of days.

Depending on the marrow's maturity, the skin will probably be edible. If you are going to stuff the marrow leave it on, to give extra support. Otherwise, it is optional. Larger marrows will definitely need to be deseeded before use, but in smaller ones the barely formed seeds are quite edible. To deseed, cut the marrow in half lengthways, then scoop out the seeds with a spoon.

COOKING By far the best way to cook marrow to serve as a side dish is to cut it into largish cubes, having skinned and deseeded it first, then tip them into an ovenproof dish, dot them with butter, add chopped herbs, salt and pepper then cover with foil and **bake** in a moderate oven (around 180°C/350°F/Gas 4) for about 30 minutes, before removing the foil and returning to the oven for a further 15 minutes to finish cooking. This boosts the light flavour of the marrow, ensuring that it is quite palatable. If you reduce the cooking time by 5 minutes or so, the marrow could be transformed into a decent gratin by mixing with a feisty tomato sauce, topping with breadcrumbs seasoned with finely chopped garlic, and plenty of herbs (thyme, finely chopped rosemary, parsley and so on) and dotted with butter, before returning to the oven to brown. Please, don't attempt the white sauce treatment. Even the best-made, slow-cooked béchamel sauce will not enhance chunks of marrow.

There are two main ways to prepare a marrow to carry a **stuffing**. The first is to cut the marrow in half lengthways (which may be impractical with monster-size marrows), scoop out the seeds, then blanch the halves in boiling water for a few minutes. If you don't have a pan large enough, which is more than likely, you will just have to cook the marrow in the oven for an extra 15–20 minutes or so, so make sure that the stuffing can take this, and protect any cheesy toppings from burning by covering with foil for part of the time. The second method is to slice the marrow into short lengths – say around 7.5–10 cm (3–4 in), then hollow out each ring of marrow with a spoon from one end to form a bowl-like container. Blanch the 'bowls' in boiling salted water for 3–4 minutes, run under the cold tap then drain well. Arrange close together in a greased baking dish before filling with stuffing.

The stuffing needs to be big and bold and full of character – the aubergine stuffing on page 162 would be just fine, but grain-, rice- or breadcrumb-based stuffings can all work well as long as they are combined with generous quantities of bold ingredients – think in terms of spices, herbs, garlic, cheese, spicy sausages such as chorizo, olives, capers, deseeded, diced tomatoes or tomato purée, Moroccan preserved lemons, chilli, nuts, currants, and so on.

* *

Marrow, ginger and cardamom preserve

Marrow preserve is supposed to be the poor northern woman's replacement for the more sophisticated melon conserves that are made in warmer, sun-drenched places where melons are cheap. In fact, it is extremely good in its own right and is definitely the most exciting thing you can do with a marrow. It needs the tingle of the ginger, but the fragrance of perfumed cardamom makes it seem positively exotic.

Note that this is a preserve rather than a jam, in other words it won't gel, so don't bother testing for setting point. The preserve is ready when the marrow becomes glassy and the syrup is thick.

Fills about 7 x 450 g (1 lb) jam jars

2–2.3 kg (4½–5 lb) marrow
1.5 kg (3¼ lb) granulated sugar
2 lemons
5 pieces preserved stem ginger, chopped
10 green cardamom pods

Peel the marrow and remove the seeds. Cut into 2 cm (¾ in) cubes. You will need 1.5 kg (3¼ lb) prepared marrow. Place in a pan of boiling water and simmer for 3 minutes. Drain and rinse under the cold tap, then leave to drain thoroughly. Now layer the marrow with the sugar in a large bowl, cover with a tea-towel and leave overnight.

Next day, scrape the sugar and marrow and juice into a preserving pan. Pare off the zest of the lemons in long thin strips, then shred finely. Add to the pan, together with their juice. Add the ginger and cardamom too. Stir over a low heat until the sugar has completely dissolved. Bring up to the boil, then reduce heat and *simmer* until the marrow becomes translucent and the syrup is thick. Draw off the heat.

Ladle into hot sterilised jars (see page 215), seal tightly and leave to cool. Store in a dark, dry place.

* *

Summer squashes

* * *

Summer squashes are, generally speaking, those edible members of the *Cucurbita* genus that mature in the summer. They usually have tender green or yellow skins and pale green or white juicy flesh. Oddly, most winter squashes, also *Cucurbita*, mature in the autumn, but they keep well into the winter. So far, so good. Until, that is, someone points out that courgettes, the best-known of all the summer squash, are really no more than juvenile marrows. Marrows mature when you let them, sometime mid–late summer and early autumn. Does this make marrow a summer squash? I guess so, though I never think of it in these terms. That may just be because I don't think about marrows much at all unless I'm landed with one unexpectedly. Anyway, the upshot of this is that I've given **courgettes** and **marrows** their own personal sections on pages 200 and 218.

The rest of this section is about three other soft-skinned squashes that occasionally pop up on the scene. There are the prettiest little **pattypan** or **scallop squashes**, white, pale green or yellow, edges curving in and out like a swollen flower. Baby pattypans, no more than 7.5 cm (3 in) across, are as tender and delicate as courgettes. Medium-sized pattypans, let's say around 20 cm (8 in) in diameter, are beginning to toughen up. Broader than that and they lose much of their taste and should be treated as if they were marrows.

Another long-standing favourite is the **vegetable spaghetti squash**. These are harvested fairly large, are an elongated oval shape and have a light flavour. What marks them out is that when cooked the flesh separates into long thin strands, just like spaghetti.

A **chayote** (a.k.a. **cho cho** and **christophene**) is not, botanically speaking, a squash, but it is a member of the broader *Cucurbitaceae* family. It originated in South America, but is grown throughout the tropics. The crisp moist flesh is like a blend of marrow, cucumber and kohlrabi all rolled into one. It's not exciting, but nor is it unpleasant. I wouldn't make a special excursion to find chayotes, but if I see them for sale (West Indian groceries often stock them) I might buy a couple just for fun.

Practicalities

BUYING Basic buying pointers apply. In other words, make sure that your squashes are firm all over, are neither wrinkly nor jaded and have no bruised soft patches. Skins should have a dull eggshell sheen, so do not expect them to be highly glossed. Vegetable spaghetti may have a matt surface.

Pattypans and chayotes should be stored in the vegetable drawer of the fridge. Vegetable spaghetti has a sturdier outer layer and can be kept for a week or more in a cool dry place, or in the fridge if that is more convenient.

COOKING Smaller pattypan squashes should be cooked whole to preserve their cuteness. This reduces your options to **boiling** or **steaming** or **microwaving**. They need only a few minutes until just tender, but drain them before they turn squishy. Serve them dotted with butter, or sprinkled with lemon oil and a scattering of fresh herbs – chives, tarragon, basil and the like. If you want something more fancy, make up a batch of flavoured butter to melt and ooze over their hot, tender youthful forms. Try a maître d'hôtel butter – butter whizzed up with chopped parsley, lemon zest and a few shots of lemon juice – or an anchovy butter (tinned anchovy fillets, butter, parsley and lemon), or an orange and ginger butter (orange zest, a knob of preserved stem ginger, a squirt of orange juice and the butter) and so on.

Of course, if you happen to have a glut of little pattypan squashes, maybe if you are growing your own, you will soon tire of boiled baby squashes, in which case you are perfectly justified in cutting them up and treating them exactly as you would a courgette – **fry, griddle, stew** in tomato sauce, whatever. They are perfect, too, for **pickling** whole.

The obvious way to use a medium-sized pattypan is to **stuff** it, using a big, bold stuffing (try the meat stuffing on page 162 or the stuffing for peppers on page 180), well seasoned to contrast with the smooth lightness of the squash. Cut off a lid carefully, angling the knife slightly downwards as you work it round the inner cone, but leaving the scalloped edges intact. Hollow out the inside a little, taking care not to break the walls. If you don't want to go as far as making a fully blown stuffing, smear the inner walls with a little butter or a slick of olive oil, then pile in a few halved cherry tomatoes, some sliced garlic and chopped anchovy and lots of pepper, replace the lid and bake at a moderate temperature (around 180°C/350°F/Gas 4) in a dish with a spoonful or so of water in it, until tender.

Vegetable spaghetti squashes are prepared much as you would expect: cut them in half lengthways, remove any large seeds, then either boil or bake. **Baking** is really the better option – brush the cut sides with a little oil, then place cut-sides down in an ovenproof dish, drizzle a little water around them, then bake until tender. Then comes the fun. Dress them with any sauce you might use on spaghetti: tomato-based sauces are probably best of all, though something as basic as butter and freshly grated Parmesan is good too. Top each half of the vegetable spaghetti with a generous helping of the sauce/dressing and then tuck in. As your fork penetrates and teases up the flesh it will separate into strands. This is the healthiest spaghetti you'll ever eat.

Chayotes are a different kettle of fish. The pale green skin is edible, but in the centre of the vegetable you will find a single, large seed. The flesh is crisp, sweetish, but pretty bland in taste. Sliced thinly, it works well in a stir-fry, adding texture in much the same way as, say, a waterchestnut. You could do no more than blanch it in boiling water, but it wouldn't wow the dinner table. Better, if you want the simple life, to **sweat** slices of chayote with a knob of butter over a low heat in a covered pan until just crisp-tender. A sprinkling of chervil or tarragon will animate it gently. As with so many of the light-flavoured summer squashes, the ideal end for a chayote is as a bearer for a good stuffing – read through the earlier paragraphs and the marrow section for more ideas on this. Chayotes can also be **candied** by simmering in a sugar syrup.

* *

Winter squashes

* * *

There comes a moment in every child's life when they realise that their parents are not the towers of perfection they had lovingly imagined. Pumpkin lust was what shattered my illusions. A subsequent incident in Cyprus confirmed it, but I won't go into that here, except to say that it involved a raincoat and a wild red tulip.

Pumpkin envy had been oozing from my mother's lips that autumn stay in France. She eyed field after field of tenderly nurtured 'potirons', ripening into their bulging, orange fullness until at last it got the better of her. My father parked the car right up close to a patch that threatened to spill out over the road. Both field-side doors were opened and my mother squatted down, looking for all the world as if she were taking a leak. But it was neither leak nor leek that she was after. She swiftly and efficiently slashed the stem of the nearest pumpkin and passed it up to my complicit father. The crime was over in minutes. That evening we ate the evidence – bowls of pale gold soup seasoned with the spice of illegality.

In mitigation, it should be pointed out that pumpkins and winter squashes were not common fare at that time back in the UK. This was in the late 1960s, at a time when trick or treating had made few inroads in Britain, and the Hallowe'en jack-o'-lantern, if carved at all, was as likely to be a large turnip or swede as a pumpkin. At least that's how it was in our neck of the woods.

Pumpkins, it must be said, are not the most desirable of the winter squash collection (unless there are no others to be had, as on that fateful day in France), and perhaps that is why it took us so long to embrace them. Not until **butternut squashes**, followed swiftly though less successfully by a host of others, appeared on the scene did we realise what exceptional vegetables winter squashes were. They do seem to have almost everything going for them. Here's a list of their virtues:

1. They keep for months when whole;
2. They come in amazing shapes and shades;
3. Their dense flesh is sweet and chestnutty (with the exception of that of the pumpkin which can be watery and thin);
4. They're easy to grow;
5. You can roast them, fry them, steam them, boil them, grill them, griddle them, braise them, mash them;
6. You can use them in savoury dishes as well as in sweet ones;
7. They are good for you;
8. You can roast and eat the seeds.

Not bad going, huh?

There are an enormous number of varieties of winter squash of varying sizes, hues and shapes, some peculiar to certain countries (Spain's 'calabaza' is an essential element in sweet pastries and puddings, the Italian 'zucca' is used in stuffings for ravioli, or in pies), but many of them are now international. An Australian colleague heard a TV chef explaining that their relatively common Jap pumpkin came originally from Japan. She checked it out. 'Nope,' said the grower, 'when I first developed that variety we already had so many other types around that we christened it the JAP. It stands for just another pumpkin.'

Our top winter squash is undoubtedly the butternut squash with its suggestive form. Always reliable, it packs plenty of sugar-sweet brilliant orange flesh, but is small enough for a couple to eat in one sitting. **Onion and red kuri** squashes are just two of the many winter squashes that come in helpful 4–6-portion sizes, giving way to massive party squashes, amongst which stands our regular pumpkin.

Practicalities

BUYING

Winter squashes are built to last. They have hard rinds to protect them, packed tight with dense flesh to cushion the tangles of fibres and seeds at their hearts. They are titans of the vegetable kingdom, magnificent and vast. Except for the miniature varieties like the **acorn squash** or **sweet dumpling**, neat single-portion winter squashes.

Regardless of how long you intend to store your squash, make sure that its skin is hard and healthy looking all over, and not marred by bruised or softening patches. These suggest that rot or mould is setting in and although you may be able to cut them out, the rest of the squash will need to be cooked and eaten straightaway. The squash should also be heavy for its size, and should smell of very little.

In markets and at greengrocers you may be able to buy wedges hacked from a massive squash. The advantage is that you can inspect the insides to make sure there's a thick layer of healthy flesh. The disadvantage is that a cut wedge must be used within a couple of days.

A whole squash will keep for several months in the right conditions. I leave mine in the garden porch where they are protected from rain and frost, but stay cool through the winter months. An airy dry shed would do the job just as well. Cut squash, on the other hand, will need to be wrapped in clingfilm to prevent drying out, then stored in the vegetable drawer of the fridge.

COOKING

Most winter squashes are pretty much interchangeable in terms of cooking. Although each type has its unique nuance of flavour, its own degree of sweetness, its particular texture, they are rarely hugely dissimilar. There are exceptions, of course. There's no point buying petite sweet dumpling squashes when you need to make a **purée** – that's just common sense. Pumpkins are usually damper fleshed and thinner on flavour than other winter squashes, which means they are particularly well suited to making **soups**, but when puréed will need plenty of draining. If you replace pumpkin with a denser winter squash you may have to add a little extra liquid. Watch out, though, for the Spanish calabaza, a beautiful big squash that collapses into threads when cooked – it's often used to make 'cabello de angelo', angel's hair, a sweet candied concoction used as a filling in pastries.

Preparation is dictated entirely by the recipe and the type of squash you have to hand. With a butternut squash, for instance, it may be enough to halve it lengthways and then scrape out the seeds and fibres, before **baking**. With other recipes you may need to remove the rind as well. For this I usually cut the squash into thick slices then pare the rind off with a small sharp vegetable knife – my vegetable peeler is quite inadequate for the job.

Don't automatically throw the seeds out, since they make a good snack. Put fibres and seeds into a bowl of water and swirl them around to loosen the seeds. Scoop out as many as you can and then drain thoroughly in a sieve. Toss with a little oil, soy sauce, a touch of sugar if you wish, and then spread out on a baking tray. Bake in a medium oven until crisp enough to eat whole – check regularly and stir about, making sure that they don't burn.

A clutch of recipes requires that you begin by making a pumpkin or squash purée, most renowned being the American pumpkin pie. Actually, straight mashed squash is a fine addition to many a meal – enrich the purée liberally with butter, and/or add the juice of an orange or two, season well with salt, pepper and nutmeg, cinnamon or ground allspice.

To make the purée in the first place, **roast** wedges of deseeded squash in oiled foil. The oven should be fairly hot, say around 190°C/375°F/Gas 5, though exact temperature doesn't matter too much. Bake until the squash is good and tender. Timing will vary according to variety and size. It could take anything from half an hour to 1½ hours. Just keep checking. Let the softened squash cool slightly, then scrape the flesh off the skin and into a sieve lined with slit-open coffee filters. Now leave to drain, covered for as long as possible – up to 24 hours. You'll be amazed by how much water drips out. Now it's ready to use. Puréed cooked squash freezes successfully, so it's worth cooking and draining plenty.

The oven is your best pal when it comes to cooking winter squashes. Not just for making purées. **Roast** squash is always a winner. To roast butternut squash halves, grease a baking dish, lay the prepared halves in it, cut-sides down, and add a squirt of water to the dish to keep them moist. Roast at around 200°C/400°F/Gas 6 (a little higher or a little lower won't matter) until tender – again timing depends on the size of the squash, but allow around half an hour. They can be served just as they are, perhaps with a knob of butter or a grating of mature Cheddar or Parmesan on them, or filled with a grain- or meat-based stuffing. At home we love fillings based on couscous, seasoned with green olive paste, sun-dried tomatoes and nuggets of goat's cheese or feta.

Any of the small one-person squashes (acorn, gem, sweet dumpling) are natural roasters. Slice off a lid and remove the fibres and seeds before cooking, then smear butter around the inner walls. Americans will add a little brown sugar and spice too, but that's optional. Plenty of pepper is probably more to our taste. Pop the lid back on and bake at around 190°C/375°F/Gas 5 until tender.

As a side dish or starter, roast thin crescents of squash, tossed in olive oil in a hot oven, 220°C/425°F/Gas 7, for some 30–40 minutes until patched with brown and divinely tender. Good served just as they are, and even better dressed up with a spoonful of crème fraîche and a drizzle of home-made pesto or salsa verde. A few drops of lemon olive oil gives them an unexpected lift.

If you slice the squash thin enough (1 cm/½in at the widest part), it can also be fried or even grilled. Dress it with lemon juice, or a drizzle of balsamic vinegar and mint or basil. Or toss into a bowl of characterful salad leaves – rocket or watercress or curly endive – and add crumbled goat's cheese or buffalo mozzarella or feta before serving.

Nobody in their right minds would ever boil winter squash in a pan of water. Not, that is, unless they were making soup. And if you are making a squash soup, which you may well be as squashes make exceedingly fine soup, do be generous with the seasonings. A tomato or two (deseeded and skinned) in the pan doesn't go amiss either – besides improving the colour, its acidity helps to balance the sweetness of the squash. A moderation of curry powder, sweated in with the onions, or else a good measure of garlic and ginger, will give the soup a vigour that can sometimes be lacking. A recipe? Sure. Turn to page 60 and replace the parsnip with winter squash.

Boiling winter squash may be a minor crime but **braising or stewing** is to be recommended. The difference is the liquid element. When stewing or braising you use or at least produce a liquid that has oodles of flavour, some of which works its way into the solid components as they release their flavour into the pot. In other words, instead of ending up with watery squash, you end up with extra tasty squash and extra tasty sauce.

The one thing to watch is that you don't overcook the squash to a pasty mush (unless you actively want this to happen in order to thicken the sauce). To avoid this, don't add the squash too early and don't cut it too small. Teensy dice will soften within a few minutes, chunkier cubes will take somewhere between 10 and 20 minutes. So, try adding chunks of squash to stews towards the end of the cooking time – they make a grand embellishment to beef stews, adding a bit of a South American touch which you can enhance with a final scattering of fresh coriander, or to pork or chicken casseroles as well. Mixed into a vegetable braise they give it a substance that may otherwise be lacking.

The best of all options for braising winter squash, however, has to be in a **risotto**. Winter squash risotto is just gorgeous. Follow a basic risotto recipe, adding cubes of squash along with the first batch of stock, and making sure that it is seasoned generously to balance the sweetness. A last-minute squeeze or so of lime or lemon juice, though unorthodox, gives a lively lift.

Warm ginger-roast butternut squash and tomato salad

I adore roast squash, just served on its own or with a salsa verde, or like this, partnered with tingling ginger and sweet-roast cherry tomatoes.

Serves 4

3/4 large or 1 small butternut squash
1 x 2.5 cm (1 in) piece fresh root ginger, grated
4 bay leaves
7 tablespoons extra virgin olive oil
24 cherry tomatoes, halved
4 cloves garlic, sliced

1/2 tablespoon fennel seeds
12 rashers pancetta
125 g (4 1/2 oz) rocket or watercress sprigs
2 tablespoons verjuice or white wine vinegar
salt and pepper

Preheat the oven to 220°C/425°F/Gas 7.

Halve the butternut squash lengthways and scoop out the seeds. Slice thickly (across the width), into pieces that are roughly 1 cm (1/2 in) thick. Remove the rind. Place the butternut squash slices in a roasting tin with the ginger, 3 bay leaves, salt and pepper. Add 5 tablespoons of the olive oil, turn so that the butternut squash is oiled all over, and slide into the oven. Cook for 20 minutes.

Meanwhile tumble the cherry tomatoes into a small baking dish or roasting tin, adding the remaining olive oil, 1 sliced clove garlic, 1 bay leaf and the fennel seeds. Season with salt and pepper and turn the tomatoes so that they are coated with oil and seasonings.

Take the squash out of the oven, having had its first 20 minutes, and add the remaining garlic. Turn the squash, then lay the pancetta over the top. Return the squash to the oven and slide the tomatoes in there too. Roast them together for another 20 minutes, until the pancetta is crisp, the squash is tender and the tomatoes are sizzling and browning at the edges.

Divide the rocket between four plates, or one larger bowl. Lift off the pancetta and reserve. Quickly spoon the hot squash and tomatoes on to the

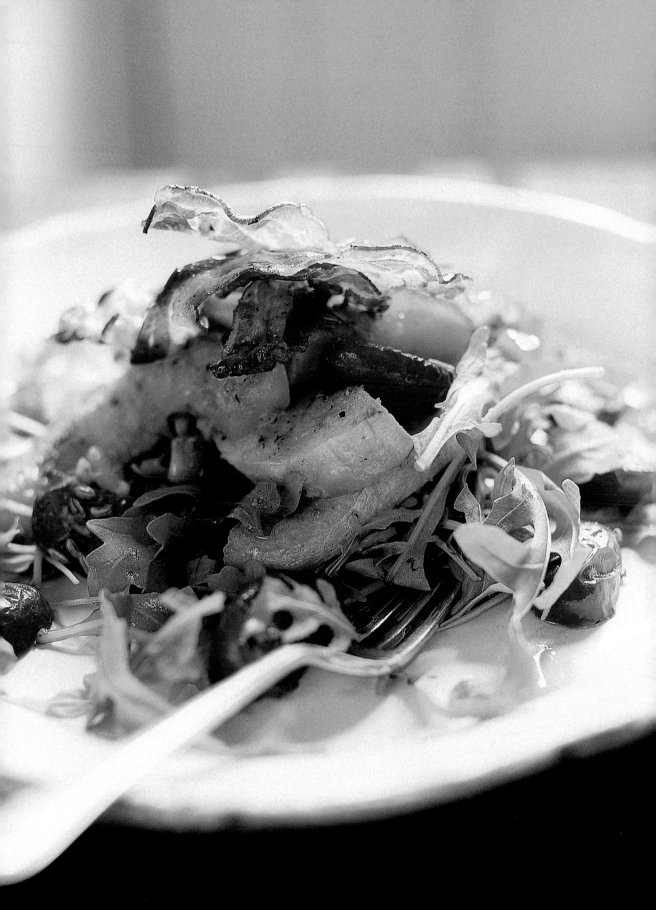

rocket. Add the verjuice to the squash roasting tin and place over a low heat. Stir, scraping in all the bits and bobs and caramelised goo until everything bubbles. Spoon this dressing over the salad. Top each salad with 3 crisp blades of pancetta and serve.

* *

Aglaia Kremezi's baked squash with garlic and walnut sauce

First the good news: this fabulous recipe, from Aglaia Kremezi's excellent book *The Foods of Greece* (Stewart, Tabori & Chang), is an unexpectedly sumptuous way to create a main course out of any kind of orange-fleshed winter squash. I've made it with both butternut and red kuri with enormous success.

Then the bad news: it looks totally vile. No getting around it. The sauce cooks to a ghastly murky brown and it is not easy to disguise. A sprinkling of chopped parsley over the top helps, but it can't work miracles. Grin and bear it, and don't serve it at a smart dinner party where you want to impress with your artistry.

Although Italian balsamic vinegar works nicely, your nearest Greek deli may stock the Hellenic equivalent, made from dried grapes.

Serves 4–6

700 g (1 lb 9 oz) winter squash, such as butternut

Sauce
5–6 large cloves garlic
1 fresh red chilli, deseeded and finely chopped
1 thick slice white bread, crusts removed, soaked in water and squeezed dry

5 tablespoons Greek balsamic vinegar or Italian balsamic vinegar
80 ml (3 fl oz) dry white wine
115 g (4 oz) shelled walnuts, finely ground
80 ml (3 fl oz) extra virgin olive oil
60 g (2 oz) shelled walnuts, coarsely chopped
salt and pepper

Preheat the oven to 190°C/375°F/Gas 5.

Cut the rind from the squash and discard any seeds, then slice thinly.

Arrange half the slices, overlapping, in an oiled baking dish (roughly 20 x 25 cm/8 x 10in).

To make the sauce, pound the garlic, chilli and some salt to a smooth paste. Now work in the bread, then the vinegar, wine, ground walnuts and pepper to form a smooth paste. Stir in half the olive oil, a little at a time. Taste and adjust seasonings, which should be strong and punchy.

Spoon half the sauce over the layered squash, and then cover with the remaining squash. Spoon the remaining sauce over the second layer of squash, then drizzle the rest of the olive oil over the surface. Cover loosely with foil and bake for 15 minutes, remove the foil and return to the oven, uncovered, for a further 15 minutes. Take out one more time and sprinkle the coarse walnuts over the top. Return to the oven for a further 10 minutes until the squash is tender but not mushy. Serve warm or at room temperature.

* *

Pumpkin and chive cornbread

This is a great way to use up the insides of a pumpkin hollowed out to make a Hallowe'en jack-o'-lantern. It takes no time at all to throw together, and is so good eaten warm from the oven, with a warming bowl or mug of soup.

Serves 8

115 g (4 oz) plain flour
175 g (6 oz) yellow cornmeal
1 level tablespoon baking powder
1 tablespoon caster sugar
250 g (9 oz) pumpkin flesh, coarsely grated
4 tablespoons chopped chives

1/2 teaspoon salt
200 ml (7 fl oz) milk
2 eggs
4 tablespoons extra virgin olive oil
  or melted butter

Preheat the oven to 200°C/400°F/Gas 6. Grease a 20 cm (8 in) square shallow tin generously.

Mix the flour with the cornmeal, baking powder, sugar, pumpkin, chives and salt. Make a well in the centre, and pour in the milk. Add the eggs and oil or melted butter, and stir all the ingredients together until evenly mixed.

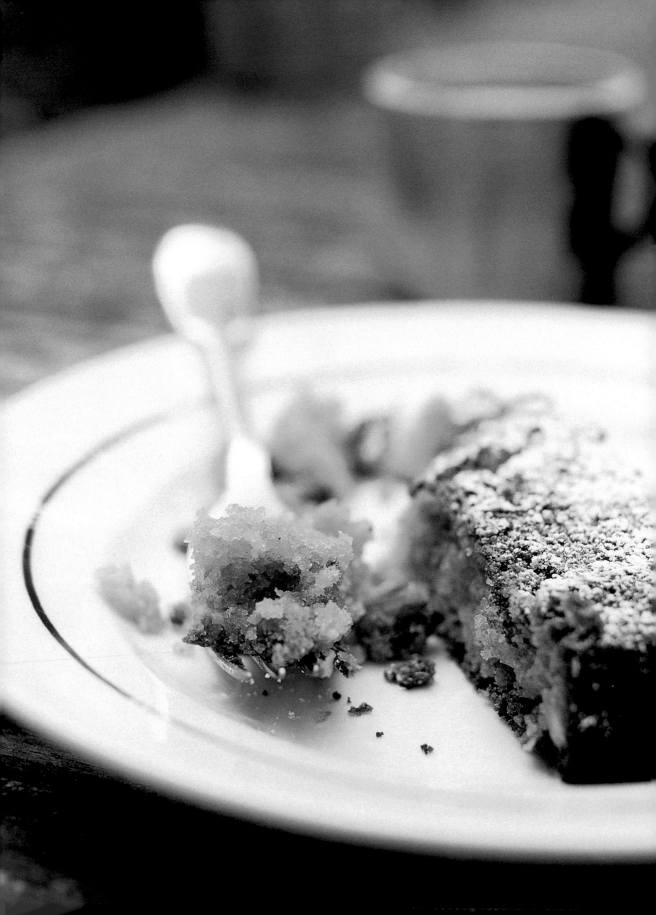

Pour into the prepared tin, and bake in the preheated oven for 20–25 minutes until firm to the touch. Double check by plunging a skewer into the centre – if it comes out clean, then the cornbread is done.

Let it rest in the tin for 5 minutes then turn out, and eat warm or cold cut into chunky squares.

* *

Squash, white chocolate, pistachio and maple syrup traybake

This is so much nicer than pumpkin pie, heretical though that may sound. The squash purée gives the crumb a pretty golden colour and keeps it moist without being soggy. I've made it using butternut squash and pumpkin and both work well.

Serves 12–16

300 g (11 oz) pumpkin purée
175 g (6 oz) butter, softened
4 tablespoons maple syrup or honey
  or golden syrup
150 g (5 oz) caster sugar
3 eggs, beaten
280 g (10 oz) self-raising flour

1½ rounded teaspoons baking powder
a pinch of salt
60 g (2 oz) shelled pistachios, chopped
150 g (5 oz) white chocolate, chopped

To finish
icing sugar

Preheat the oven to 180°C/350°F/Gas 4. Base-line a 30 x 23 cm (12 x 9 in) tin with baking parchment, and grease the sides.

Put all the ingredients except the nuts and chocolate into a bowl and beat together until evenly mixed. Fold in the nuts and chocolate and pour into the prepared tray. Smooth down lightly.

Bake in the preheated oven for about 40–45 minutes until firm to the touch. Cool in the tin. Dust with icing sugar and cut into squares.

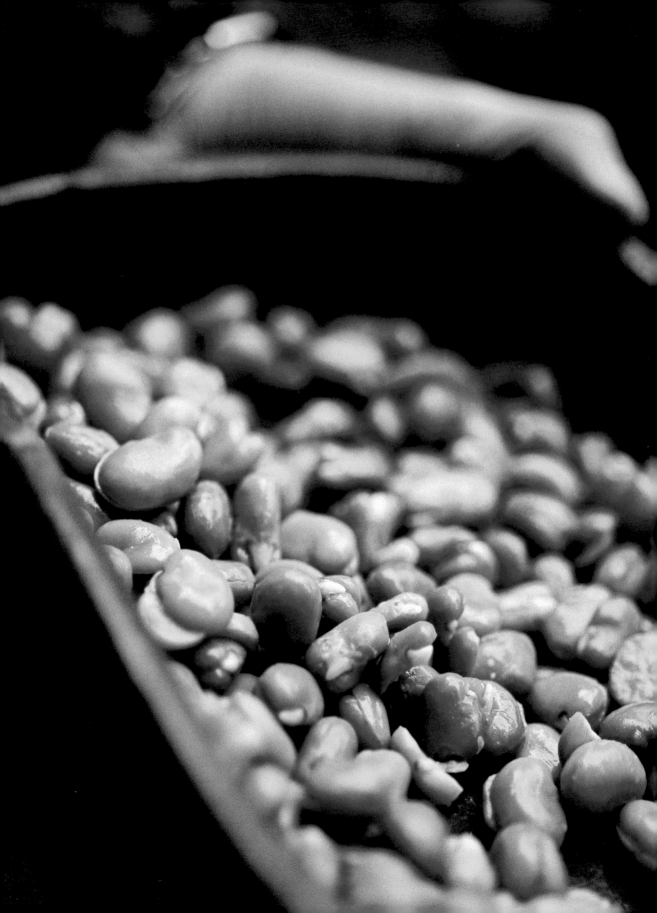

Pods and seeds

* *

Broad beans Edamame **Green beans** Mangetouts and sugarsnaps **Peas and pea shoots** Runner beans **Shelling beans** (borlotti, flageolet and cannellini) **Sweetcorn**

Broad beans

* * *

The broad bean is a vegetable that rewards patience. It hides its virtues well, cloaking them under thick layers of green and grey, so that only those gifted with quiet determination will find them. I admit to hesitating when I see a pile of burly broad beans in their pods for sale. Not because I doubt their excellence, but because I need to assess whether I will find the time to pod them first, then skin the podded beans one by one. Only then are the vivid emerald green beanlets revealed to the world and it is these that make broad beans the most subtle and elegant charmers of the bean brethren.

Unlike kidney beans and haricot beans that come originally from the New World, broad beans are our own native European beans and have been grown here since neolithic times. Both ancient Greeks and Romans ate them, or deliberately avoided them. Romans, for instance, believed that they housed the souls of the dead, so ate them at funerals, while Pythagoras forbade his followers to consume them because he considered they were made from the same base substance as humans had been created from. Luckily this doesn't seem to have put subsequent generations of bean-eaters off their stride. The broad bean lives on victorious, embedded in the cuisines of the entire Mediterranean basin (they originate from the eastern end, apparently), creeping their way up north to find a welcoming home in the British Isles.

So at home have they become here, that I find it hard to think of them as anything but a quintessentially British vegetable. I'm wrong, of course, but even so, they have, over the centuries, made themselves as indispensable to our idea of early summer bounty as the first new potatoes or little green peas. Mind you, the former come from the Andes, the latter from the eastern Mediterranean, so what's new?

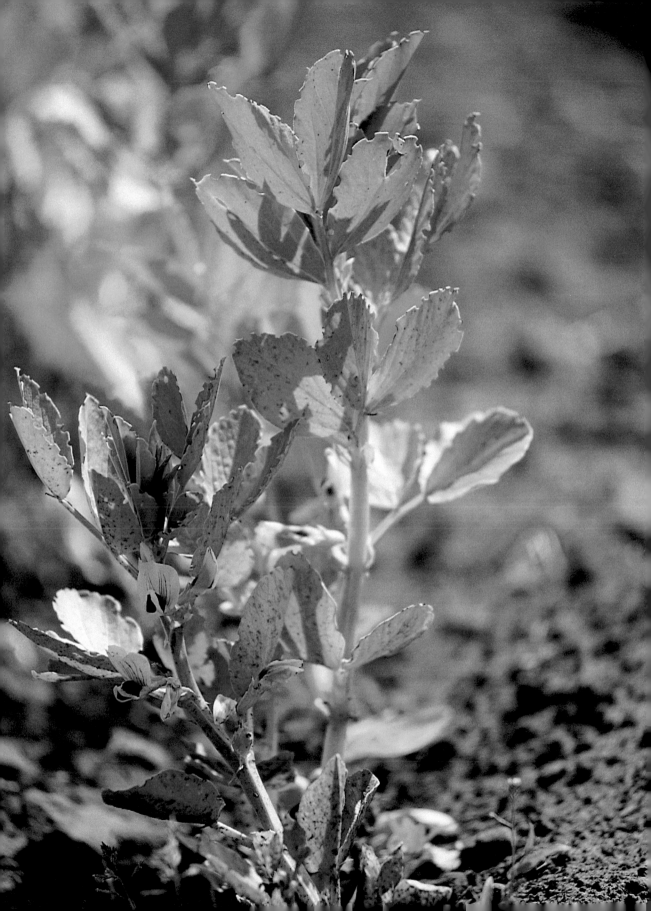

Practicalities

BUYING There are two choices when it comes to buying broad beans: fresh in their pods, or frozen podded (or shelled). Tastewise, fresh are likely to be superior, but only if they are newly picked, and not horrendously large. Frozen broad beans are a brilliant year-round standby.

Fresh broad beans are in season from early summer right through until late August by which time the few latecomers are often big and mealy. Better then to make the most of them in June and early July. Look for pods that are of medium stature, bulging here and there but not bursting at the seams. Small brown blemishes are to be expected, but discard any beans that have evidence of rot, or that are obviously drying out. Bean to pod ratio is relatively low – buy a good 400g (14oz) of beans in their pods per person, as you'll be throwing away up to three-quarters of the weight.

The blanket-thick pod keeps its cargo of beans fresh for 4 or 5 days, but don't let them tarry at the back of the fridge for any longer than that.

To pod or shell the beans, press the seams of each pod together firmly until they crack open, helping the process along with your fingernails if necessary. Pull the pod right open and take out the beans. Most people, most of the time, cook and eat the beans at this stage. This is fine when the beans are small and their grey-green skin is still delicate. In fact when they are extra small and impeccably fresh you don't even need to cook them – in Italy they are served raw with Parma ham as a first course.

COOKING However, it doesn't take long for the greyish skin to thicken and gain the bitterish taste that puts so many people right off broad beans altogether. It doesn't have to be like this, not if you are prepared to spend more time on those beans. You'll be glad you did in the end. To remove the skin, drop the beans into a pan of boiling water. Bring back to the boil and simmer for 1 minute, then drain and run under the cold tap. Now the bean can be slit open (use a small knife or fingernails) and the joyous pure green beanlet popped straight out. These beanlets will need a few minutes' more cooking to bring them to full tenderness, but boy, will they taste good.

If you are using **frozen broad beans**, which will already have been blanched at the processing factory, all you need do is leave them to thaw, then skin them as you would fresh ones. Job done.

Once they've been skinned you can finish the cooking by **simmering** for a further 2–3 minutes in boiling salted water, or take a different tack by **frying** them gently in olive oil or butter, over a low heat, with a little chopped garlic and/or sliced spring onion if you will, until they soften to the right degree. It is almost universally acknowledged that salted cured pork works a kind of magic on broad beans, so if you have some to hand, add strips of pancetta or prosciutto crudo (e.g. Parma ham) or high-quality bacon to the frying pan as well. One of the best broad bean dishes I've ever eaten was based on this combination: a plate of spaghetti, tossed with broad beans, pancetta, garlic and the olive oil they'd been finished in, sprinkled with parsley and freshly grated Parmesan. Bliss.

PARTNERS The key herb for broad beans is summer savory with its warmth and hint of bitterness, but failing that, a sprinkling of chopped parsley, fresh thyme or marjoram, or a final scattering of shredded fresh mint are also winners.

There has been, in the UK, a feeling that broad beans are good dished up in a pool of white sauce. I'm not convinced. It strikes me that this may have originated as a bid to disguise over-large broad beans in their bitter tough skins. If so it was not successful. What does work is to moisten either very young broad beans in their skins, or patiently skinned broad beanlets, in a very, very, very good parsley sauce. Dish this up with very, very, very hot gammon or ham and you have a match made in heaven. To make a v.v.v. good parsley sauce, begin by stewing lots of chopped parsley in butter over an extremely low heat for about 20 minutes, before adding flour to make a roux, followed by milk in the usual way. Make the starter sauce quite thin and runny, and then cook it gently for at least 20–30 minutes to mellow out the floury taste and thicken it gently. Remember to stir it frequently so that it doesn't stick. Now stir in some double cream and a squeeze or two of lemon juice, or crème fraîche, season and it's ready.

Oddly, broad beans are not improved by a home-made tomato sauce. It's just too overwhelming for the little mites. The subtler approach is to toss some diced deseeded tomato, along with fragrant summer herbs, in with broad beans just before serving so that they have time to warm through but no more than that.

Broad beans and rice are a coupling that turns up all around the Mediterranean. In Rome, for instance, one traditional family dish is a soup/stew of beans and rice in a tomato broth, while further north, broad bean risotto is a spring-time delicacy. Working round to the eastern and southern sides we find gentle pilaffs of broad beans and rice (see page 244), or broad beans stewed with minced meat and rice. Here too, and in Italy, fat end-of-season beans are dried for winter use. In Egypt, falafel are made of dried broad beans, rather than the chickpeas of countries like Israel, while in Sicily they tuck into a thick, warming dried broad bean soup called 'maccu'.

Fresh broad beans, too, make a heavenly soup, but only if they are a) young or b) skinned individually. Add them to a soup base made by sweating chopped onions, potatoes and celery in butter, along with light chicken or vegetable stock, simmer until tender, then add chervil or a little tarragon and parsley and liquidise before reheating with lemon zest and a small slick of cream. If you haven't the patience to skin enough broad beans to thicken a creamed soup, instead throw a couple of handfuls into a minestrone.

In summer months, for smart dinner parties, or for a special treat, my mother used to serve artichoke bowls (see page 141) filled with a rich and creamy broad bean purée, made by liquidising broad beans with cream and butter. We pulled off the outer leaves, dipped those little nuggets of flesh at the base into the purée and chewed them off together. A wonderful combination but to make adequate supplies of the purée you have to pod and skin an awful lot of beans. For me, that reduces it to a dish to be made for no more than four people at the outside. Even if I don't go as far as creating the artichoke cups, I still occasionally make a bean purée, sometimes eking out the beans with a little potato, to serve as a side dish to liven up something like plain grilled lamb chops.

A final note for those of you who grow your own broad beans or know someone who does. Unless the blackfly is excessive, save the leafy bean tops that you pinch out in the late spring. They can be eaten just as they are, tossed into a salad perhaps along with handfuls of rocket or watercress and leaves of little gem lettuce, or if you have enough of them, blanched lightly and eaten like spinach, or used to make a soup. Waste not want not.

Broad bean, yoghurt and mint soup

This soup turns out the most cool, pale green, so pretty when it is flecked with darker green mint and bright green, skinned beans.

Do not reheat the soup once you have mixed in the yoghurt. If it gets too hot it will curdle in a most unattractive manner.

Serves 4

450g (1lb) shelled broad beans, thawed if frozen
1 onion, chopped
1 stick celery, thinly sliced
30g (1oz) butter
2 tablespoons pudding rice
1 generous sprig summer savory or thyme

1 litre (1¾ pints) chicken stock, or vegetable stock
115g (4oz) Greek yoghurt
a handful of mint leaves, chopped
4 small sprigs mint
a little paprika or cayenne pepper
salt and pepper

Blanch and skin the beans as usual. Take about one-eighth of them, chop roughly and set aside. Sweat the onion and celery gently in the butter in a covered pan over a low heat, for about 10 minutes until very tender. Add the rice and savory or thyme, and cook for another minute, uncovered. Now add the beans, stock, salt and pepper, bring up to the boil and simmer for about 10 minutes until the rice is tender. Remove the savory stem, and then liquidise the soup in batches.

Shortly before serving reheat thoroughly, then draw off the heat. Stir in a tablespoonful of the yoghurt, together with the reserved beans and the chopped mint. Mix in a second tablespoonful of yoghurt, and continue stirring in a spoonful at a time, until all is incorporated. Taste and adjust seasoning, and serve quickly while still warm, floating a sprig of mint and a light dusting of paprika or cayenne on the surface of each bowlful.

Broad bean, dill and saffron pilaff

This looks like Easter, said a friend of mine, and I know just what she means. Shades of fresh spring green, yellow and white all coming together in one plate. To get it at its best Pascal prettiness, you do have to take a little time over preparing the broad beans, but they'll taste all the better for it.

Serve this pilaff as a gentle main course on its own, or as a side dish (in which case you don't really need the yoghurt).

Serves 4–6

500g (1lb 2oz) broad beans in their pods,
 or 350g (12oz) shelled broad beans
a big pinch of saffron threads
400g (14oz) basmati or long-grain rice
45g (1½oz) butter
1 onion, finely chopped
2 cloves garlic, finely chopped

750ml (1¼ pints) vegetable or chicken stock
3 tablespoons chopped dill
salt and pepper

To serve
thick Greek-style yoghurt

Pod the broad beans if fresh. Drop the beans into a pan of boiling water and simmer for 1 minute. Drain and slit open each bean to squeeze out the brilliant green beanlet inside. Discard the skins. (If you are using frozen broad beans, just thaw them out, then skin as for fresh beans.)

Soak the saffron in a tablespoon of very hot water. Rinse the rice if using basmati and leave to drain until needed.

Melt the butter in a saucepan and fry the onion and garlic gently in it. Now add the rice and stir to coat each grain in buttery juices. Add the stock, dill, salt and pepper, bring up to the boil, then stir in the broad beans. Cover tightly and reduce the heat to a teensy thread. Cook for exactly 10 minutes, without lifting the lid.

Draw off the heat, remove the lid and stir – the liquid should by now have been completely absorbed. Stir in the saffron water, then taste and adjust seasonings. Serve straightaway with the yoghurt.

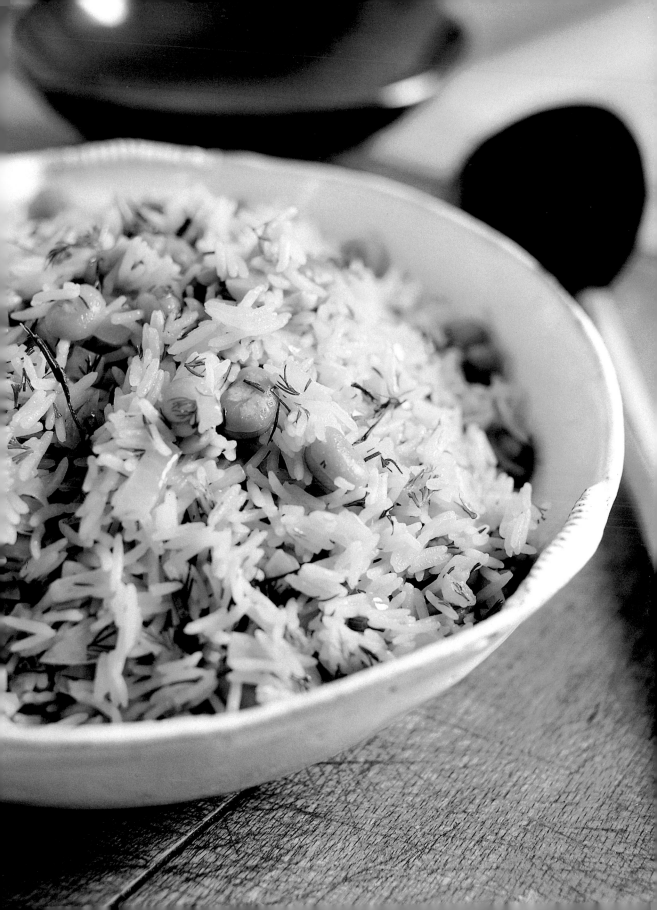

* *

Two bean, chickpea and tomato salad

This salad is a pretty way to show off a small amount of fresh broad beans at their best.

Serves 4

200 g (7 oz) French beans or string beans, topped and tailed
250 g (9 oz) shelled broad beans, cooked and skinned
115 g (4 oz) cooked chickpeas
150 g (5 oz) cherry tomatoes, halved
1½ tablespoons finely chopped parsley
1½ tablespoons finely chopped basil
1 tablespoon finely chopped mint

1 tablespoon chopped chives
salt and pepper

Dressing
juice of ½ lemon
½ teaspoon caster sugar
1 teaspoon tomato purée
3 tablespoons extra virgin olive oil

Simmer the green beans in lightly salted water for about 4–5 minutes, until just cooked. Drain, run under the cold tap to set the colour, then drain again. Cut into 2.5 cm (1 in) lengths. Mix with the broad beans, chickpeas, cherry tomatoes and herbs.

To make the dressing whisk the lemon juice with the sugar, tomato purée, salt and pepper, then gradually whisk in the olive oil. Pour over the beans and toss together. Serve at room temperature.

* *

Edamame

* * *

I like the word 'edamame'. It rolls off the lips and tongue with an exotic rhythm that promises something special. They are, too. Edamame is the Japanese for fresh soy beans, cooked in their pods, and whilst they may be an everyday sort of delicacy in Japan, in Europe they are still an unexpected treat. Until relatively recently the only place you might get them would be at a Japanese or Chinese food store and probably only frozen even there. More recently, however, I've spotted them for sale in both a supermarket and a greengrocer. Admittedly it was a pretty fancy greengrocer, but there they were in their fuzzy green pods looking fresh and dewy and very enticing.

COOKING

In my all-too-meagre experience of Japanese food, edamame are eaten as a preamble to the main meal, a light mouthful to get the gastric juices flowing. Cooking them is elementary – just drop them into boiling lightly salted water and cook for 4–6 minutes. Drain them and quickly toss with flakes of sea salt (not fine salt, nor solid crystals) and place in the centre of the table, within everyone's reach. To eat them, squeeze the beans out of the pod with your teeth and discard the pod. Delicious.

* *

Green beans and wax beans

* * *

Don't you just love those glorious mistranslations on foreign menus? My top examples remain the 'fragrant crap curry' discovered in Bangkok and the 'boiled buttered string' offered on a cross-Channel ferry some three decades ago. The curry was indeed fragrant, though the crap's claws were sticky and hard to crack, while the string turned out to be nothing more exciting than overcooked string beans. So more a sin of omission than of mistranslation.

That's not so likely to happen today, now that what were once called string beans so rarely have a string to their name. When my mother first taught me how to prepare **green beans** (and runner beans), you topped and tailed them both, carefully pulling away the long tough fibres that ran down their edges. Now you could waste hours searching for any fibres at all. This welcome improvement has come, as far as I can tell, without discernible loss of taste. Hurrah.

Despite dispensing with one name, I still find myself hesitating over what to call these most delicious long slender tubes of green. 'Green bean' always seems too vague – lots of beans are green, after all – but the term **'French bean'** appears to have been redefined to denote particularly slim green beans, though these may also be sold as **'fine beans'**. I wonder if there's a note of cross-Channel xenophobia creeping in here? It wouldn't be the only time we've reclaimed something from the French – think of crème brûlée, which we now know was British in the first place and should properly be called 'burnt cream', and when did you last hear anyone refer to a contraceptive as a 'French letter'? Even French kissing is on the decline, nominally at any rate.

Back to green beans. Not only do we have fine beans, occasionally French beans, but supermarkets also sell **bobby beans**, chunkier than the other two, but still comparatively svelte in the bean world, and more recently, pretty **yellow wax beans** have started to appear on the shelves. The latter have, incidentally, long been a regular fixture on the French summer scene. Ultimately, there seems no alternative but to stick with 'green bean' as the umbrella name for all of them, despite the canary brightness of this latest addition to the British bean world.

Practicalities

BUYING

I'm sorry to bang on about freshness yet again, but it makes such a difference to a humble green bean. Packaged and prepared and ready to go straight in the pan, they will taste absolutely fine, but get them newly plucked from the plant, fresh as daisies, and tangled up in an unruly heap, and the difference is startling. Suddenly they leap into a state of total gorgeousness, taking the number two spot in the league of high summer vegetables. Number one spot obviously goes to the perfect sun-ripened tomato.

If you are not growing your own, then July and August are when to go in search of locally grown, ultra-fresh green beans. Trawl your farmers' markets and farm shops and greengrocers and buy plenty whenever you see them.

Remember that they are part of nature's bounty, which means that they will not often be ramrod straight and pristinely unblemished. Curves are good. The beans themselves will be firm fleshed and should snap in half cleanly.

Green beans will keep in a tolerably good state for as much as a week in the vegetable drawer of the fridge, *but* just think what you are losing. Every day the apex of taste perfection recedes a little further into the past. Cook them whilst still in their prime and you'll have everyone coming back for seconds.

Preparation is simple if not speedy. Nip the stalk end off each bean – I use a knife to do this, my cousin uses the kitchen scissors, but you can just as well do it with your fingernails. Time-honoured tradition has it that you should also remove the other end – top and tail – but it struck me recently that there is no good reason for this now that stringiness is so rarely an issue. So unless you have bought 'heritage variety' or overlarge end-of-season beans, burdened with stringiness, don't bother. If you are in a tearing hurry, then slice the ends off a whole bundle of beans at one go, but be aware that this can be a wasteful method of topping.

COOKING

Green beans should be **boiled** or **steamed** or possibly **microwaved**. It is possible to cook them in other ways, but they are mostly pretty impractical. Imagine trying to keep them lined up on a grill rack, for instance, without falling through the wires. Once in a while I might **deep-fry** them as a special treat (the recipe on page 251 is extraordinarily good) but it's not the stuff of everyday meals.

So, it's back to basic methods, essentially. The important thing is to keep the timing brief. So, I reckon that for average-sized green beans, 4–5 minutes in simmering water is quite long enough to soften them. More than that and they become soggy and lose flavour. Drain quickly, tip into a warm serving dish, dot with butter if you wish, and serve straightaway.

If you are not serving them straightaway, maybe because you want to use them in a salad, or you want to reheat them later with other seasonings, run the newly drained steaming green beans under the cold tap for at least 30 seconds, longer if your patience holds, in order to stop them cooking further in their own heat. Then leave to drain and cool.

Here are a few of the ways I like to dress up green beans. Sometimes I will fry shallot or onion in a little butter in a wide frying pan until almost tender then add a shake of brown mustard seeds. As soon as they begin to pop (you may need to raise the heat a little), I tip in the beans and cook until heated through. When I want more spiciness, I'll replace the mustard seeds with a teaspoon or two of curry paste or powder. For a softer taste, I'd fry flaked almonds in butter until they turn golden, before adding the beans. Or I might fry chopped garlic in olive oil until beginning to colour, add the beans, stir for a minute or two, then throw in some diced, deseeded tomato and chopped parsley or basil or coriander to finish. Or simply fry garlic and fresh deseeded, chopped red chilli in olive oil, then add the beans and, when hot, fresh parsley or coriander.

PARTNERS Green beans also make a fantastic salad, either on their own or with other ingredients. For the best flavour, dress them with a vinaigrette as soon as they have drained while still warm. As they cool, they'll soak up some of the dressing. As the main ingredient of the salad, on their own, you can get away with no more than a straightforward wine vinegar and olive oil vinaigrette, but play the changes with tarragon vinegar or avocado oil once in a while. Anchovy and green beans go well together – add some anchovy essence to the dressing, but not so much that it over-salts the salad.

Toss the dressed beans with toasted flaked almonds or chopped toasted hazelnuts, fresh soft-leaved herbs such as tarragon, chervil, parsley, coriander, marjoram and so on. I'm not so keen on mint or basil with green beans. I love to seed a salad of green beans with diced, deseeded tomatoes, or a more ample supply of halved or quartered cherry tomatoes.

Green bean and new potato salad is always a winner. I like them turned with a bright vinaigrette spiked with plenty of coarse-grain mustard. For a main-course version, add sliced garlic sausage or even good-quality frankfurters, finely diced hard-boiled egg and cornichons or gherkins and lots of chopped parsley. Another fine match with green beans is chicken – mix them with a light mayonnaise and serve on a bed of shredded cos or little gem lettuce for a summer lunch, or enclose between slices of bread to make a cracking sandwich.

Sichuan green beans

This exceptional way to cook green beans is one that I first came across not in Sichuan, sadly, but in a deli in Toronto, many years ago. I would never in a blue moon have imagined that deep-fried green beans could be so incredibly good, let alone beans that have been deep-fried and then simmered. Dried shrimps and Sichuan pepper are available from Chinese supermarkets. The Sichuan pepper could be replaced by black peppercorns, but there is no substitute for the dried shrimps.

Serves 4 as a first course or side dish

2 tablespoons dried shrimps
sunflower or vegetable oil for deep-frying
500 g (1 lb 2 oz) green beans, topped
2 cloves garlic, thinly sliced
½ teaspoon Sichuan peppercorns, coarsely crushed
2.5 cm (1 in) piece fresh root ginger, peeled and cut into matchsticks

½ teaspoon salt
1 tablespoon caster sugar
1 tablespoon dark soy sauce
2 teaspoons rice vinegar
1 tablespoon sesame oil

Cover the shrimps generously with boiling water and soak for 20 minutes. Drain and reserve the liquid. Chop the shrimps finely.

Heat a panful of oil to 190°C/375°F and deep-fry the beans in batches, for 5 minutes, until tender and patched with brown. Drain on kitchen paper.

Heat a wok over a high heat until it smokes. Add 1 tablespoon oil, swirl around then add the garlic, Sichuan pepper and ginger and stir-fry for a few seconds. Then add the shrimps and stir-fry for another 20–30 seconds. Now add the salt, sugar, soy sauce and 5 tablespoons of the shrimp water.

Finally tip in the green beans. Toss in the sauce to coat well, then cover and, keeping the heat high, cook until virtually all the liquid has been absorbed. Check after 1 minute – the sauce should have caramelised and the beans should be several shades darker, even verging on black. Toss and if necessary, cover again for a further 30 seconds or so to finish cooking. Remove from the heat and mix with the rice vinegar and sesame oil. Serve hot or at room temperature.

Ratatouille of green beans, broad beans, courgettes and peppers

The success of a great ratatouille depends on two things. The first and most obvious is excellent ingredients: vegetables in their exact prime, fruity and fragrant olive oil. The second, almost as critical, is time. This is not a dish to attempt in a hurry. No point taking shortcuts, either. Whether you are tackling a classic ratatouille or a modified version like this (aubergine replaced with green beans and courgettes), take it at a leisurely gait, allowing plenty of time for each batch of vegetables to mellow down and release its particular gift.

The corollary is that a wise cook settles down to the creation of a fine ratatouille the day before the guests arrive for the barbecue. Although you can serve it hot, ratatouille tastes best (and after all that loving attention, how could you demand anything less) warm or at room temperature.

Note, too, that a divine ratatouille is not a handful of vegetables swimming in vats of tomato goo, but a blessed balance and coming together of equal partners. Enough tomato, but not so much that the other vegetables lose their importance.

Serves 6–8

extra virgin olive oil
450 g (1 lb) courgettes, halved lengthways
 and thickly sliced
2 red peppers, deseeded and cut into strips
2 large onions, halved and thinly sliced
6 cloves garlic, sliced
2 teaspoons coriander seeds, coarsely
 crushed
600 g (1 lb 5 oz) ripe fleshy tomatoes,
 skinned, deseeded and roughly chopped

1 bay leaf
2 generous sprigs thyme
3 tablespoons chopped parsley
a pinch or two of caster sugar (optional)
250 g (9 oz) French beans, topped and tailed,
 then cut in half
250 g (9 oz) shelled broad beans, thawed if
 frozen (see introduction)
salt and pepper

Heat 3 tablespoons oil in a wide, deep frying pan. Fry the courgettes in the oil until lightly patched here and there with brown. Scoop out and leave to drain on kitchen paper. Now fry the peppers briskly until touched with brown here

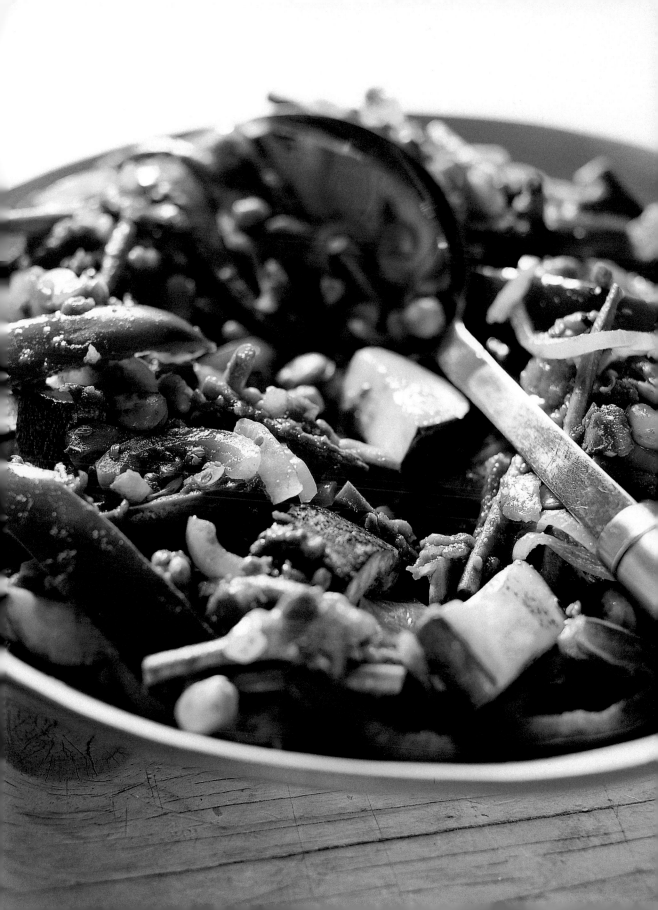

and there. Scoop them out, and add to the courgettes.

Turn the heat down and add a further 3 tablespoons oil to the pan. Fry the onion slowly until tender, without browning, allowing a good 10 minutes. Add the garlic and coriander and fry for another 2 minutes. Tip in the tomatoes, bay leaf and thyme tied together with string, half the parsley, a pinch or two of sugar if your tomatoes are not perfectly flavoured, salt and pepper. Cook gently, covered, for about 10 minutes, then add the green beans, cover and simmer for a further 5 minutes. Now add the thawed broad beans, the courgettes and peppers and simmer for a final 5–10 minutes, this time uncovered, until the stew is thick and fragrant. If at any time you fear that the ratatouille is about to burn, stir in some water. Conversely, should it turn out at all watery, keep right on cooking for a further 5–10 minutes until all wateriness is banished. Taste and adjust seasoning and leave to cool.

Just before serving, stir the mixture and spoon into a serving dish. Sprinkle with the remaining parsley and drizzle over a filigree of extra virgin olive oil to give fresh gloss and flavour.

* *

Green beans with pears

In Germany it is relatively common to combine fruit and vegetables in one pan, and it's something we should consider taking up here. We've already absorbed sweet and sour red cabbage cooked with apple, but this is simpler, quicker and just as good. If you have slightly under-ripe pears all the better (though not essential), as the natural tartness adds an extra stab of flavour.

The only slightly tricksy thing about this recipe – and it's not much of a problem – is getting the timing right. Vigilance is your best ally. You need to catch the pears and beans just as the last of the water has evaporated, but before anything starts to burn.

Serves 4–6

250g (9oz) green beans (French beans, bobby beans)
350–400g (12–14oz) pears

30g (1oz) butter
salt and pepper

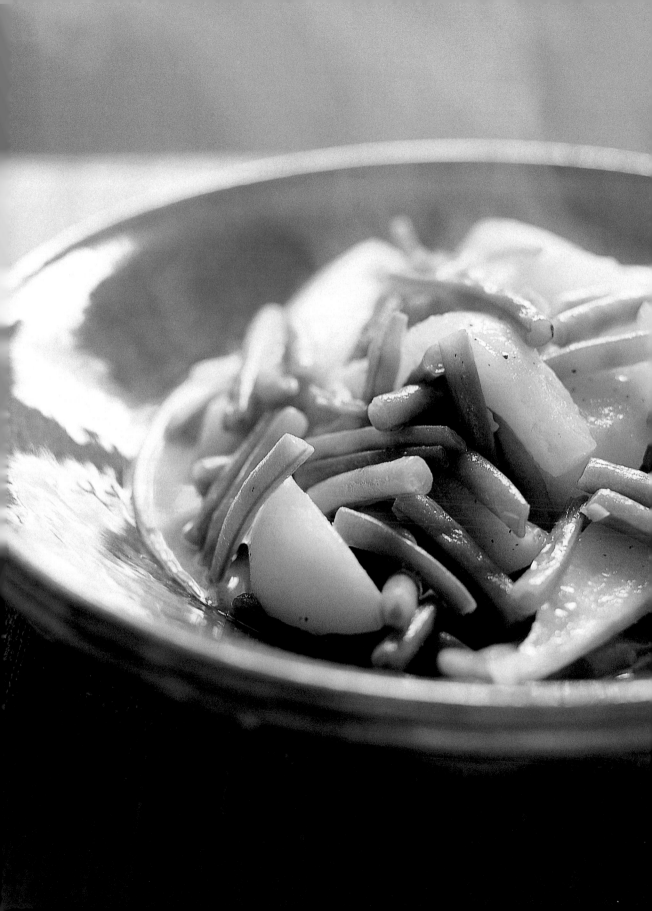

Top and tail the green beans and cut in half. Peel, quarter and core the pears, then cut each quarter into halves or thirds. Place beans and pears in a pan, add the butter, salt and pepper and about 300ml (10 fl oz water. Cover and bring up to the boil. Uncover and then bubble for around 5–8 minutes, stirring occasionally until the water has virtually all evaporated, leaving behind the buttery juices to season the beans and pears. Taste and add more salt if needed, and then serve.

* *

Mangetouts and sugarsnaps

* * *

You know those moments in kids' cartoons where Tom or Taz or Bugs gets run over by a steamroller, then wobbles up squished and flat, but still going in a bemused kind of a way? That's a mangetout moment. **Mangetouts** are no more nor less than steamrollered peas in their pods. Not literally of course, though the notion conjures up rather fine images of the cartoon variety, but they work in much the same way, except that they don't reinflate at any point. The nearest thing to a reinflated mangetout is its close relation, the **sugarsnap**, fatter than a mangetout, yet far slimmer than a full pea pod. Like the mangetout, the sugarsnap is eaten in its entirety, pod and all.

Practicalities

BUYING Use your common sense when buying mangetouts or sugarsnaps. They've got to look keen and lively and beaming with healthiness. So you want a sprightly green colour and a firm texture. When they are being sold loose, not so common these days, insist on being able to taste before buying, so that you can be sure that they carry their full complement of crisp texture and leguminous, sweet flavour. Signs of tiredness or decay (flabbiness, dullness, withering stems or tips) mean they are not worth buying. Blemishes are a problem in mangetouts or sugarsnaps, unlike in other chunkier vegetables where they can easily be cut out or ignored.

Mangetouts and sugarsnaps often come fully prepared, but if stems are left on, or a little thread hangs from the opposite tip, just snap or snip them off. There is no point cooking either mangetouts or sugarsnaps when you are going to use them in salads, unless you positively want to soften them. Most of us like the crisp juiciness just as it is. Cutting them into narrower strips is thoughtful, but not necessary, either. Use them wisely and with restraint and they will bring texture and colour to most salads, but don't just chuck them in willy-nilly. I wouldn't, for instance, mix them into a potato salad, but I might well add a handful to a bowl of cherry tomatoes, cos, and mozzarella. This is no more than personal preference, but before you go wild with raw mangetouts, pause and consider whether they will enhance, or distract or dominate.

COOKING Cooking brings out the fuller flavour, giving it more depth, but it takes only a few minutes. Overcook sugarsnaps or mangetouts and they soon turn slimy and soggy and shed everything they had going for them, including their colour. They should be exposed to heat for no more than 2–4 minutes at most. So, either **blanch** them in boiling salted water or **steam** them literally minutes before serving, then dress them with a little butter if you wish, or even nicer, **stir-fry** for a few minutes in a wok over a high heat. Keep it pure adding just a spot of oil to keep them moving, or go oriental and add chopped garlic, ginger, chilli, spring onion, soy sauce and/or sesame oil. When you are making a mixed stir-fry, add mangetouts towards the end, when the other vegetables are almost ready. Flaked toasted almonds, or chopped toasted hazelnuts, go well with mangetouts and sugarsnaps, boiled, steamed or stir-fried.

Neither mangetouts nor sugarsnaps take kindly to most other cooking methods. You could, I suppose, thread bits of either on to a skewer, between other more substantial ingredients (cubes of chicken, monkfish or prawns) but I'm not sure that it would be worth the bother. In other words, don't try getting too fancy with these flattened peas. They appreciate the simple life.

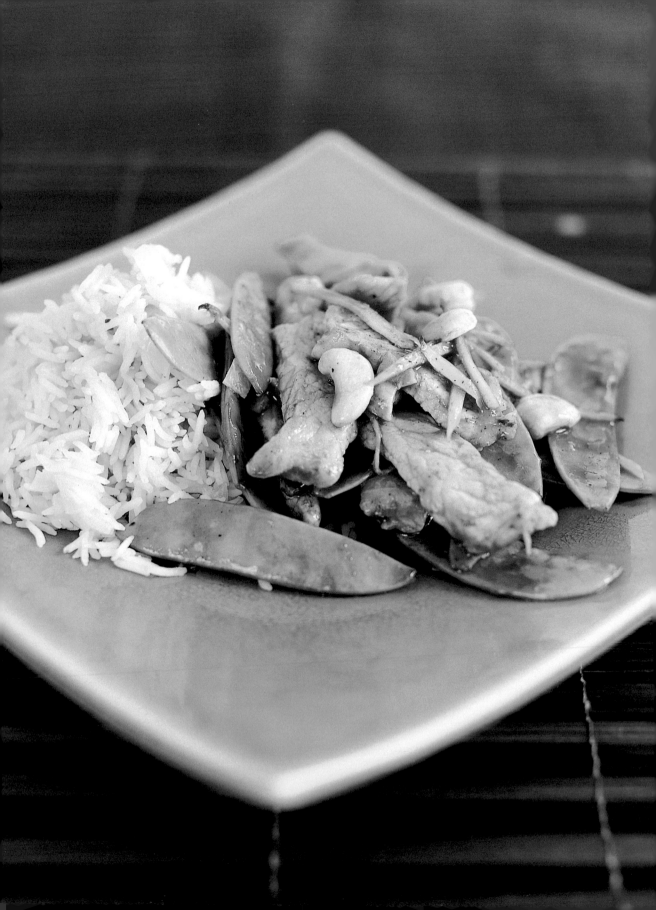

* *

Stir-fried pork with mangetouts and yellow bean sauce

Mangetouts are obvious candidates for stir-frying, on their own, with other vegetables or as in this recipe with meat to produce a quick, satisfying main course.

Yellow bean sauce is now widely available in supermarkets as well as Chinese foodstores. It is made with fermented soy beans and has a sweetish flavour.

Serves 4

400 g (14 oz) pork steaks
2 tablespoons vegetable oil
2 cloves garlic, chopped
2.5 cm (1 in) piece fresh root ginger, cut into batons
175 g (6 oz) mangetouts, topped and tailed

25 g (scant 1 oz) flaked almonds or cashews
3 tablespoons yellow bean sauce
1 teaspoon sesame oil
1 tablespoon soy sauce

Trim the fat off the pork steaks, then cut them into thin slices. Prepare and measure all the remaining ingredients and gather them all together around the stove.

Put a roomy wok on to heat through. Once it starts to smoke, add the oil. Swirl once, then add the garlic and ginger. Stir-fry for a few seconds, then add the pork and carry on stir-frying for about 2 minutes until the pork is almost cooked through. Next add the mangetouts and almonds and carry on stir-frying for another 2 minutes. Stir in the yellow bean sauce, sesame oil and soy sauce. Give it all another minute or so until everything is mixed together and steamingly hot and fragrant. Taste and adjust seasoning and add more soy or yellow bean sauce if needed. Serve immediately with rice.

Peas and pea shoots

* * *

Peas, carrots and sweetcorn – the three vegetables that even the most recalcitrant children will eat. Our top national vegetable trio, excluding the potato which exists in a popular-vegetable nirvana all of its own. I've learnt over the years that if I am to have any chance of getting my children's friends to eat vegetables when they stay for lunch or supper, it has to be one of the above. Colour, I am sure, plays an important part in this. Neither carrots nor sweetcorn are green, which instantly earns them mega-likeability points with any child. Peas, however, are green, so their appeal must lie with their small stature and their taste. The one common denominator for this trio is an inherent sweetness. Sweetcorn takes the sugar trophy, but peas come a determined second. That, I imagine, is their trump card.

Later on, as tastebuds mature, sweetness is no longer the be-all and end-all quality of a vegetable for most of us, but peas still remain a constant favourite. They do have a remarkable, unique taste which doesn't resemble other legumes, is more complex and interesting than the sugariness of sweetcorn, less earthy than the sweetness of carrots. They also freeze well. I'm not suggesting that frozen peas are as good as the best fresh peas. They are different, but similar, that's all. They can't compare with the divine burst of pea sweetness unleashed on the tongue as you eat a just-picked just-podded raw pea. That's a rare and amazing pleasure. However, as frozen vegetables go, peas are pretty damn fine.

Practicalities

Buying fresh peas ought to be a joy. It's all too often a disappointment. Nearly all the commercially grown peas are picked at their peak of perfection then scooted straight off to the processing plant to be frozen within hours. The tiny remainder are what end up in the shops, several days later. They may be too large and they will certainly have lost the immediate burst of brilliant gorgeousness of a freshly picked pea.

So what does the person who wants to embrace the short pea season do? There are two options. The first is to grow your own peas, and that will guarantee that you get the very best, young, fresh juicy peas as they should be. The second is to make a beeline for farmers' markets or the local pick-your-own when peas are in season, and keep your fingers crossed. It's true that some supermarkets sell trays of fresh podded peas at other times of the year and these are pretty tasty. They are also expensive, which is not surprising given the work involved and the distance they will probably have travelled. On the whole, I'd rather enjoy more local peas when the time is right, and stick with frozen when the season is over. Bear in mind when buying peas in their pods that you will end up with about half their weight once shelled, although if the pods are tender, you could make a soup with them, or at least add them to a vegetable stock.

So, only buy peas in the pod when you can be fairly certain that they are young and picked locally. Disregard pods that look old, dry, papery. To shell fresh peas, simply crack open the pod, then run your finger down the inside to release the peas into a bowl. Try not to eat all of them at once.

Really fresh new peas are lovely raw – toss them straight into salads just as they are. If you want them hot, then cook them just long enough to heat through. A minute or so in **boiling** salted water with a couple of sprigs of mint is quite enough. Ignore old-fashioned recipe books that instruct you to cook them for 10 minutes – what a crime! They just don't need it. Drain well, add a few knobs of butter and voilà – one of early summer's finest offerings. When the last of the season's asparagus overlap with the first of the peas, add blanched asparagus cut into short lengths to make it even more delicious. You could even cook asparagus and peas together in a little home-made stock, together with mint, and then serve in soup plates, with the stock, a poached egg and a scoop of soft cheese perched on top – a marvellous celebration of the purest of foods.

We know that peas make a welcome side dish, we can doll them up with the addition of flavoured butters, with a touch of chilli, with pesto and so on, though to be honest there is little to beat mint and butter. Why is it, then, that we don't include them more often in more complex dishes? It must be no more than over-familiarity. Peas, fresh or frozen, are so easy to incorporate in all manner of foods, from pasta to stews or even soufflés.

Peas and pasta are great together. I often add a handful or more of frozen or fresh peas to a tomato sauce as it nears the end of its cooking time, only minutes before tossing with spaghetti or whatever shapes are in the offing. Grill bacon or pancetta or prosciutto crudo until crisp, then crumble over the pasta, too, and it's even nicer. When it comes to lighter sauces, the oil or butter ones that barely need cooking, I throw the peas into the water with the pasta for the last couple of minutes before draining. For a rich and simple sauce, simmer cream until reduced by a third, cook the peas with the pasta, drain, then combine with the cream, flaked tinned tuna, finely grated lemon zest, and lots of freshly grated Parmesan.

I've always loved peas and eggs together, in an omelette (blanch peas first, then sprinkle over the egg mixture as it cooks in the pan, together with crumbled goat's cheese, and a little chopped fresh mint), or stirred into buttery scrambled eggs with shreds of good smoked salmon, spooned on to toasted English muffins for an uplifting breakfast. An Italian-style frittata is also a good host for lightly blanched peas, their sweetness mitigated by a generous helping of freshly grated pecorino or Parmesan.

Although I wouldn't put peas in a big, dark, beef stew, they have a natural home in the lighter quicker style of casserole, say in a chicken stew with a creamy or tomatoey sauce, or with pork, or perhaps with spring lamb, before it is mature enough to swamp their more delicate taste.

It would be odd if I didn't suggest that peas are good for making soups and purées. They are, but be careful that their flavour doesn't become too insistent. A helping of fresh peas in a minestrone is ideal, but when making a pea soup, it is wise, I think, to add a softening element, such as rice, and to season it carefully. The same goes for pea purées, which I love, but need to be handled with care. A straight pea purée – literally just peas and cream or butter or a little stock for a lighter turn – is good in small quantities, almost as a sauce rather than a vegetable aside, but not as an alternative to, say, mash. Better, I think, to purée equal quantities of peas and potatoes together if you want to make more of a feature of a pea purée. Remember, though,

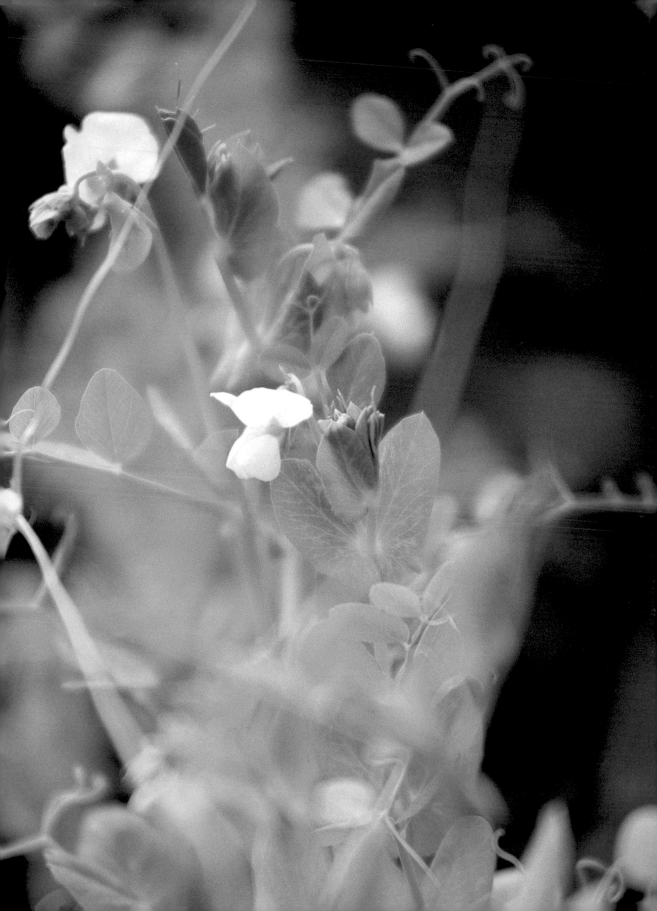

that processor-puréed potatoes turn gluey, so it's better to pass both through a vegetable mill (mouli-légumes) or potato ricer, before beating in warm milk, butter and/or cream, along with lots of freshly grated nutmeg, salt and pepper.

The latest addition to designer salads is the humble **pea shoot, or tendrils**. If you grow your own peas, you will have plenty of these to hand to add to your salads whenever you fancy. If not, then buy a pack at least once to give them a try. Not only do they look charming with their curlicues of green, but they add a bright, fresh sweet note that is very welcome. Balance their sweetness with a few peppery leaves nipped from the nasturtiums and you transform a humble green salad into a tasteful fashion icon. Now there's something you don't see that often.

* *

Crushed peas with mustard

The caterers who keep the opera-goers' stomachs from rumbling during the second half of the performance at Oxfordshire's Garsington Opera served this unexpectedly good side dish a few summers ago. Clever idea, excellent with gammon or steak.

Serves 4

200 g (7 oz) shelled peas
½ teaspoon honey
2 teaspoons coarse-grain mustard
15 g (½ oz) butter
salt

Cook the peas in boiling salted water for a few minutes until tender. Drain well and return swiftly to the pan. Add the remaining ingredients, stir them in and then mash the whole lot roughly with a potato masher. Taste and adjust seasoning, adding a little more salt if needed. Serve swiftly while still hot.

Petits pois à la française

Adding the shredded lettuce and spring onion to the peas as they cook gives them an unrivalled flavour, especially if they are fresh and young. There's no better way to cook peas in the early summer. You shouldn't need to add any more water, as the lettuce will give out a surprising amount, but check once or twice as they cook, just to be on the safe side. Because the peas are semi-steamed, they do, for once, need to be cooked for as much as 15 minutes.

To turn this into 'petits pois à la crème', stir 4 heaped tablespoons of crème fraîche into the peas once the liquid has boiled away, then simmer for a minute or so more, before serving.

Serves 4

30 g (1 oz) butter
500 g (1 lb 2 oz) shelled peas, thawed if frozen
1 round lettuce, shredded
6 spring onions, sliced
4 tablespoons chicken or vegetable stock or
  water
salt and pepper

Melt the butter in a saucepan then add the peas, lettuce and spring onions and salt. Stir so that the peas are all coated with butter, then add the stock. Place over a low heat, clamp the lid on and cook for around 10–15 minutes, stirring once or twice. Take off the lid and, if necessary, boil hard for a couple of minutes until virtually all the liquid has evaporated. Taste and adjust seasoning, and serve.

* *

Spaghetti with prosciutto, peas and shallots

Peas and Parma ham, peas and spaghetti, peas and cream. All good pairings and all together here in one fell swoop. This is a quick and easy and luxurious supper dish, best made with first-class fresh peas, but almost as good with frozen (thaw them out before adding to the pan).

Serves 4

400 g (14 oz) spaghetti
2 large shallots, halved and thinly sliced
  (about 65 g/2 oz prepared weight)
85 g (3 oz) prosciutto crudo (e.g. Parma ham)
  or pancetta, cut into thin strips
30 g (1 oz) butter

250 ml (9 fl oz) double cream
200 g (7 oz) shelled peas, thawed if frozen
a handful of basil leaves, roughly shredded
30 g (1 oz) Parmesan, freshly grated
salt and pepper

Bring a large pan of well-salted water to the boil. Add the spaghetti, stir and boil until al dente. Drain.

Meanwhile, fry the shallots and prosciutto in the butter until tender. Add the cream, peas, salt and pepper. Simmer for 2 minutes or so until lightly thickened. Pull off the heat. Pour over the spaghetti, add the basil and toss together. Serve at once, sprinkled with Parmesan.

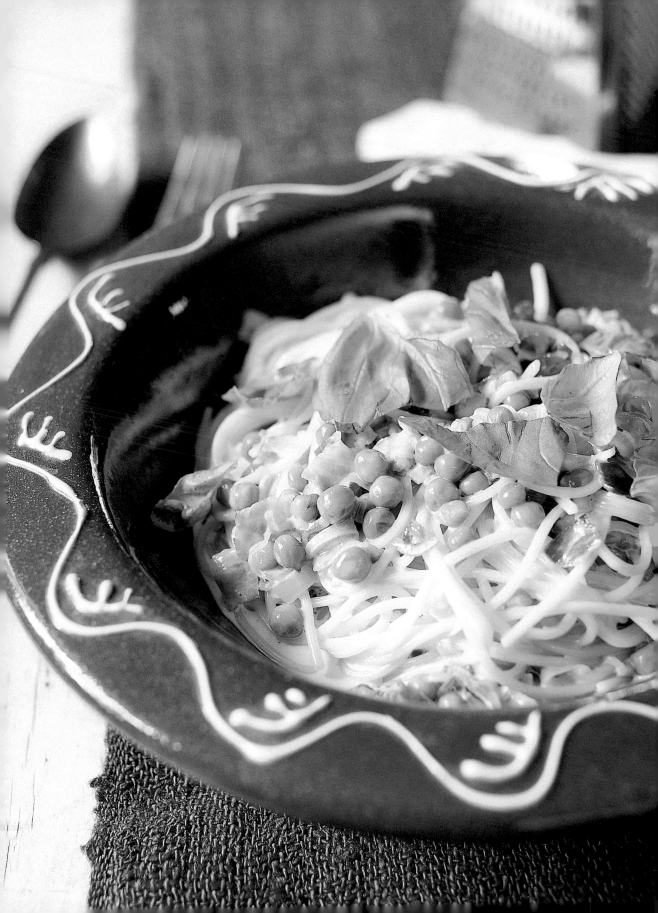

* *

Runner beans

* * *

I'm an appalling snob when it comes to runner beans. I blame it on my parents, at the same time worrying about what my children will eventually blame on me. It's too optimistic to believe that it will be nothing worse than a spot of vegetable snobbery. Actually, I don't know whether my father had any prejudices against runner beans, but my mother certainly did. She exhibited few positive leads for me to follow in this respect. Green beans were undoubtedly superior in her vegetable hierarchy. I feel much the same, and like her I would suggest that this is not entirely unreasonable, any more than it is unreasonable to suggest that asparagus are superior to leeks. What is unreasonable is to look down on leeks or runner beans as a result. Just because they are not the best, does not mean that they are not good.

My mother also loathed the habit of cutting runner beans into fine strips. This, I think, is unreasonable, but unfortunately I've inherited her stance. I can see no logical reason why one shouldn't shred runner beans if one feels like it, but I blench at the thought of eating them. How ridiculous is that? Like all vegetables, runner beans are at their best when ultra-fresh and when picked at a moderate stage in their development. Left to spread to monster proportion, they become chewier, with a tough flat inner lamina and a rough-tough outer surface. Flower-show prize-winning runner beans can be epic in stature, but they fall flat at the cook's first hurdle. Now there's a thought. Could that be why my mother dismissed shredded runner beans so categorically? Could it be that the shredding was intended to disguise the shortcomings of outsize runner beans? Was that the problem, being forced to consume shredded monster beans as a child? Even if you outwit nature by shredding away the toughness, you can't hide the overgrown coarseness of taste so readily. Well, I never. It's my grandparents I should be blaming for my runner bean snobbery, not my mother at all.

Practicalities

BUYING High summer vegetables that they are, there is no point buying runner beans out of season. If they are not brilliantly fresh, newly picked and of a moderate size they are not worth eating. Out-of-season imports will never be fresh enough, so unless you have a total obsessional passion for runner beans, just ignore them. The price should be enough to put you off, anyway. Wait until summer, wait until every gardener in Britain (or so it seems) has a glut of runners, then make your move. If you grow your own, you will know all this, but please, don't foist the whoppers that you don't want on unsuspecting friends. Have the kindness to pick pods young and tender, both for your family and your friends' sake.

In the right place at the right time, non-gardeners will be able to lay their hands on a bag of runners for a song. If no-one gives them to you, head straight for farmers' markets to get the best price for the freshest runners. A really fresh runner bean will be firm of form, with a pleasingly uneven surface, not yet so old that it has become distressingly rough and bumpy.

Store your beans in the vegetable drawer of the fridge and eat them up as soon as possible. Once they start to show signs of flabbiness they are no longer worth toying with. You've left it too late.

COOKING To prepare them for cooking, top and tail them as required – in other words cut or snip or break off the stalk end and the opposite end if you think it necessary (if it looks damaged or browned). Then cut the beans up into manageable lengths. If you like them shredded, go for it – you can buy runner-bean shredders to speed up the task.

The standard way to cook runner beans is to **boil** or **steam** them – 5 minutes' simmering should be quite enough to soften them without overcooking them to a slimy state. Shredded runners need only a couple of minutes. If you steam them, allow a minute or so longer.

I love **stir-fried** runner beans, too. Cut them on the diagonal into diamonds a centimetre or two wide, heat a wok until it smokes, add a slug of oil, some chopped garlic and sliced shallots, toss and stir-fry for a few seconds then add the beans and carry on stir-frying for a further 2–3 minutes. If they were young beans, this will be enough, but with more mature beans you may need to add a few spoonfuls of water, clamp a lid on and leave to simmer for another 1–2 minutes to finish cooking. Before serving, season them with a teaspoon or two of sesame oil, or Chinese black bean or plum sauce.

Runner beans have a natural affinity with tomatoes. This could mean something as simple as tossing freshly cooked beans in hot olive oil together with diced deseeded tomatoes and chopped coriander or mint, or perhaps braising them gently in a tomato sauce until tender. This latter method is a big favourite in Turkey, where the tomatoey beans will be served at room temperature as part of a meze.

When runner beans are at their most prolific, dress them up by tossing them with toasted flaked almonds and a little butter, or giving them a last-minute sizzle in olive oil with chopped garlic and rings of fresh red chilli, then serve with crumbled goat's cheese scattered over the top, or stir-fry with red or yellow peppers, throwing in a few chopped black olives to heat through just before serving.

Runner bean chutneys can be good, though their purpose is mainly to use up gardeners' inevitable gluts. If you do boil up a batch, slice or shred the pieces of runner beans up fairly small, so that they absorb more of the sweet-sour flavours and be sure to boil it down well to prevent watery dullness.

* *

Loubia bi zeit
Lebanese runner beans braised in tomato sauce

Whenever we visit our local Lebanese restaurants, we make a meal of the myriad little dishes that are offered as appetisers. It was here that we discovered that deep-fried cauliflower is surprisingly good, and we've developed quite a taste for these slow-stewed beans in a dill-scented tomato sauce. They're usually served at room temperature but are just as good hot.

Serves 6

500 g (1 lb 2 oz) runner beans, topped, tailed
  and strung
1 large onion, halved and sliced
5 cloves garlic, smashed and halved
4 tablespoons extra virgin olive oil

1 tablespoon tomato purée
3 tablespoons chopped dill
3 medium tomatoes, skinned, deseeded
  and roughly chopped
salt and pepper

Cut each bean into 5 cm (2 in) lengths. Soften the onion and the garlic in the
oil over a gentle heat until very tender, without browning too much – allow
a good 10–15 minutes to develop their full sweetness. Now add the beans
and fry for a further 3–4 minutes. Next stir in the tomato purée, dill, enough
water to just cover, salt and pepper. Bring up to a simmer and simmer gently
for another 15–20 minutes, until the beans are very tender and bathed in
a sauce. Stir in the tomatoes, and cook for a final 2 minutes, then taste
and adjust seasoning. Serve warm or at room temperature.

* *

Cousinat

'Cousinat' is a confusing blighter of a name. In one area of France it means
a chestnut soup but in the area around Bayonne in south-west France, it is
a vegetable stew. That's the version here. You can use all kinds of vegetables,
though ones that survive long cooking are best. It should, naturally, be made
with Bayonne ham, but since that is hard to find, substitute either pancetta
lardons, or jamón de Serrano or some other raw cured ham.

Serves 6–8

3 globe artichokes
1/2 lemon
175 g (6 oz) raw cured ham, diced
30 g (1 oz) lard, or 2 tablespoons extra virgin
  olive oil
cloves from 1 head garlic, separated and
  peeled
500 g (1 lb 2 oz) carrots, thickly sliced
250 g (9 oz) runner beans, topped and tailed,
  cut into 2.5 cm (1 in) lengths

300 g (11 oz) shallots, peeled but left whole
2 fennel bulbs, trimmed and quartered
400 ml (14 fl oz) vegetable or chicken stock
150 ml (5 fl oz) dry white wine
400 g (14 oz) ripe tomatoes, skinned,
  deseeded and roughly chopped
1 tablespoon tomato purée
chopped parsley
salt and pepper

First prepare the artichokes, rubbing cut surfaces with the halved lemon as you go along, to delay browning: snap the stems from the base and discard. Break off the outer layer of leaves, trim the base, then slice off the top of each artichoke about 1cm (½in) from the base itself. Quarter, then use a teaspoon to remove the choke from the centre of the artichoke. Drop into a bowl of water acidulated with the rest of the lemon juice.

Fry the ham in the oil or lard in a heavy casserole until lightly browned. Add all the vegetables except the tomatoes, and plenty of pepper (the ham can be quite salty, so don't add salt until the very end of the cooking time and then only if it needs it). Pour over the stock and wine and bring up to the boil. Cover and simmer gently for 30 minutes. Remove the lid, stir in the tomatoes and tomato purée, and simmer for a further 30 minutes or so, until the sauce has reduced and thickened and the vegetables are very, very tender. Taste and adjust seasoning. Serve hot or reheat gently when needed, sprinkled with parsley.

* *

Shelling beans
(borlotti, flageolet and cannellini)

* * *

You don't see fresh shelling beans for sale often enough. Not that you would expect to find them throughout most of the year. These are strictly summer legumes with a comparatively brief season around July and August. Even more specifically, I would limit them to summer holidays and summer weekends, when you have time to shell them at leisure, enjoying the repetitive, soothing process, ideally sitting out in the garden in the sunshine.

I've found them now and again in farmers' markets and farm shops at home, but I have to wait until our summer trip to France to get a reliable source. Here I've come across borlotti and cannellini beans. Over the Channel we have a choice of **borlotti**, yellow-podded '**michelet**' and if we are lucky, **flageolets**.

Like the beans themselves, the pods of borlotti beans are streaked with scarlet or purple against a creamy background. As they cook they become almost brown skinned and have a meaty taste to them. American **cranberry beans** are virtually the same as borlotti. **Cannellini** and michelets are straightforward white beans, with a lighter tone, whilst flageolets are the most refined and delectable of the group. The taste of these fresh beans is, as you might expect, brighter and fresher than that of their dried form, with a creamy texture that makes them enormously appealing. Whenever you see them for sale, hand your money over with alacrity.

Practicalities

BUYING Although freshness is always a good thing, with fresh beans, it is not as critical. We all know that they dry easily and cleanly to produce the long-life dried beans that have sustained families well into winter in the past. So don't dismiss fresh borlotti with pods that are beginning to develop a touch of papery dryness here and there. They may even have been picked like this, as these beans will begin to dry out on the plant. Ideally, however, the pod will be almost leathery and supple, and you will be able to feel the fully formed beans within it.

Don't be put off by the odd dry blemish, either. It's damp, mouldering pods that should put you on your guard – it's disappointing and more than a little infuriating to spend half an hour shelling beans only to have to throw half of them out.

Although their very nature tells you that they can be kept for some weeks, in a cool airy place, out of their plastic bag, where they will just gently lose moisture and dry, there seems little point in this. Cook them soon to get the maximum benefit from their short-lived freshness. To prepare, all you need do is squeeze the pods between your fingers to crack open, then remove the beans, discarding any that are under-formed or show signs of deterioration.

COOKING In **boiling** water, unsalted, beans in their first freshness should take around 20–30 minutes to cook, but this varies according to age and size, so check regularly. The best way to check that they are adequately cooked is to taste a bean – it should be soft and creamy, though not yet disintegrating to a mush. As soon as they are done, drain them and either serve swiftly, tossed with melted butter and salt or a shake of best extra virgin olive oil, and lots of chopped parsley, or run them under the cool tap to halt cooking and leave to drain and cool.

Fresh beans like having a fuss made over them and being starchy they can take a lot of it. So toss hot cooked beans, or reheat cold ones in a mixture of garlic lightly coloured in olive oil, together with plenty of chopped tinned anchovies for their piquancy, for instance, adding diced ripe red deseeded tomato for good measure. Or frizzle garlic and chilli in oil, then toss into the beans together with lots of chopped spring onion and coriander. Or mix them with sautéed cubes of red pepper and courgette, together with lots of fresh marjoram. For a direct substitute for mash, crush beans roughly and reheat with butter and cream and plenty of seasoning. Very nice with barbecued sausages or lamb chops on a cooler summer's evening.

If you have time for the shelling, or a few extra hands around the house to help out, it's worth cooking large amounts of fresh borlotti or cannellini so that you can enjoy some hot straight from the pan, and save the rest for a salad next day, or a creamy, garlicky purée like the brandade below, or to add to a minestrone-style soup.

PARTNERS Like fully dried pulses, fresh beans make lovely salads. You need do little more than turn them in a sharpish vinaigrette (wine vinegar, olive oil, mustard, salt and pepper), preferably while still warm, then leave to cool. Add finely chopped shallot and chopped parsley and it's ready to put on the table. Everyone loves that old Italian salad of beans, onion or shallot, tinned tuna and maybe some diced deseeded tomato, or halved cherry tomatoes. There's no reason not to get more playful with bean salads, adding other vegetables, cooked or raw as appropriate: fried courgettes, blanched green beans, roasted tomatoes, confit tomatoes, raw tomatoes, crisp lettuces, rocket, bitter lettuces, especially curly endive, grilled peppers, grilled or roasted red onion wedges, marinated onion rings, roasted or fried carrots, raw coarsely grated carrots, chopped spring onions and no doubt many more. Garlic, chilli, parsley, thyme, rosemary, marjoram, tarragon, chervil, lovage, summer savory, and other warm-scented herbs suit beans too.

For a summer version of baked beans, not from the tin, simmer up a pan of tomato sauce, cook the beans separately, then mix the two together and reheat thoroughly together. Flavour the sauce with sage, lots of it, and you more or less have the delicious Tuscan 'fagioli al'uccelletto', another of the finest bean dishes around.

* *

Cannellini and coriander brandade

The classic brandade is a rich and creamy purée of salt cod, much enjoyed in the south of France. This purée is made in the same way, but takes soft fresh cannellini beans as its base. Serve it with hot toast as a first course or snack, or try it alongside grilled lamb chops.

When you can't get fresh beans, use dried cannellini or haricot beans – soak 200 g (7 oz) beans overnight, then cook until tender in plenty of unsalted water.

Serves 6–8

300 g (11 oz) podded fresh cannellini beans
2 cloves garlic, chopped
3–4 tablespoons coriander leaves, chopped
100 ml (3 1/2 fl oz) extra virgin olive oil
100 ml (3 1/2 fl oz) single cream

juice of 1/2 lemon
salt

To serve
hot, crisply griddled slices of bread

Bring a large pan of water to the boil and add the beans (no salt yet). Simmer until tender – about 20–30 minutes, depending on freshness. Drain well, reserving a little of the water. Transfer the beans to the processor with the garlic, coriander, some salt and 2 tablespoons cooking water.

Heat both the olive oil and the cream until hot in separate saucepans. Process the beans and seasonings to a rough purée, then with the blades still whizzing round, trickle in first a slurp of olive oil, then a slurp of cream, continuing until both are entirely incorporated. Now add the lemon juice. Taste and adjust seasoning. Serve warm or at room temperature, with a trickle of fresh olive oil drizzled over it, and with a pile of hot griddled bread.

* *

Flageolets in rich tomato sauce

A second rich and luscious bean dish, but totally different in nature to the brandade. Though it goes very nicely with all kinds of main course, it's particularly good with lamb.

Serves 4

200 g (7 oz) podded fresh flageolet beans
4 cloves garlic, unpeeled
1 bouquet garni (1 bay leaf, 2 sprigs parsley,
 1 sprig rosemary, tied together with string)
½ onion

Tomato sauce
½ onion, chopped
15 g (½ oz) butter
1 x 400 g can chopped tomatoes, or 450 g
 fresh tomatoes, skinned, deseeded and
 chopped
1 tablespoon tomato purée
1 large sprig rosemary
½ teaspoon caster sugar
150 ml (5 fl oz) double cream
salt and pepper

Put the flageolets, unpeeled cloves of garlic, bouquet garni and onion in a pan and add enough water to cover generously. Bring up to the boil and cook for 20–30 minutes until the flageolets are tender. Drain and pick out the bouquet garni, cloves of garlic and onion. Save the garlic but throw out the bouquet garni and the onion – they've done their job now.

To make the sauce, cook the onion gently in the butter until tender, then add the chopped tomatoes, the tomato purée, rosemary, sugar, salt and pepper. Bring up to the boil and simmer for about 10 minutes. Throw out the rosemary. Squeeze the garlic from the flageolets out of the skins and into the sauce. Liquidise and rub through a sieve, or pass through a vegetable mill (mouli-légumes).

Return the sauce to the pan together with the cream and the flageolets. Simmer gently for a few minutes to heat through. Taste and adjust seasoning and serve.

Sweetcorn

Frozen sweetcorn is fine, canned sweetcorn is mushy, but eclipsing them both are the fresh cobs of corn that pile into farmers' markets and farm shops towards the end of the summer. I always long to buy bags full of them, but I limit my purchases to what we will eat within the next 24 hours while they are at their sugary best.

It's well known that the sugars in sweetcorn start turning to starch as soon as the cobs are snapped from the plant, although modern supersweet varieties are not half as prone to this as the more traditional varieties. The 'sh2' varieties are supposed to hold their full load of sweetness for up to a week, but even if that's true, you have to wonder what happens to the actual flavour of the kernels. Call me suspicious, but...won't it just disappear leaving a heavy yellow sugar rush and little else? 'Sh', by the way, stands for 'shrunken gene', which I find an unfortunate bit of jargon as it conjures up images of the grotesque shrunken heads in the Pitt Rivers Museum in Oxford. And that starts me thinking in Frankensteinian-style, imagining the evil science lab empire of the sweetcorn development moguls, torturing innocent ears of sweetcorn into sweet soulless submission. Surely not...

You might have noticed that supermarkets haven't gotten a look in so far. It's not that I never buy sweetcorn from the big boys, but until they date-stamp their sweetcorn and rush it from stem to store like the first Beaujolais nouveau, there's no telling what it will be like on the plate. For the best you have to bide your time, waiting for the season to begin, go a mite out of your way, and then make the most of it while the going is good. If you want to buy imported sweetcorn at other times of the year, fair enough, but it becomes more of an everyday sort of a vegetable, nothing to write home about and to be frank, you might just as well go with the convenience of frozen corn kernels, as faff around with out-of-season corn on the cob.

Practicalities

BUYING Perfect **fresh corn on the cob** is easy to spot. It should look well-padded, the cob completely enclosed in a pale green, pliable husk, with a few fine, silky threads peaking out at the end. An intelligent seller will have one semi-peeled cob on display so you can see the kernels inside. They will be a pretty primrose yellow, snuggled up tight together, neatly swollen and full. As they march towards the tip, the kernels will get smaller and smaller, showing that this is a youthful tender cob.

The higher the temperature, the quicker the sugars in the kernels turn to starch, so don't buy beautiful fresh sweetcorn then leave it sweltering in the car while you finish the rest of the shopping and have a coffee. If the sun is shining take a cool bag out with you, complete with a few frozen ice packs in order to keep your sweetcorn cool and sweet. As soon as you get home, transfer it to the fridge until you are ready to cook it, hopefully that day or the next.

To prepare, pull off the husk and those soft silky tresses, and trim off the stem. Pause before you throw out the husks – in Mexico they are used to wrap 'tamales', packages of delicious corn-based dough, that are cooked over the embers. One of these days, look up a recipe or two in a Mexican or American cookbook or on the internet and give it a go. It's a great idea for a barbecue, though rather time-consuming to prepare.

COOKING Once dehusked, a properly fresh cob of corn needs only minutes in a pan of **boiling** salted water before it is ready to eat. I give mine a mere 3–4 minutes after the water comes back to the boil. Those raw kernels are so sweet and juicy that they barely need more than heating through. Drain well and then serve with plenty of butter (I prefer salted to soften the sugariness) to slather on the hot cobs and dribble down your chin and fingers as you bite off the golden kernels.

When I want to make more of a fuss of corn on the cob, I'll whiz the butter with some piquant flavourings before serving. I love black olive butter (use a good-quality black olive purée, or stone good olives yourself, but don't make it with those horrid soapy ready-stoned canned olives) with them, or an anchovy butter (canned anchovy fillets, squeeze of lemon juice, parsley), or coriander and lime and chilli butter.

Those flavoured butters are good with **barbecued** or **grilled** corn too.

There are two ways to tackle barbecued corn. The first is to soak the whole cobs, still in their husks, in a bucket of cold water for at least an hour, before laying them on the barbecue or under the grill. Not only does the damp husk protect the kernels from the full fierce heat, but it creates its own mini-sauna inside to steam-heat the kernels. Turn the cobs every 3 or 4 minutes, until the outer layer of the husk is charred, then serve while hot. The second method is to strip off the husks and silks as normal, then brush the cobs with protective oil before laying them over the coals or under the grill. The advantage with this method is that you get direct, smoky heat on the surface of the cob. However, the kernels will brown here and there, becoming chewier than usual. I like this quite a lot, but it's not to everyone's taste – if there's a party going on, then it's probably best to cook them both ways so everyone stays happy.

When sweetcorn is plentiful, try adding chunks of corn on the cob to chicken or beef **stews** as they do in many South American countries. Quartering the cobs demands a spot of brute force and a sharp sturdy knife, but the whole pieces will impart their softening, subtle fresh flavour to the stew in a way that no other vegetable can. Add them about 8 minutes before serving the stew, so they just have time to make their light mark, but not long enough to overcook.

Most of the time, however, most of us cook sweetcorn kernels off the cob. They are the nation's second favourite vegetable, apparently, tottering in behind carrots. To get them at their finest, you will slice them straight from a fresh cob of corn: cut a thin slice off the stalk end so that it can be stood firmly upright, then use a sharp small knife to slice downwards from the point, taking off the kernels in narrow sheets. Possibly the nicest way to cook these newly released kernels is to pile them into a saucepan, then scrape the cobs over it to release the last of the corn juice into the pan, and add a little cream, salt and pepper. Stir this over a gentle heat, letting the cream bubble gently, for 3 minutes or so before serving. Wow, that's good.

The other option is to drop them into a pan of boiling salted water and **blanch** for 2–3 minutes until hot and barely cooked through, before draining and adding a knob of butter. In other words, just the same way as you would cook **frozen sweetcorn**, one of the lifelines of the busy parent with clamouring hungry children at their heels. If I'm serving plain sweetcorn, then I cook frozen according to packet instructions. For most other recipes I let it thaw out before using.

Sweetcorn kernels, fresh or frozen, have a kaleidoscopic range of culinary possibility. I suspect it is probably non-u to add sweetcorn to pasta sauces, or to home-made pizza toppings, but I do both. More acceptable foodie ways of using sweetcorn might include adding it to thick chowders or Chinese chicken soup, or for making crisp sweetcorn fritters, either by stirring lightly cooked kernels into a light beer batter, or by whizzing the kernels with egg, flour and a little milk together in the processor to form a batter. I vary them by adding chopped herbs, small cubes of cheese, roughly chopped prawns and so on. They are just gorgeous topped with a dollop of crème fraîche or soured cream and a small spoonful of herring roe caviar or even better, the real thing. Or with smoked salmon or smoked eel.

* *

Sweetcorn and saffron mash

This is the most glowing mashed potato you'll ever come across with its streaks of orange gold from the saffron and the nuggets of sweetcorn in it.

Serves 6

1.2 kg (2 lb 11 oz) large baking potatoes
200–250 ml (7–9 fl oz) milk
1 or 2 generous pinches saffron threads
45 g (1½ oz) butter

180 g (6½ oz) lightly cooked sweetcorn
  kernels
salt

Bake the potatoes in their jackets in a hot oven (around 200°C/400°F/Gas 6) until cooked through – about 1–1½ hours. Meanwhile, bring 200 ml (7 fl oz) milk up to the boil, draw off the heat and stir in the saffron. Set aside.

When the potatoes are done, cut in half and scoop their flesh out into a saucepan. Mash with the butter and plenty of salt, and set over a gentle heat. Beat the saffron milk in a good slurp at a time. Stop and assess the texture. If you prefer it softer and runnier, add more milk. Stir in the sweetcorn, taste and adjust seasoning, and then serve.

Sweetcorn soup with red chilli and garlic cream

It starts off as a soothing soup, then gets a kick up the derrière with a shot of chilli and garlic. This is a terrific way of using fresh corn when it is plentiful.

Serves 4

4 cobs fresh sweetcorn
2 sprigs parsley
1 bay leaf
2 sprigs thyme
30 g (1 oz) butter
1 large onion, chopped
1 medium potato, peeled and diced small
1 leek, sliced

150 ml (5 fl oz) milk, or milk and cream
salt and pepper

Red chilli and garlic cream
1 fresh red chilli, deseeded and roughly
  chopped
1 clove garlic, roughly chopped
1 tablespoon lime or lemon juice
100 ml (3 ½ fl oz) double or whipping cream

Slice the kernels from the cobs and set aside. Put the cobs into a saucepan with the herbs and enough water to cover generously. Bring up to the boil and simmer for 20 minutes. Strain off the stock and bin the cobs and herbs. Measure out the stock, adding more water if necessary to give 600 ml (1 pint).

Melt the butter in a saucepan and add the onion, potato and leek. Cover and sweat over a very low heat for 10 minutes. Now add the measured stock, salt and pepper and half the corn kernels. Bring up to a boil, reduce the heat and simmer for some 15 minutes or so, until the vegetables are all tender. Liquidise with enough of the milk to give the consistency of runny double cream. Taste and adjust seasoning.

To make the cream, put the chilli, garlic and a good pinch of salt into a mortar and work to a purée, then stir in the lime or lemon juice. Mix in the cream, then transfer to a large bowl and whisk until it just holds its shape. Set aside until needed, and stir once more just before using.

Just before serving bring the soup up to the boil and add the remaining corn. Simmer gently for 2 minutes, then taste and adjust seasoning. Ladle into warm bowls and float a spoonful of chilli cream in each one.

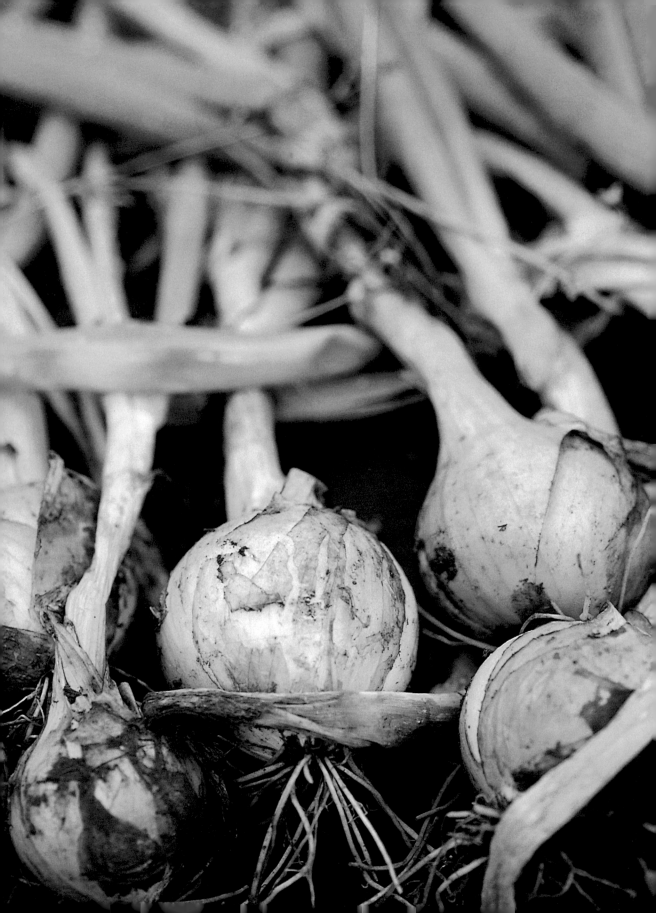

Onion family

* *

Garlic Garlic scapes
Leeks Onions **Shallots**
Spring onions Wild garlic

* *

Garlic

* * *

You could argue that garlic is not truly a vegetable. A seasoning, a base note, a herb, an essential, maybe, but a vegetable? That implies a certain substance, that as a foodstuff it can stand alone and make a solid contribution to a meal. And it can. The joy of garlic is that it plays both ways, given the chance. In modern times we take garlic for granted even in northerly countries where once it seemed a fearsome foreign intrusion. It's there, it goes into a thousand and one dishes along with the onion. Chopped up small and imperceptible, it disappears into the whole and no-one gives it a second thought.

The only way for garlic to get noticed is to resist the knife. Whole cloves of garlic on the plate are hard to ignore. To the uninitiated they are scary, to those in the know they promise moments of subtle gastronomic delight. Yes, I do mean subtle. Cooked whole, garlic is mild and enticing, with none of the fiery pungency of sliced or chopped raw garlic. The reason for this is no mystery. That extraordinary wham of garlicky power is not actually enclosed within the whole garlic clove. It doesn't exist at all until the knife blade slices into the clove, breaking and bruising the cell walls. In an infinitesimally short split second, enzymes within the garlic set in motion a chain reaction, resulting in the release of the rich, lingering, trenchant scent of newly cut garlic.

So, a whole clove of garlic, cell walls unbreached except for perhaps the tiniest scratch at the base, are the vestal virgins of the garlic scene, mild and pure and untainted. That is why no-one need be scared when confronted by a mêlée of whole cooked garlic cloves on their plate. Rejoice and consume.

Practicalities

BUYING Most of the year there is only one form of garlic to be had – the familiar firm bulbs encased in papery skin. You may be able to choose amongst varieties – **purple** or **pink** or **elephant garlic** – but the essential qualities remain the same: firmness and an absence of smell. When buying garlic to use as a vegetable I hardly need point out that it pays to pick bulbs formed of large cloves – the swell of the skin is your guide here. If it undulates too much the cloves are probably small, but if the curves are full and wide the prognosis is good. Elephant garlic has particularly large cloves.

Garlic does not keep well in the kitchen where the warm moist air soon attacks it. For the kitchen, buy an earthenware garlic pot to hold the head of garlic currently in use, and keep other heads somewhere cool and airy and dry. Do not keep garlic in the fridge where it will taint other foods.

During the early summer, for a brief period, **fresh or wet garlic** makes an appearance in shops and markets. It's one of the new crop of vegetables I look forward to, though not with quite the anticipation of, say, asparagus or new potatoes. Wet garlic invites us to treat it as a vegetable proper, cooking it whole, the tender skin so soft in the centre that it can be eaten, or at least sucked clean with supple ease. Despite this, I'm always a little disappointed by it. The taste is not extraordinarily different to that of the semi-dried garlic we have all year round. A little juicier perhaps, but not so much more than that. The biggest difference is that it takes longer to cook, particularly when baked. Wet garlic should be used swiftly, within a couple of days, and should never ever be stored in the fridge. A cool, dry airy place is what it needs, but of course, here it will begin to dry out.

My friend, Sam, who cooked the food for the photographs in this book, tells me that when she needs dozens of cloves of garlic, but can't face peeling them, she trots into her nearest Indian food store where she buys bags of ready-peeled garlic cloves for a snip. Worth remembering if you want to make garlic pickles, though I can't help feeling that they won't taste quite as good as when you peel them all yourself.

COOKING Treating garlic as a vegetable effectively means either poaching it or roasting it. **Poaching** (or braising or simmering – they all boil down to the same thing here, if you'll excuse the pun) demands fully peeled cloves of garlic (usually). This is tedious, but there's nothing to be done about that. If you want to inject a little fun into the proceedings, try separating the cloves as follows: snip off any remaining tough stalk, set the head of garlic root-end down on the work surface, cover with a tea-towel folded in four, then hit it with your fist. Voilà! Cloves all tumbling apart.

For **purées**, poach the peeled cloves for 2 minutes in boiling water then drain (this draws out any bitterness, softening the flavour). Then cook in fresh water or milk until tender. The cloves can then be puréed, perhaps with a little of their milk, or with a knob of butter or a slurp of cream. Seasoned with salt, the purée can be used just as it is (try it with grilled lamb chops), or combined with mashed potato, or swirled into soups, added to sauces and so on. It's pretty mild and won't offend anyone.

Braised whole peeled cloves of garlic are good in casseroles and pot roasts of all kinds. The most obvious is the classic French chicken with 40 cloves of garlic (opposite), but there's no reason why you shouldn't throw a handful of garlic cloves into practically any sauce-heavy dish that is to be cooked for at least 40 minutes or so, allowing plenty of time for the garlic to soften. Don't worry about blanching the cloves in advance – the other ingredients will cover any mild bitterness. To make a soothing garlic and potato soup, sweat plenty of whole cloves of garlic with cubed potato, chopped onions and a bouquet garni in butter or oil, then add stock and simmer until tender, before liquidising.

Roasting is a harsher method of cooking and those sweet little cloves need protection. Keep them in their skins. Whenever I'm roasting a tray of vegetables, I nearly always add a big handful of unpeeled garlic cloves, so that they too can roast to a seductive, melting tenderness. My children fight over them, so it pays to be generous. Depending on the softness of the garlic when it hits the plate, either pull the skin off, or suck out the molten flesh, or squeeze it on to toast or bread. So very delicious.

Roasted whole heads of garlic make a terrific first course, but only if you are fairly certain that your family and friends can cope with the concept. Arrange the heads, trimmed of excess papery skin, in an ovenproof dish with a few spoonfuls of water, a drizzle of olive oil, twigs of thyme or rosemary or both, cover with foil and bake in a hot oven for half an hour. Remove the foil, baste and carry on cooking for another 20 minutes or
so until softly roasted. Serve a head a piece, spooning some of the fragrant juices over it, together with griddled country bread. I partner them with a cream made of beaten goat's cheese and crème fraîche, flecked with green herbs. To eat, squeeze the garlic out of each clove on to the bread. Messy and convivial. Provide napkins.

You may also consider, when roasting chunks of lamb or even lowly chicken portions surrounded by a mess of vegetables, throwing in a couple of heads of garlic that have had their top knots lopped off to reveal a tight rose of cut cloves. As long as both cut and uncut surfaces are coated with oil, they will turn out well – a little chewier than whole heads, of course, but more handsome to behold.

SEE ALSO GARLIC SCAPES AND WILD GARLIC (PAGES 284 AND 290).

* *

Chicken with 40 cloves of garlic

Please, please, please, try this recipe. It is brilliantly simple and brilliantly good. Don't baulk at the thought of ramming 40 cloves of garlic into a dish for four – cooked gently in the wine and chicken juices, they soften down so beautifully that you may wish you'd added another handful.

You'll need three or four heads of garlic altogether and naturally, it doesn't matter whether you count out the cloves with mathematical precision, or err marginally one way or the other. Still, there is something rather pleasing about that nice round number – just like Ali Baba's 40 thieves, but more appealing.

Serves 4

1 free-range chicken, cut into 4 portions,
    or 4 free-range chicken portions
2 tablespoons extra virgin olive oil
150 ml (5 fl oz) dry white wine

1 bouquet garni (2 sprigs parsley, 4 sprigs
    thyme, 1 bay leaf, tied together with string)
40 garlic cloves
salt and pepper

Preheat the oven to 180°C/350°F/Gas 4.

Heat the oil in a heavy casserole over a medium heat. Brown the chicken pieces in the oil, then take out. Pour off excess fat, then add the wine. Bring up to the boil, scraping in the brown bits stuck to the bottom. Return the chicken pieces to the pan along with the bouquet garni, 100 ml (3½ fl oz) water and all 40 peeled cloves of garlic. Season with salt and pepper.

Cover the casserole and transfer to the preheated oven. Cook for 40–45 minutes, then check to make sure that the chicken is cooked through. Remove the bouquet garni. Taste and adjust the seasoning, and serve straightaway, with a mountain of mashed potato, and a pile of spring greens or spinach or purple sprouting broccoli.

* *

Sweet-sour garlic and oil preserve

Press-gang friends or family into a garlic-peeling bee so that you can make these excellent olive oil and garlic preserves. They'll have to wait a couple of weeks before they can taste the results, but they'll be glad they pitched in when tasting day arrives. Eat them (the pickles, not your family and friends) with farmhouse cheeses and bread, or as part of a mixed antipasto.

Fills 1 x 500 ml (18 fl oz) jar

4 large or 8 small heads garlic
300 ml (10 fl oz) white wine vinegar
300 ml (10 fl oz) water
150 g (5 oz) caster sugar
2 teaspoons cumin seeds

2 teaspoon coriander seeds
2 whole star anise
2 dried red chillies
extra virgin olive oil
sunflower oil

Separate the cloves and peel the whole lot of them.

Put the vinegar, water, sugar and spices into a pan and bring up to the boil, stirring until the sugar has dissolved. Simmer for 5 minutes, then add the garlic cloves and reduce the heat. Simmer for 10–15 minutes until barely tender. Lift the cloves out with a slotted spoon, bringing as many of the spices with them as you can. Leave to drain in a sieve.

Pack into sterilised but cold jars (see page 215). Pour in enough olive oil, or olive oil mixed with sunflower oil, to cover completely. Let them stand for an hour or so to settle, then top up with oil if necessary. Seal tightly, label, then store in a cool dark cupboard for at least 2 weeks before using.

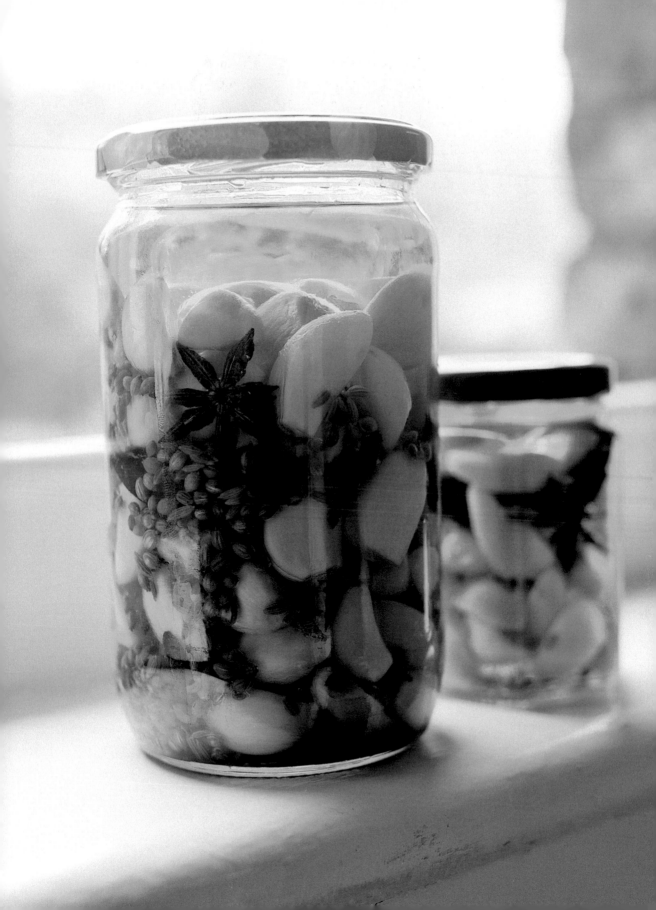

* *

Garlic scapes

* * *

Now here is something brand new and extraordinarily delicious. The appearance of a new vegetable is not a common event and I admit that it may take a few years for garlic scapes to grace vegetable displays the length and breadth of the country, but I'm pretty certain that they'll make it soon.

Garlic scapes are the flowering stems of one particular variety of garlic. The scapes shoot up in teasingly curly and rambunctious form towards the middle and late weeks of spring, at their tender best for only a few short weeks, before the garlic is harvested. Eaten raw, they are pungent and sharply garlicky, excellent finely chopped in, say, a potato salad, or whizzed to a vivid green paste with basil and pine nuts or toasted hazelnuts or walnuts, Parmesan and olive oil to make a spring pesto. To my mind, though, their full glory is brought out only when they are cooked. Just a few minutes in the pan is all it takes to tame the pungency, releasing the inherent flavour that lies somewhere between that of asparagus and fresh green beans, with most pleasing mild undertones of garlic.

Do not imagine, as I did before I actually got my hands on some scapes, that they are just the hollow green shoots that push up out of poorly stored garlic that's been ignored at the back of the vegetable rack. No, garlic scapes are solid through to the core, juicy and firm and cool to the touch. Keep a look out for them and if, when, you are lucky enough to spot some for sale, grab plenty to keep you going for the next fortnight or so.

Practicalities

BUYING Store garlic scapes in the vegetable drawer of the fridge, but wrap them up in several plastic bags to prevent their garlic aroma penetrating milk and butter and eggs. They keep nicely for at least 2 weeks stored in this fashion, but like any vegetable, they are best eaten as soon as possible.

Early season scapes will be shorter, with a gentle curve to them. As the weeks progress, they extend and grow into fantastical pigs' tail curls, stretching out to well over half a metre long (that's around 1½ feet) whilst the diameter is roughly 5 mm (¼ in). Only the lower portion, below the flower bud, is worth eating. Above the slightly paler green bulge of the incipient flower the scape hollows and becomes fibrous, and is better on the compost heap than in the pan.

COOKING Although you can cook them in one great tangled mass – an impressive sight on the plate, to be sure – it is easier in most instances to cut them into shorter lengths. Quite how long is up to you.

Raw scapes are powerfully garlicky so treat them with respect. Sliced thinly they make a good addition to salads and salsas, or can be thrown into the processor along with herbs, nuts, cheese, mayonnaise or oil and lemon juice or wine vinegar to make dressings and sauces.

They take very little time to cook, and the transformation is remarkable. I've **steamed** them and **blanched** them quickly in boiling salted water; 3 or 4 minutes is quite enough time to bring them to perfect tenderness. After that you can serve them just plain as a side dish, perhaps with a little butter, or dressed with lightly toasted sesame seeds and a shake of soy sauce, or give them treatment royal by keeping them long and serving as a first course on their own with a hollandaise sauce, or melted butter sharpened with lemon juice, just as if they were the finest asparagus.

Even more addictive are **fried** scapes. Either shallow-fry them in olive oil in a frying pan over a high heat, or nicer still, stir-fry them with or without other vegetables. A simple stir-fry of chicken and scapes, finished with a light coating of black bean or oyster sauce, would make a brilliantly quick supper dish, served on a mound of steaming rice. If you feel that you need a greater shot of luxury, replace the chicken with fresh scallops – scapes work very well with the sweetness of shellfish.

Fried scapes are gorgeous tossed with pasta, a little chopped chilli and freshly grated Parmesan, or dressed with a little vinaigrette then left to cool and mixed with halved cherry tomatoes to make a cheery salad. When it comes down to it, there are infinite possibilities for this bright, new vegetable. It's just a question of finding it to carry out your own experiments.

SEE ALSO GARLIC AND WILD GARLIC (PAGES 284 AND 323).

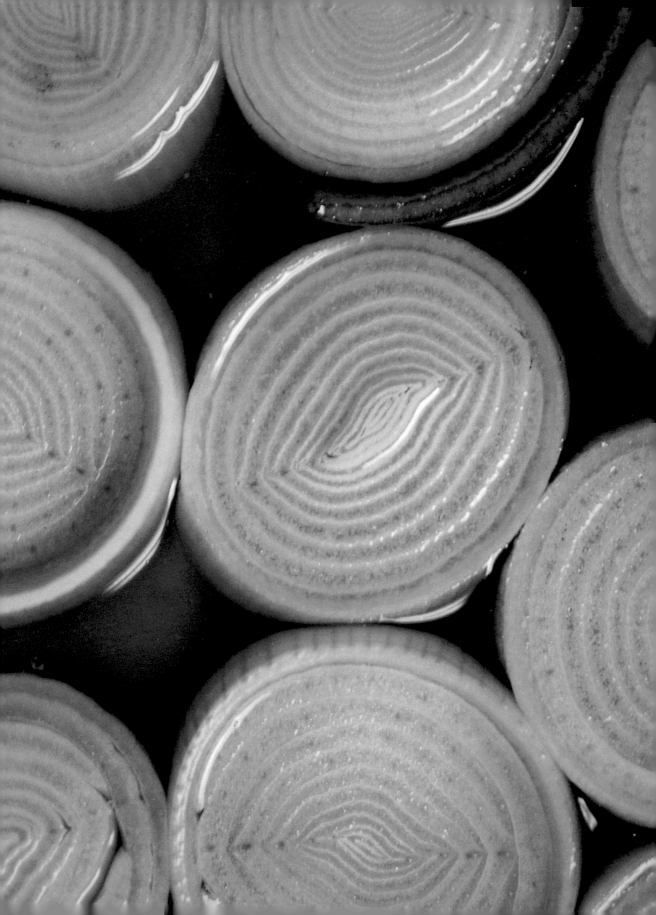

Leeks

'She sits amongst the peas and leeks' or 'She sits amongst the leeks and peas'. Oh, how that used to make me laugh when I was a child. If it hasn't raised so much as a slight smirk, try saying it aloud. And if that doesn't work either, forget it. We're on a different humour wavelength. I'm sorry mine is still so childish. You are obviously far more sophisticated.

A good leek (enough of the mirth, please) is only as good as the way it is cooked. Multitudes of children have been alienated from leeks by being forced to eat them overcooked and subsumed in a pool of gluey white sauce. No fun there. Still, somehow the leek has hung on, despite such maltreatment. One of our basic winter vegetables, though now with us all year round, which is not entirely helpful to its cause. In summer it looks lacklustre beside all the tomatoes and courgettes and peppers, and my inclination is to pretend it just isn't there. Magically, I make it reappear sometime in early autumn. I realise that this is a very old-fashioned attitude, but I'm not about to peddle the oh-for-the-days-of-seasonality line. Leeks just work better for me in autumn and winter food. That's where they belong, that's where they shine.

Practicalities

BUYING Check the extremities first. Are the roots white and fresh? Are the dark green leaves at the other end firm and fleshy? Good. Next cast a glance at the white parts. Splits are not a good omen, and worse still are pink-brown streaks which suggest inner rot has set in. I'm not a stickler for perfection but with leeks it pays to be fussy. Size matters, too. Very thick chunky leeks will be blessed with full flavour (excellent for stock and stews), but tend to be tough and stringy. Too thin, and you'll discard a greater proportion when preparing and spend longer at it, too. Mini-leeks are cute, but are they much more than outsize spring onions? In my experience, they can be just as stringy as larger ones.

It is important, when preparing leeks, to be conscientious. Gritty leeks are not nice to eat. So, trim off the roots, then cut off the dark green portions. Now, using a sharp knife, quarter the upper end towards the stalk for a distance of around 3–4 cm (1½ in). Under a running tap, splay out the cut ends, rinsing off any scraps of earth that are embedded amongst the layers. Dry the leeks and then carry on with any further preparation. With larger leeks the outer layer may be tough and stringy – use it to flavour a stock, or as a neat wrapper for a bouquet garni of fresh herbs: wrap a length of leek around a bundle composed of bay leaf, thyme sprigs and parsley, or whatever herbs you are using, then tie them together with a piece of string. Easy to find and extricate when all their flavour has been extracted.

COOKING The best way to cook sliced leeks is to put them in a saucepan with a knob of butter and just a small splash of water and a little salt. Cover and cook over a low heat for 4–5 minutes, checking once or twice to make sure they are not burning. They should, all being right with the world, end up a tender mass bathed in butter, nothing to drain off. If there is too much liquid, remove the lid, raise the heat and blast it off for a minute or two. If there is too little and they have browned, that's fine. If there is too little and they've burnt, your heat was way too high, so chuck them in the bin and start again.

Sliced leeks were never meant to be boiled in a saucepan of water. **Steaming** is preferable, giving you slightly more leeway before they descend into sliminess – 3–4 minutes will be quite enough. Whole leeks, or even leeks that have been halved lengthways, are robust enough to cope with being dunked into a pan of boiling water, as long as you have removed the tougher outer layers. They will need to be drained extremely well – no-one likes watery leeks. You might serve them hot, with a touch of butter, but in general I think this treatment best reserved for that joyous French dish, leeks vinaigrette, also known as poor man's asparagus. In other words, boiled, perfectly drained leeks, dressed while still warm with a lively vinaigrette (white wine vinegar, Dijon mustard, salt, pepper and olive oil), then served cold, sprinkled with chopped hard-boiled egg, as a first course.

It's hard to think of a vegetable that can't be turned into a good soup, but leeks are more important to the soup cook than any others except onions, carrots and potatoes. It is an all-but-essential component of any home-made stock for a start. Not only are leeks and potatoes the main ingredients of one of the most famous classic chilled soups, Vichyssoise, but they also bring a more rounded flavour to many other vegetable soups. I'll often add a leek to a carrot or tomato soup, for instance. No-one will detect it when they eat, but they will think it a particularly fine bowl of soup.

I know several people who blench at the mention of leeks in white sauce, but put together with a little attention to detail it should be delicious. **Braise** the leeks in butter instead of boiling them, then nap with a white sauce that has had at least 15 minutes simmering quietly and has been seasoned with nutmeg, or chopped dill. Sprinkle generously with freshly grated Parmesan, before finishing under the grill if all the ingredients are still hot, or baking in a hot oven until browned if not.

Leeks are excellent sliced and braised in a tomato sauce, flavoured perhaps with orange or coriander seeds, and served hot, warm or even at room temperature. Or cook in scraps of bacon or pancetta and a sprinkling of chilli flakes for more vigour. Good on its own, as a side dish, or tossed with pasta.

I love to find leeks nestling in a chicken pie (replace the Jerusalem artichokes with leeks in the recipe on page 43, but cook them only lightly before enclosing in pastry), or in a stew of practically any sort, be it fish, fowl or beast. Generally, the rule in all of these is that the leeks should be popped in only some 10–15 minutes before the end of the cooking time. All good rules have exceptions. Here the exception comes with dishes like the pot-au-feu below, where whole leeks, other vegetables and meat are stewed for hours on end. Excess proves beneficial – the sodden leeks develop a beautiful flavour, though the texture is not appealing to everyone.

Deep-fried strands of leek have become a fashionable garnish for dishes and when done well, that's a good thing. The oil must be hot, but not too hot (around 180°C/350°F) and the leeks frizzled for just a few seconds until they begin to colour. A couple of seconds too long will render them bitter instead of sweetly crisp and curly. Pile them high on bowls of steaming soup, or on main-course salads or any other dish that has bold enough flavours to support a thatch of golden leek threads.

Creamed leeks with orange

Over the years this has been the most requested and appreciated recipe in my entire repertoire. I came up with it for my first vegetable book, originally to serve with roast pork, though it goes well with fish or chicken too. Without apology, I repeat the recipe here, in the hope that you will enjoy it as much second time around.

Serves 4–6

5 large leeks, trimmed
40 g (1½ oz) butter
juice and finely grated zest of 1 orange
40 g (1½ oz) plain flour

300 ml (10 fl oz) milk
a squeeze of lemon juice
salt and pepper

Cut the leeks into 4–5 cm (1½–3 in) lengths, then shred finely. Melt the butter in a wide pan and add the leeks. Stir to mix then add the orange juice and a little salt and pepper. Cover and simmer gently together for 10 minutes or so, stirring occasionally, until the leeks are tender. Uncover and boil off most of the watery juices until all that remains are a few tablespoonfuls of buttery liquid.

Now sprinkle with the flour and stir to mix evenly. Gradually add the milk, stirring, and then the orange zest. Bring to a simmer and cook for 3–5 minutes until very thick and creamy. If absolutely necessary, add a little more milk. Season with salt and pepper and stir in the lemon juice. Taste and adjust seasoning. If not using immediately spear a small knob of butter on the tip of a knife and rub over the surface to prevent a skin forming. Reheat gently, stirring frequently to prevent catching, before serving.

Smothered leeks with parsley and lemon

Smothering in this case means cooking in the minimum of liquid for far longer than you would normally dare. It takes the leeks past the point of 'overcooked' into the realms of wonderfully soft and silky. Every last drop of flavour is concentrated back into the leeks, along with the buttery juices. Never has al dente seemed so far away.

Serves 4

4 medium leeks, trimmed and cut
  into 5 cm (2 in) lengths
30 g (1 oz) butter
4 tablespoons chopped parsley

finely grated zest of 1 lemon
juice of ½ lemon
salt and pepper

Cut each chunk of leek in half lengthways. Melt roughly two-thirds of the butter in a wide sauté pan. Add the leeks, parsley, lemon zest and juice, salt and pepper. Stir, then pour in just about enough water to cover the base of the pan. Cover tightly, then cook over a very gentle heat for some 40 minutes, stirring once in a while, until the leek is very tender. You shouldn't need to add any more water – unless the heat is too high, or the lid doesn't fit properly, in which case you may evaporate off too much. If this does happen, just add a splash more water before everything burns. Conversely, if the leeks end up tender but swimming in water (they will release plenty of liquid into the pan as they cook), take off the lid towards the end of the cooking time and let the excess water boil away. What you are aiming for is a mellow mess of soft leeks and parsley, bathed in the smallest amount of buttery juice.

    Once you've reached the right point, just taste and adjust the seasoning, stir in the reserved butter, then serve.

Leeks with lentils, chorizo and eggs

Cooked lightly in with the chorizo-spiced lentils, the leeks retain just enough crispness but don't taste raw. The eggs move the whole into the realms of a main course, with no need to add anything else to the plate.

Cooking chorizo looks like a firm red-brown sausage but is a little softer than the sort sold ready sliced. It may be 'piccante' (hot) or 'dulce' (mild). Choose whichever one suits your tastes best.

Serves 4

4 leeks, trimmed and cut into rings roughly 1 cm (½ in) thick
250 g (9 oz) brown or green lentils (Puy are just the ticket here)
1 onion, quartered
1 bouquet garni (2 sprigs parsley, 2 sprigs thyme, 1 bay leaf, tied together with string)

4 cloves garlic
2 tablespoons extra virgin olive oil
250 g (9 oz) good-quality cooking chorizo, cut into 2 cm (scant 1 in) chunks
4 eggs
a little chopped parsley

Rinse the leeks thoroughly, then set aside to dry.

Put the lentils into a pan with the onion, bouquet garni and one of the cloves of garlic, peeled and sliced. Do not season at this point. Add enough water to cover generously and bring up to the boil. Simmer for about 25–35 minutes until the lentils are just tender, but not mushy. Stir in the leeks and simmer for a further 2 minutes. Drain, reserving a little of the cooking water. Discard the bouquet garni.

Chop the remaining cloves of garlic. Heat the oil in a frying pan and add the garlic and chorizo. Fry until the chorizo and garlic are tinged with brown. Now tip in the well-drained lentils and leeks and turn and stir so that they take on the gorgeous flavour of the chorizo and garlic. Stir in 2–3 tablespoons of the lentil cooking water to moisten. Season with salt and pepper, and stir until steaming hot. Meanwhile, poach or fry the eggs and keep warm.

Pile a big heap of lentils, leeks and chorizo on each plate and top with an egg. Sprinkle with a little parsley and serve.

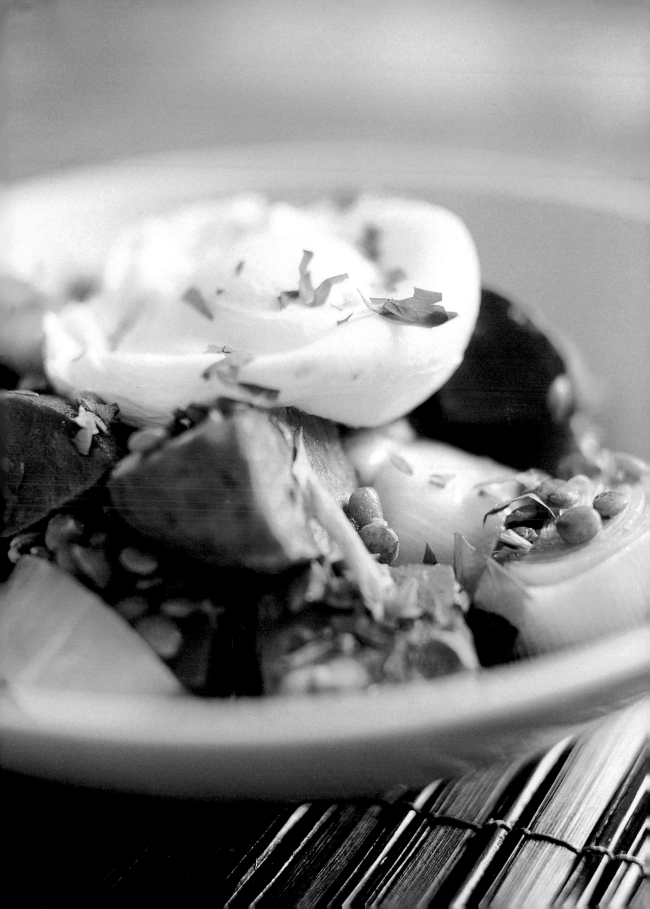

Petit pot-au-feu

A veritable pot-au-feu is a magnificent two-course dish of several slow-simmered cuts of meat. This version is 'petit' only in that I use just one type of meat – silverside – but it still tastes terrific, especially with the horseradish aïoli, which is my addition to the classic.

The first course is a simple bowl of the broth from the pot, padded out with, perhaps, some pasta or croûtes of toasted bread to soak up the delicious juice. The beef itself follows this, with that particular tenderness that comes only from long cooking, sliced and moistened with its own stock, and the vegetables, soft and tender with masses of flavour.

You may prefer to save half the leeks to add nearer the end of the cooking time (say about 20 minutes or so), so that they retain their form and texture.

Serves 8

1 x 2.5 kg (5½ lb) piece boned, rolled
  silverside
1 onion, studded with 4 cloves
1 bouquet garni (6 sprigs thyme, 2 bay
  leaves and 5 big sprigs parsley, tied
  together with string)
700–800 g (1 lb 9 oz–1¾ lb) medium carrots
1 kg (2¼ lb) leeks, trimmed and washed well
400–500 g (14–18 oz) small turnips, peeled
4 sticks celery, cut into 7.5 cm (3 in) lengths
200 g (7 oz) vermicelli or spaghetti,
  broken into short lengths
chopped parsley
salt and pepper

Horseradish aïoli
1 clove garlic, crushed
2 tablespoons creamed horseradish
2 teaspoons white wine vinegar
1 egg
250 ml (9 fl oz) sunflower oil
50 ml (2 fl oz) extra virgin olive oil

Unless you have a very long thin casserole, begin by cutting the meat in half, to create two smaller joints. Put them in a large pan together with the onion and the herbs. Add enough water to cover by about 5 cm (2 in). Bring up to the boil and then reduce the heat so that the water just burbles gently. Leave to simmer quietly for the next 2 hours. Keep skimming off the dirty-looking brown scum that will rise to the surface, until all that materialises is pure white foam. This will blend back into the pot-au-feu in time. Once you reach this stage, season with salt, three-quarters cover with a lid, and leave to simmer for the remainder of the cooking time.

While it simmers, prepare the horseradish aïoli. Put the garlic, horseradish, vinegar, egg and a little salt into the jug of a liquidiser. Whiz together until smooth then, blades still running, pour in first the sunflower oil and then the olive oil in a steady stream. Not too fast, mind, but nor do you have to be painfully slow about the process. Once the mayonnaise is thick and unctuous, taste and stir in more vinegar, salt or horseradish if you think it needs it.

Tie up the prepared leeks in two bundles with a couple of lengths of string. After the first 2 hours of simmering, tuck all the vegetables in around the meats, adding more hot water if necessary, then leave the whole caboodle to simmer for another 1–1½ hours until the meat is very tender.

Lift the meat and vegetables out on to two warm plates. Spoon over a little of the broth, cover and keep warm. Skim off as much fat as you can from the broth. Quickly add the pasta to the pan. Simmer for another 8–10 minutes until al dente, then serve bowlfuls of broth and pasta, sprinkled with parsley, as a first course.

Carve the meat and serve with the vegetables (snip the string off the leeks, before dishing up) and the aïoli as a main course.

* *

Onions

* * *

'Life is like an onion; you peel off layer after layer and then you find there is nothing in it,' wrote James Gibbons Huneker, American music and art critic in the early 20th century. Now you could interpret this as a lesson in the miserable futility of life, but those of us who appreciate our onions will see it in a different light: enjoy the layers for what they are and quit worrying about elusive inner meanings. That's far more useful, and no-one, not even Mr Gibbons Huneker, could deny that the onion is one of the most useful vegetables you are ever going to come across. It is one of the triumvirate of culinary gods – along with the potato and tomato – without which our meals would be infinitely the poorer. Like the potato and tomato, its popularity is worldwide yet it retains a humble modesty, preferring to shelter in the wings, rather than hog the limelight. Three cheers for the unassuming onion.

What else can I tell you about a vegetable that you know so well? Begin at the beginning, I suppose, though the origins are pretty vague. Food historians tell us that the onion seems to have originated in central Asia, that its use is recorded as far back as 3500 BC in Egypt and that they were being grown in the doomed gardens of Pompeii – excavators found no mummified bulbs, just the rows of bulb-shaped cavities in the earth where they had been growing. Jainism is the only religion that actively excludes the consumption of onions – they are considered root vegetables and to eat them would violate their strict laws of respect for life of all types. They are replaced in many recipes by a pinch or two of the foulest-smelling of all spices, asafoetida, which mellows on being cooked to a surprisingly subtle background oniony scent.

In most other cultures, a vast swathe of recipes begin with the common act of chopping an onion. Though it may melt into the background, it undoubtedly blesses savoury foods with an essential supportive structure, a foundation if you like, for other more obvious ingredients to rest on. Perhaps more important, however, is that the onion is such an extraordinarily versatile and multi-faceted creature. Raw, its overwhelming characteristic is an aggressive tear-jerking bite, often obliterating an underlying natural sweetness. Recently developed varieties may be milder, but I'm not sure that I totally approve – that tongue-tingling contrast of flavours is not altogether unpleasant when used in the right way.

Bring heat into the equation and everything changes. Gone is the bar-baric punch, and from its ashes emerges, if not a phoenix, at least a gentler, equally persistent beast. A mark, I think, of an experienced cook, is that they can manipulate the taste of cooked onions to boost the dish they are creating. Boiled, baked swiftly or slowly fried, deep-fried or caramelised, braised or grilled – each method reveals different facets of the humble onion.

Practicalities

BUYING The world of onions can become confusing if you delve deeply, but broadly speaking onions proper fall into three main categories: 'white' and 'yellow' globe (everyday spherical onions), red globe, and tiddly pearl or pickling onions. Spring onions and shallots, though related, are different enough to earn sections all of their own (see pages 318 and 312 respectively).

White or yellow globe onions are the everyday ones you are going to keep a permanent supply of to grab at a moment's notice. Small ones weigh in at around 115 g (4 oz) each, with larger ones reaching double or even treble that weight. Where size is not specified in a recipe, opt for a medium onion of around 150 g (5 oz). The precise hue of the inner layers or indeed the outer skin is no indicator of strength of flavour.

Included in this category are what were once known as 'Spanish onions', which are larger yellow-fleshed onions, and other varieties such as the American Vidalia which is relatively mild and sweet. French Roscoff onions are the first of the clan to gain an 'appellation d'origine contrôlée', in other words strict regulations regarding both where and how they are grown. With their pinkish tint, these are the onions that were once hawked around the south of England by Breton 'onion johnnies' on their bikes.

Look out, too, for the Italian 'cipolline' onion, a flattish variety that in

Sicily is roasted to a perfect sweetness to use in salads alongside sun-ripened tomatoes. Smaller versions of this onion are sold as 'borettane' onions, delicious preserved in a sweet-sour marinade to serve with cheese or cold meats.

Red onions are the fashionable ones, usually but not always milder than common yellow onions. With their dark purple-pink skins and rings of similar hue, they are undoubtedly handsome creatures. They look and taste great in salads (particularly with that store-cupboard standby of canned tuna and cannellini beans, dressed with lemon, olive oil and chopped parsley, or of a warm summer's day with ripe, sweet tomatoes and black olives, drizzled with red wine vinegar or balsamic vinegar and yet more olive oil – in winter replace the tomatoes with slices of sweet orange for an almost-as-good, season-friendly variation). Slow-roasted in quarters, doused with oil and seasoned with salt, they make a fine vegetable on their own, or again can be cooled and tossed into a salad. Effectively, however, it's the colour you are paying for when you splash out almost twice as much as you would on a bog-standard round onion.

Pickling, pearl, button and silverskin onions are much smaller, some 2–3 cm (around 1 in) in diameter. These little darlings are, as their name suggests, brilliant for pickling, and that doesn't have to imply an appallingly violent assault on the senses when consumed. If pickling isn't your thing, don't just ignore them. I use them frequently in stews, especially rich and robust beef stews, as a vegetable rather than a backdrop seasoning. They are also a classic element in a proper coq-au-vin, browned first in butter, before simmering briefly alongside the bird in its wine-rich sauce. Like shallots, they are delicious cooked in a sweet-and-sour bath of a marinade, or simply caramelised slowly, to serve as a blend of vegetable side dish and relish. Add them to mixed vegetable kebabs, or string between chunks of lamb and whole bay leaves on skewers to be grilled at the next barbecue.

Unlike most of the miniature onions, silverskins have a papery white skin. To minimise the tedium of peeling any of this clan, top and tail them first, then cover with boiling water for a minute or so, before draining. Now the skins will slip off like a glove.

Keep onions in a cool, dry, dark, airy spot that is not the refrigerator. Onions, especially cut onions, tend to pass their scent around everything else in the fridge, which doesn't matter much in some instances, but doesn't do any favours to, say, the milk you stir into your tea or pour over your morning bowl of cereal. A lone unused onion half can be wrapped in clingfilm to diminish cross-contamination but it doesn't necessarily work that well. Better I find, to leave it, clingfilmed, on the work surface so that you remember to use it up next day.

Tears

Uncontrollable weeping in the kitchen is usually, hopefully, the by-product of chopping onions. We've all been there. Some onions are worse than others, for no better reason than that they are juicier. As we cut into the flesh of the onions, enzymes go swiftly to work, releasing various sulphuric compounds into the air, amongst them a volatile substance called allicin. Mingling with the dampness of our eyes, it is transformed into a mild solution of sulphuric acid. No wonder we weep.

Over the years I've come across a multitude of ways to minimise the tears. The most common seems to be the absurd suggestion that you peel and chop the onions under running water. Dangerous? Impractical? Well, I'd have said so. What does seem to help is occasionally holding the insides of your wrists under the cold tap. Apparently the chill swiftly transfers to your nasal passages, where the blood vessels constrict, thus somehow reducing the opportunity for noxious onion fumes and watery tears to combine. I've also found that stuffing a tiny knobble of mauled bread under your upper lip impedes the tears, but it does make you look very silly. Perhaps the best advice is to sharpen your knife up properly before you start – that way the whole process will be so much easier and swifter, that a few tears shed along the way is neither here nor there. Get on with the chopping, and stop pratting around with time-wasting trifles.

SEE ALSO SPRING ONIONS AND SHALLOTS (PAGES 318 AND 312).

Braised sausages with chestnuts and onions

For this dish, I used plain, free-range pork sausages – chunky ones that benefit from slow cooking rather than slender chipolatas – but if you wanted to substitute fancier flavoured sausages, why not? The only restraint I'd suggest is that you ignore sweeter ones (such as those with added apricot or apple) as both the onions and the chestnuts provide hints of sugar. A good savoury banger is the optimum choice.

Unless you are a kitchen saint, use ready cooked and peeled chestnuts, but not the ones that are soggy from being canned in brine. Vacuum-packed cooked chestnuts are infinitely superior.

Serves 4

4 onions
2 tablespoons extra virgin olive oil
8 free-range pork sausages
2 cloves garlic, chopped
150 ml (5 fl oz) decent red wine
250 ml (9 fl oz) chicken stock

1 tablespoon tomato purée
6 sage leaves
3 bay leaves
250 g (9 oz) cooked, peeled chestnuts
salt and pepper

Peel and quarter the onions, doing your best just to slice the merest sliver off the root-end, so that the quarters each hold together. It doesn't matter too much if they fall apart, but it does make the next stage a touch fiddlier.

Take a heavy-based frying pan, wipe a touch of oil over the surface, then place over a high heat until violently hot. Lay the onion quarters in it and sear until patched with brown on all sides. Reserve.

Take another wide frying pan (or clean the first one to get rid of the blackened residues), and place over a moderate heat. Add the oil and fry the sausages fairly briskly until browned. Reserve with the onions. Next fry the garlic in the same oil.

Return the sausages and onions to the pan, and add all the remaining ingredients except the chestnuts. Bring up to the boil, then reduce the

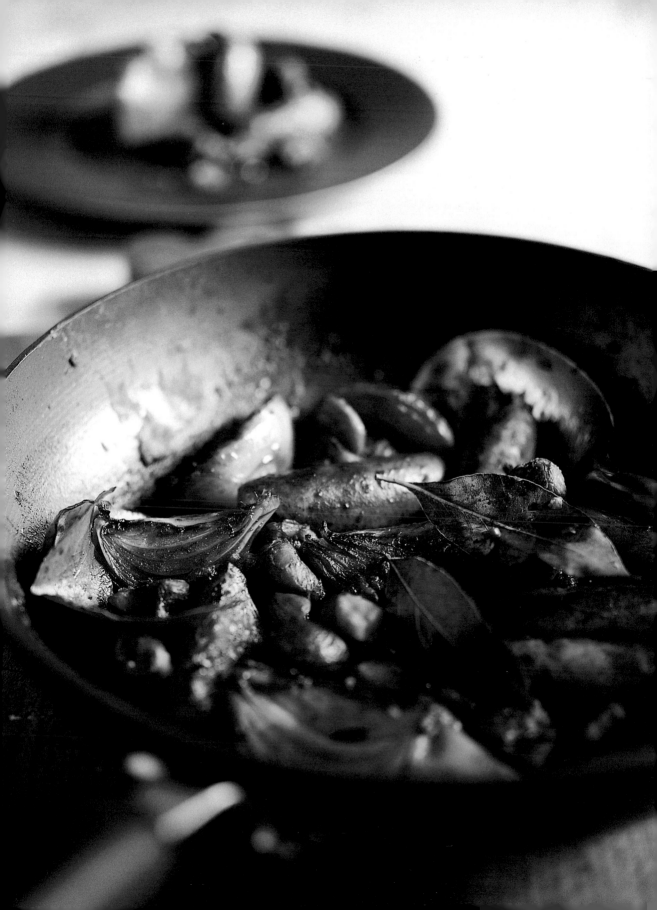

heat and simmer for about 20 minutes, uncovered. Stir in the chestnuts and simmer for another 5 minutes or so. Taste and adjust seasoning.

Serve with lots of mashed potato.

* *

Chicken Yassa

I just adore this African dish of chicken cooked in a stew of sweet soft onions and sharp, aromatic lime juice. Grilling the chicken before braising brings a hint of smokiness that you just can't get by browning it in the pan. Clever cooking with simple ingredients.

Serves 4

1 chicken, cut into portions
juice of 6 limes
4 large onions, sliced
2 tablespoons sunflower or groundnut oil

3 sprigs thyme
1 bay leaf
1/2 teaspoon cayenne pepper
salt and pepper

Marinate the chicken pieces in the lime juice for at least 2 hours, turning occasionally. Preheat the grill thoroughly.

Take the chicken pieces out of the marinade, reserving the marinade. Pat the chicken dry, then grill until browned all over.

Meanwhile, fry the onions gently in the oil until tender – this should take a good 15 minutes or so. Now add the thyme, bay leaf, cayenne, some salt, the marinade, and 60ml (2 floz) water. Lay the chicken on top, season with a little more salt and cover the pan tightly. Leave to simmer gently for 20 minutes or so, stirring once or twice, until the chicken is cooked through. Taste and adjust seasoning. Serve with roast yams or rice.

* *

Chilean tomato salad

This version of tomato salad from Chile seems unremarkable at first glance, but as with so many simple dishes, it is the balance of ingredients, allied with one small trick – in this case soaking the raw onions to soften their blow – that makes all the difference.

Serves 6–8

400 g (14 oz) finely sliced onion
800 g (1¾ lb) finely sliced tomatoes
  (around 10)
juice of 1 lemon

3 tablespoons olive oil
a big handful of roughly chopped coriander
salt and pepper

Cover the sliced onion with cold water and set aside for an hour. Drain well and pat dry.

Toss the onion with the tomatoes, and season with 1 teaspoon salt, some pepper, the lemon juice and oil. Top with the coriander and serve.

* *

Roasted onion flowers

This is such an easy and effective way of using onions as a vegetable all on their own, that I don't know why it isn't more well known. As they roast in the oven the 'petals' of the onions open out and soften in the heat. The result, the roasted onion flowers, are great with a steak, as their natural sweetness sets off the deep savouriness of the meat.

Serves 4

4 small onions, weighing around 115 g (4 oz)
  each
3 tablespoons olive oil
3 tablespoons balsamic or sherry vinegar
salt and pepper

Preheat the oven to 180°C/350°F/Gas 4.

Slice off the root of each onion very near to the base so that it holds together. Slice off the top as usual, then peel. Now cut each onion into 8 wedges, without cutting right through to the base: the knife should stop about 5–10mm (¼–½ in) from the root end, give or take.

Place the onions, root end down, in an oiled roasting tin, leaving plenty of space between each one so that the 'petals' can open out. Drizzle over olive oil and season with salt and pepper. Roast for 20 minutes until tender, and opened like a flower. Baste with juices and drizzle over the vinegar. Return to the oven and carry on cooking for another 10–15 minutes. Serve hot or warm.

* *

Soupe à l'oignon gratinée

Way, way back when I was a student, we used to make something that we called French onion soup. Well, I suppose it did have similarities to the real thing (onions and lots of them, principally) but it wasn't until I tasted the vrai chose in the heart of Paris, that I realised what a truly glorious creation it is. Whenever I go back to Paris in cool weather I make a point of searching out a fine soupe à l'oignon gratinée to stave off cold and fill me with a sense of warmth and wellbeing. It's like being snuggled up in the softest, most luxuriant, cashmere stole but on the inside.

There are differences between the Parisian version and the Lyonnais version, but the undoubted key to both is a spot of patience. That huge heap of raw onions needs time, and plenty of it, to cook down to the essential pulpy, sweet, semi-caramelised state. This is what bequeaths proper soupe à l'oignon its magical powers. Second most important is a tolerably good beef stock. A fabulous one is the ideal, but since beef stock is not something I ever make at home, it's not really on the cards. Instead I've tasted my way through a slew of mostly repulsive 'instant beef stocks' and tinned beef consommés and finally come to the conclusion that the only ones worth buying are the concentrated bouillons that come in wobbly plastic sachets. I use them diluted a little more than recommended and the result is pretty darn good.

Although cooking the onions takes at least an hour, the basic soup can be made in advance and reheated just before serving.

Serves 6

100 g (3½ oz) butter
1.5 kg (3¼ lb) large onions, sliced
2 teaspoons caster sugar
100 ml (3½ fl oz) dry vermouth
1.5 litres (2¾ pints) beef stock

2 bay leaves
1 baguette, thickly sliced, or 6 thick slices
    sourdough bread
300 g (11 oz) Gruyère cheese, grated
salt and pepper

Melt the butter in a large pan and add the onions. Stir, then cover and leave to cook very gently, stirring from time to time, until the onions are utterly tender. This will take around half an hour. Stir once every 10 minutes or so. Remove the lid, stir in the sugar, raise the heat a little and simmer until almost all the liquid from the onions has boiled away. Another 20 minutes or so. Stir more frequently towards the end of this time. Now carry on cooking, with you dancing all-but constant attendance on the pan. Once the bulk of the liquid has boiled away, the onions will start to take on a delectable golden hue, but this requires frequent stirring and scraping of the base of the pan to prevent burning, which is definitely not an advantage. I find it takes roughly another 10 minutes or so to develop a deep golden brown colour, which is what you are aiming for.

Now add the vermouth, bring up to the boil, and boil until all trace of it has disappeared – just a few minutes this time. Pour in the stock, add the bay leaves and season, making sure that you add plenty of freshly ground pepper. Leave to simmer comfortably, half covered with the lid, for a final 20–30 minutes.

Sometime during all that sweating and simmering of the onions, preheat the oven to 180°C/350°F/Gas 4. Arrange the slices of bread on a baking tray and bake until dry and lightly browned, around 20–25 minutes, depending on thickness. You can do everything up to this point a day or even two in advance.

Preheat the grill. Shortly before serving place a couple of pieces of bread in the base of each bowl, ladle over the soup including plenty of onions, then scatter a thick layer of grated Gruyère over the top. Slide under the grill until the cheese is melting and sizzling, and serve immediately.

*

Shallots

* * *

Shallots look like onions, they're built like onions, but they are not onions. Not quite. They grow differently, for a start, in clusters joined together at the base, rather than as individual orbs. To the cook, however, the main difference lies in the taste. Shallots are ladylike compared to rough-tough onions. In other words, they have a true oniony flavour and oodles of that innate sweetness but none of it masked by the bullish aggression of the onion. They are used extensively in the upper regions of cuisine, when chefs want depth of flavour without the reek of crude onion, especially in raw or lightly cooked dishes. For those of us peddling in lowlier styles of cuisine, they work just as well.

Just as onions vary enormously in size, so do shallots. The **purplish-pink shallots** used by Asian cooks tend to be relatively small, no bigger than a walnut, beside which the European **banana shallot** looms like Goliath. More varieties weigh in somewhere between these two extremes. It is for this reason that recipes will often specify a weight of chopped shallot, rather than numbers of whole shallots.

What if you don't have any shallots? Can you substitute onions directly? Yes, but.... Several yes-buts, in fact. Yes-but 1) you must remember that your average shallot is a good deal smaller than your average onion – let's surmise that '2 medium shallots, chopped' is roughly the same in volume as '⅓ medium onion, chopped'. Yes-but 2) the flavour of onion is raunchier so in any dish where shallots are left raw, chop onions extra small or slice paper thin, and use less. Yes-but 3) in dishes where subtlety is of major importance (e.g. a classic beurre blanc), onions may unbalance the whole slightly. Yes-but 4) when shallots are used whole, or halved (as in the upside-down tart below), you may be able to get away with using pearl onions, but they are a real pain to peel.

Practicalities

BUYING Select the best shallots just as you would the best onions. In other words, they should be firm, smooth skinned and dry. If labels have gone astray, the shallot is the one with the concave curve on one side, or a tip-tilted root end, where it has clustered up close to its fellow shallots as it grew.

Like onions and garlic, shallots will have been cured after picking, in other words, hung up to dry a little so that they keep through the winter. Sometimes their stems will have been neatly bound together to form a string which can be hooked up anywhere that is dry and not too warm (nor too cold – they don't like frost) for storage. Your kitchen is unlikely to be suitable. I keep strings of any of the edible alliums in my porch. Loose shallots are best tumbled gently into a vegetable rack in a cool, dry place. Do not store them in the fridge. Not only is it too cold, but their scent will creep sneakily into your milk and yoghurt and cream.

COOKING Preparation of shallots is the same as for onions. As with onions, check the inside as you prepare them, and discard any parts where brown rot has crept down the length of a layer of stalk into the centre of the shallot. Then carry right on, leaving them whole, or halving or slicing or chopping as appropriate. Shallots rarely induce tears, in me at any rate, though they may affect those with sensitive waterworks.

Shallots are ideally sized to cook whole. They are fabulous **in casseroles** where you will probably brown them first in oil or butter, before adding to the main stew. Try them with beef in a red wine or beer casserole, or add to chicken being cooked with red wine, mushrooms and a touch of tomato. And as an addition to a meat-free vegetable stew they give it a substance that can sometimes seem lacking. Don't think, however, that because whole shallots are entering the mix you can do without the fried chopped onion base which gives the depth of flavour to the sauce. You need both. 'Echalotes confits', shallots cooked in a sweet-sour sauce until deeply tender, is another classic use of whole shallots, so good served with meat dishes, or with a fine hunk of cheese. You might also consider adapting a recipe for **pickled** onions, turning it into an altogether more subtle venture by using shallots and wine vinegar in place of pickling onions and malt.

Sliced or chopped shallots are good for pepping up salads and salsas, where they work as substitutes for spring onions or onions. Scatter rings of fresh pink shallot over tomato salads in summer, or over discs of orange, adding a few black olives, a sprinkling of mint and a light dressing in winter. Use them, too, in marinades for fish and chicken.

They star in sauces, particularly cream- or butter-based sauces where the taste of onions might be too big. And they feature regularly in Asian cooking, especially South-East Asian cooking. **Stir-fried** they can be used lavishly to build up a foundation layer of flavour along with chopped fresh ginger and garlic. Sliced shallots, **fried** in plenty of oil until browned and crisped, are used as a delicious final garnish for both hot dishes and room-temperature salads.

It's worth noting that shallots are not always a good replacement for onions. Wherever onions are employed to give that crucial base note – in stocks, in stews, in soups – shallots are really too lightweight to do the job properly.

* *

Upside-down shallot tart with thyme and orange crust

When you want a meat-free main course to delight and to rev up all those taste-buds, this is one to go for. As you turn it out, the sight of all those glistening, caramelised shallots is enough to make you shout for joy. The taste is good too, with the short, spiced-up cheese pastry mollifying the sweetness of the shallots.

Serves 6

400 g (14 oz) shallots, halved lengthways
85 g (3 oz) butter
60 g (2 oz) caster sugar
juice of 1 large orange
2 tablespoons balsamic vinegar
salt and pepper

Pastry
190 g (6½ oz) plain flour
85 g (3 oz) unsalted butter
85 g (3 oz) Parmesan, freshly grated
2 teaspoons thyme leaves
finely grated zest of 1 orange
½ teaspoon cayenne pepper
½ teaspoon salt
1 egg

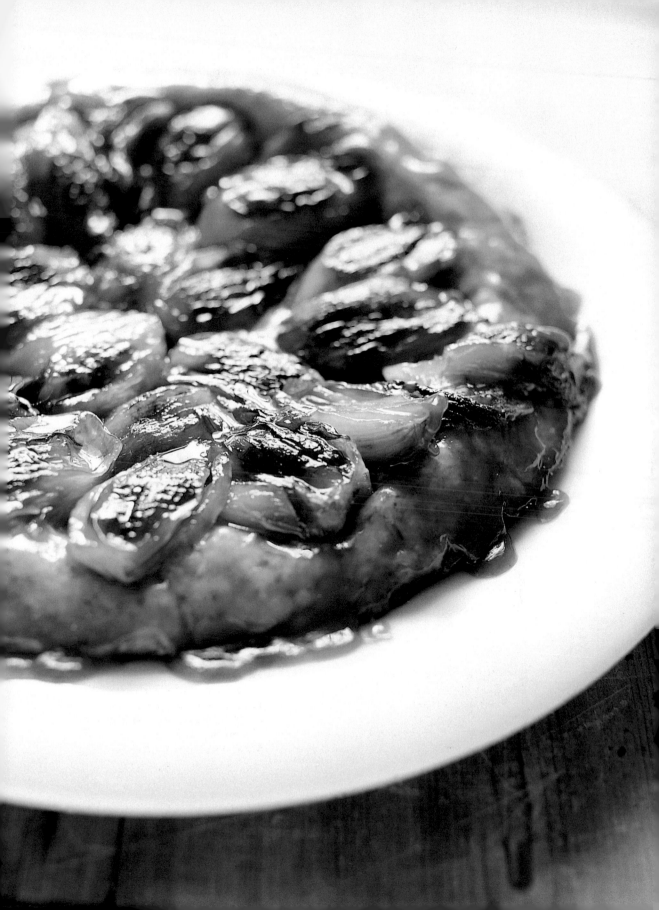

First make the pastry. Put the flour into a mixing bowl and rub in the butter until the mixture resembles a pile of fine breadcrumbs. Now stir in the Parmesan, thyme, orange zest, cayenne and salt. Make a well in the centre and break in the egg. Mix to a soft but not sticky dough adding just enough icy water to bind – I used 1 tablespoon. Wrap in clingfilm and chill for half an hour.

Preheat the oven to 180°C/350°F/Gas 4.

Prepare the shallots, halving them lengthways through their widest part. Cut the butter into thin slivers and lay them over the base of a heavy-based ovenproof frying pan or special tatin mould, with a diameter of 25 cm (10 in). Season with salt and pepper, sprinkle over the sugar, then pack the shallots into the frying pan in concentric circles, curved sides down. Drizzle orange juice and vinegar over the shallots.

Set the pan over a gentle heat, so that the butter melts without burning. Once the buttery juices start bubbling up around the sides, continue cooking until the juices have thickened to a rich syrup that is just beginning to caramelise – in other words beginning to gather a touch of brown. This will take around 20–25 minutes.

Roll the pastry out on a lightly floured board to form a circle with roughly the same diameter as the frying pan. Lay on a baking sheet and return to the fridge to chill until you need it.

As soon as the shallots are ready, take them off the heat and quickly lay the pastry over them, tucking the edges down inside the pan. Transfer to the oven and leave to cook for a further 25–30 minutes until the pastry is browned.

Take out of the oven, let the tart settle for 2–3 minutes, run a knife around the edge to loosen, then cover with an upturned serving dish. Turn pan and dish over swiftly and, all being well, you will hear the tart dropping satisfyingly on to the plate. Lift off the frying pan and there it should be, glistening tantalisingly. Inevitably, the odd piece of shallot will have stuck to the frying pan. Just ease it off and pop it back where it should be on the tart. Serve hot or warm.

* *

Thai stir-fried beef with shallots and basil

A few summers ago, I cooked Thai stir-fried beef with shallots and basil twice a day for 18 days – not consecutively, I hasten to add. I had been engaged to give a series of demonstrations, and at each one, this was undoubtedly the star turn, particularly with the men. Both shallots and basil feature more heavily than one expects in a stir-fry, to create a fully flavoured showstopper of a dish, streaked with the red of chillies.

To carry the bold seasonings, you really need to buy first-class beef, that has been properly hung to develop its full flavour – the kind of beef you find at a good butcher or a farm shop or a farmers' market.

Serves 4

2–3 tablespoons sunflower, peanut or vegetable oil
8 medium shallots, thinly sliced
4 cloves garlic, chopped
3 red chillies, deseeded and thinly shredded
1 cm (½ in) piece fresh root ginger, finely chopped

450 g (1 lb) rump or fillet steak, thinly sliced
2 kaffir lime leaves, very finely shredded
60 g (2 oz) basil leaves
2 tablespoons fish sauce
2 teaspoons palm sugar or dark muscovado sugar

Heat a wok over a high heat for a couple of minutes until it smokes. Add the oil. Swirl around once or twice, then add the shallots and stir-fry for about 1 minute. Now add the garlic, chillies and ginger and stir-fry for another 30 seconds.

Next add the beef and stir-fry until it loses its translucent, raw look. Sprinkle over the kaffir lime leaves, and toss for another 20–30 seconds. Pile in most of the fresh basil leaves, the fish sauce and sugar. Stir-fry for a final 30 seconds or so.

Scoop into a warm serving dish, top with the reserved basil and serve with rice.

* *

Spring onions

* * *

Spring by name, all-year-round by market forces. I suppose there was a time when spring onions really were available only in the spring, but have you ever heard anyone bemoaning the passing of spring onion seasonality? No, me neither. Though I wonder whether growers or supermarket buyers are anxious in case a retrograde spring-onion backlash breaks out? Could that be why they've renamed them salad onions?

Spring onions are quiet and unassuming, as vegetables go. Not prone to making a loud, crashing entrance, nor to taking a major role on our plates. Spring onions are generally seen as incidentals. Just a handy way to inject a crisp, oniony zip, without the chunkiness of genuine onion. Fresher tasting, easy to handle, fun to play with, bracing enough to liven up a salad or salsa without dominance. So very handy, that it's no wonder we love to have them on tap all year round.

Over recent years there's been a little play on the basic spring onion. I've had a momentary pash on the charming **'red' spring onion**, actually more of a pinky purple, fading into the usual green of the upper leaves. They don't taste different, but like purple basil, they make a decorative change every now and then. We've also seen an influx of chunkier **salad onions**, which have a genuine bulging little onion at the base. The brave of mouth will no doubt bite off the bulge in one go, but I've never been one for whole mouthfuls of raw onion, even of the softer salad style.

Practicalities

BUYING Fresh spring onions are lively, firm leaved, pearly skinned, healthy looking. Say no to wrinkles, wilt, dryness. Spring onions are, by their very nature, slender, but avoid extra thin stems – more waste and more work.

I've always stored spring onions loose in the vegetable drawer of the fridge, with no evidence of onion-scented infiltration of the milk, eggs or butter. Stored in the cool, they will keep nicely for up to 4 or 5 days. Preparation is minimal. Trim off the roots and the tougher top inch or two (3–5 cm) greenery. If the outer layer looks a little dry, pull it off. Now chop or not as the recipe demands.

COOKING Here's the list of dishes that I use spring onions in most often: salsas, salads, champ (Irish mashed potatoes), stir-fries, sauces, soups (as a final garnish), kebabs, mayonnaise, savoury pancakes, scrambled eggs, omelettes. I may well have left a few out.

The renowned South or Central American **tomato salsa** is a natural home for the spring onion. I love it, everybody loves it, with grilled chicken or beef or pork, in hot tortillas, with fish, even on fried eggs. All you do is mix finely diced, deseeded tomatoes with a little crushed garlic, a little deseeded, finely chopped chilli, lots of chopped coriander, lime juice and chopped spring onions, then season with salt and pepper. A modern classic. If you want to get fancy, add diced avocado, replace some or all of the tomatoes with mango or fresh pineapple or fresh sweetcorn; for an Italian salsa cruda, replace the coriander with basil, tone down the chilli, replace lime with lemon, but keep that spring onion just as it is.

Spring onion **in salads** should be sliced or shredded, but massive great big chunks of spring onion can be overwhelming. Think of them as a way to bring a notion of onioniness without taking over. Champ, one of the best of Irish creations, is no more than beautifully mashed, buttery potatoes, improved by having plentiful chopped spring onions that have been softened in a little more butter, stirred through it. Handsome and soul-satisfying.

Spring onions can get double billing **in a stir-fry**, being thrown in right at the start to scent the oil along with garlic and ginger, as well as making a comeback as a final addition, either stirred in to the hot vegetables and meat or fish so that they soften just a fraction, losing a little of their raw hiss, or scattered on to the dish as it is served to retain more of that raw character.

In paler gentler sauces, hot sauces that is, the spring onion should go in relatively early on so that it has time to soften and sweeten, whereas in a more strongly flavoured darker sauce (I'm thinking in particular of tomato sauce) they make a good addition stirred in right at the end of the cooking time so that they are not instantly lost. In mayonnaise, where no heat takes part, chop the spring onion more finely before stirring in. Like an elder cousin of chives, they also make a terrific garnish for a soup, perhaps scattered over just before serving together with a handful of herbs, or crisp croûtons, or crumbled crisp bacon or pancetta. Like chives, again, they have a natural affinity with eggs, stirred into creamy scrambled eggs, or whisked into the egg mixture for making an omelette.

Spring onions warm very well to a spot of **grilling**. Whole perhaps (see the recipes below), or cut into 3–4 cm (1½ in) lengths and strung on to kebabs between chunks of chicken, or pork or monkfish, or other vegetables to provide a counterpoint to the main element.

SEE ALSO ONIONS (PAGE 302).

* *

Grilled spring onions with Romesco sauce

A much anticipated treat every spring in Catalonia in Spain is the arrival of the first 'calçots'. These are a form of fat, juicy spring onion. They are grilled until streaked with brown, and eaten hot and tender in vast quantity with Romesco sauce. So to get something of the taste of this, buy the thickest, perkiest, handsomest spring onions and light up the barbecue (or preheat the grill – not half as romantic, I know, but grilled spring onions are good too).

Romesco sauce is one of Catalonia's great creations, a brick orange cream of dried local peppers ('ñoras') and toasted nuts bound together with punchy olive oil. The trouble with trying to reproduce it here is precisely those excellent and most important peppers, which are not so easy to find. So I cannot honestly say that the recipe I give here is for a true Romesco, but it does, I think, capture something of the glorious flavour which marries so well with grilled spring onions, as well as chicken, or fish and even baked potatoes.

This is not a dish to eat smartly with knife and fork. No, not at all. Pick the grilled spring onions up with your fingers, dip into the Romesco and then bite and chew and suck and slurp.

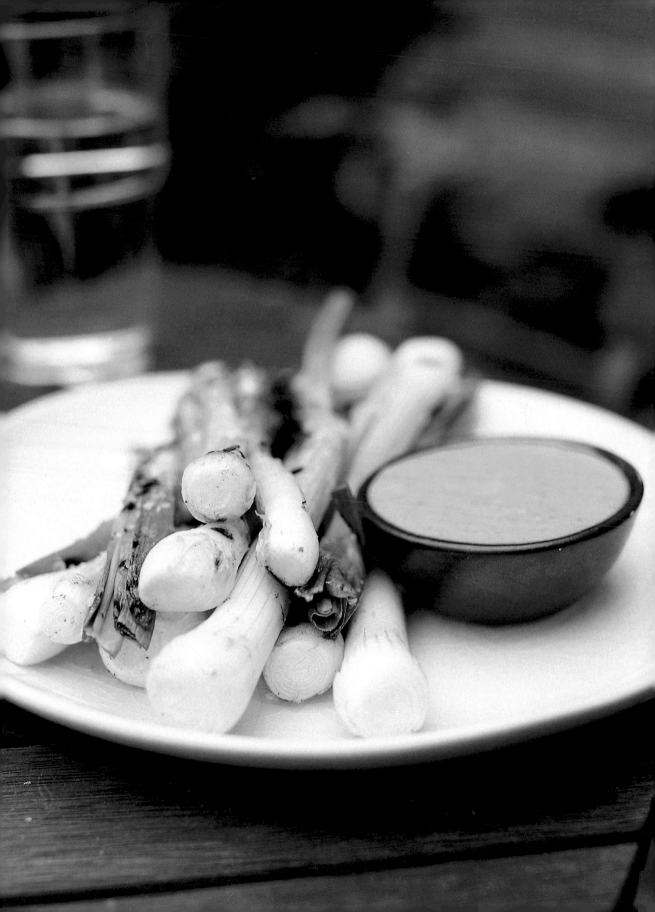

Serves 4

16–20 thick spring onions
olive oil
salt and pepper

Sauce
1/2 thick slice white bread, slightly stale
225 ml (8 fl oz) extra virgin olive oil
3 cloves garlic

85 g (3 oz) grilled, skinned red peppers
1 tablespoon red wine vinegar
40 g (1 1/2 oz) shelled whole almonds, toasted
40 g (1 1/2 oz) shelled hazelnuts, skinned
 and toasted
1 teaspoon smoked paprika (pimentón)
1/4 teaspoon cayenne pepper
salt and pepper

To make the sauce, first fry the bread in 2–3 tablespoons oil until golden brown. Drain on kitchen paper, then break into pieces and drop into the bowl of a processor.

Slice 2 of the garlic cloves and fry in the same oil, adding a little more if needed, until lightly browned. Chop the third one roughly. Add the fried and raw garlic to the bread. Add the peppers, vinegar, nuts, smoked paprika, cayenne, salt and pepper too. Process together until finely chopped to a thick paste, scraping down the sides with a spatula. Keep the motor running, and gradually trickle in the remaining oil, and 4–5 tablespoons hot water. Taste and adjust seasoning. Scrape into a bowl and cover until ready to serve.

Shortly before eating, preheat the grill thoroughly or light the barbecue. Trim the spring onions, but leave whole. Toss in a little olive oil – just enough to protect them under the heat of the grill. Grill or barbecue for around 7–8 minutes, turning until streaked with brown. Serve immediately with the Romesco sauce.

Wild garlic

* * *

The trouble with wild garlic is that you have to track it down. The good thing is that once you do, you'll be blessed with a copious supply every spring forever and anon, and all for the price of a walk in the woods. You could, I suppose, buy it, if you happen to shop at some very fancy greengrocery, but personally I object paying through the nose for something that grows profusely in the wild. Half the fun of cooking with the stuff is that you've gathered it all yourself. Anyone who is unlucky enough to have a garden riddled with wild garlic will know that, unlike so many other wild plants, this one is not in any danger of disappearing in the near future. Once established, wild garlic is extremely hard to eradicate and spreads copiously. Although its white flowers and broad tulip-like leaves are charming to the eye, the smell can be overwhelming, which is not every gardener's idea of perfection.

Obviously if you are going to pluck and eat a wild plant, you do need to be absolutely sure that you are dealing with the right thing. In this case, a relatively easy task. The leaves are pretty distinctive, putting in an appearance from mid-April through to the summer, but it is the strong reek of garlic that seals the identification. In fact, I'd even go as far as to say your nose is the optimum tool for tracking down wild garlic, especially on a warm spring day – as we did one sunny May afternoon last year. Driving back from the Peak District, windows wound down, the smell assaulted us unforgivingly. Whoa there – stop the car at once. Sure enough, hidden away behind a low dry-stone wall, lay a tumbling bank carpeted with wild garlic, in full bloom. I picked as much as I could hold, wrapped it tight in a plastic bag, and bore it home in triumph. That evening we sat down to a supper of wild garlic and new potato risotto – a rare and unexpected treat.

Practicalities

STORING Wild garlic is best used within a day or two of picking, when it is still at its freshest and liveliest. The fridge is probably the best place to store it BUT make sure you wrap it really, really, really well. Otherwise that garlic smell will migrate to milk, eggs, cream, and whatever else lurks in the chilly portals of the fridge.

Wash wild garlic leaves thoroughly before using. Organic they may be, but who knows what creatures have lingered near them whilst they grew. I always make a point of picking well away from paths, in the hope that less wild-life will have left its trace on the leaves, but that may just be wishful thinking.

COOKING In their first flush of youth, say in April or the first few days of May, the leaves are tender enough to use raw in salads, shredded or torn up into smaller pieces. As they begin to mature, however, they toughen, and are better cooked to tenderise them. Sadly, they lose a good deal of their pungency in the heat of a pan, but a gentle trace still lingers on. Wild garlic can be **cooked like spinach** – either wash and shake off excess water, then cram into a pan with a knob of butter, cover and cook over a moderate heat for a few minutes, stirring once or twice, until wilted, or **stir-fry** them (the best method for both vegetables, I find) with just a little oil in a brilliantly hot wok for 30–60 seconds, or however long it takes for them to begin to wilt.

I love them in mashed potatoes, a sort of halfway house between cooked and raw. Shred plenty of wild garlic and stir into a pan of steaming hot buttery mash just before serving – fabulous with beef stew, or even a juicy grilled slab of rump steak. I also use them **as wrappers** for fish or little parcels of other foods – blanch the leaves literally for seconds in a pan of boiling water to soften them, then drain and wrap before using.

For a **wild garlic sauce**, shred the leaves and soften in a little butter until tender, then add a spot of stock and some double cream or crème fraîche and simmer until thickened to the degree that takes your fancy. Very good with pink-roast lamb. And for a simple starter or nibbly thing before a main meal, you could even dip them in a light batter and fry until crisp – delicious and unusual.

SEE ALSO GARLIC AND GARLIC SCAPES (PAGES 284 AND 290).

Wild garlic and new potato risotto

Wild garlic and new potatoes are a fortuitous pairing, matched in season and in flavour. Plunged into a risotto together, they make a warming, soothing dish for a fresh spring evening. With good home-made stock, this is a lovely dish. I like it as the recipe runs below, but my children insist that it is better for the addition of a handful of roughly chopped sun-blush tomatoes, stirred in with the wild garlic.

Serves 3–4

75–100 g (2½–3½ oz) wild garlic leaves
1.4 litres (2½ pints) chicken or vegetable
  stock
40–60 g (1½–2 oz) butter
1 onion, chopped
250 g (9 oz) risotto rice
1 bay leaf

2 sprigs lemon thyme
250 g (9 oz) freshest new potatoes, scrubbed
  and cut roughly into 1 cm (½ in) cubes
150 ml (5 fl oz) dry white wine
40 g (1½ oz) Parmesan, freshly grated
salt and pepper

Remove the larger stalks of the wild garlic, then shred the leaves roughly. Put the stock in a pan and place over a moderate heat to warm through.

Melt 30 g (1 oz) butter in a wide pan. Add the onion and fry gently until softened without browning. Now add the risotto rice, bay leaf, thyme, salt and pepper. Stir around for a minute or so until the rice becomes slightly translucent. Add the new potatoes and white wine. Simmer, stirring, until the wine has virtually all evaporated.

Add a good ladleful of hot stock, and carry on stirring until most of the liquid has been absorbed. Add another ladleful of stock and stir some more. Carry on in this way, adding more stock every time the last batch has all but disappeared, stirring more or less continuously, until the rice is just tender but still retains a mild bite. It's at this moment that you stir in what will look like a mountain of wild garlic, which soon wilts to a more manageable and less disturbing volume. Draw off the heat and stir in the remaining butter and the Parmesan. Taste and adjust seasoning and serve straightaway.

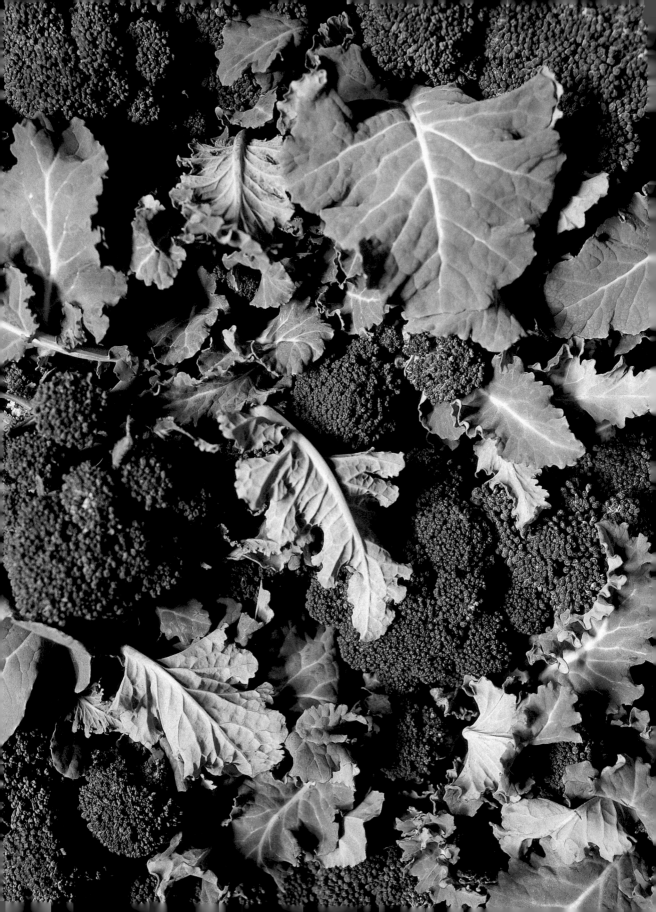

Brassicas

* *

Broccoli, calabrese
Broccoli, sprouting
Brussels sprouts
Cabbage **Cauliflower**
Red cabbage

* *

Broccoli, calabrese

* * *

There is a criminal mastermind at work in the fields of Britain, or in the packing houses adjacent to said fields. Someone, somewhere is stealing broccoli stems. You must have noticed that more and more broccoli is arriving in shops with no more than the bare minimum of stem, just enough to hold the florets in place. Why? Many of us actually prefer the sweet juiciness of the stem to the fall-apart florets. Perhaps our criminal mastermind goes a step further. Could he be obsessed with the stems and so determined to harvest them for himself alone? I wonder.

Or it could be a conspiracy. Everyone loves a good conspiracy theory. A cluster of evil executives, huddling in office corners, wondering how to demoralise a nation in the subtlest of ways? I dare say there is some totally boring explanation lurking around somewhere, but even so I'm lodging a complaint. Broccoli stems are unbeatable and I want my fair share. Actually, what I like is the best of both ends, the contrast in one small vegetable of the foamy florets and the smooth, succulent but firm stem. It is for this reason that I have taken greatly to a recent introduction, the svelte **tenderstem broccoli**, where stem is the raison d'être and never needs peeling, while the floret is a little token of tenderness stuck on the end.

Calabrese, calabrese broccoli and **broccoli** are all the same thing. When fat-stemmed broccoli was introduced to this country in a big way, back in the middle of the last century, it needed to be distinguished from the then more common purple sprouting broccoli. The appendage 'calabrese', meaning from Calabria, did the job nicely. Now that it has become the dominant broccoli, the term is dropped more often than not.

Practicalities

BUYING Any hint of yellow, normally such a sunny welcome colour, is a warning beacon in broccoli. It's beaming out the message 'old and past it...old and past it'. Fresh broccoli is an enticing, dark blue-green on the top, astride a stem of paler clear green. Firm from top to bottom and not a hint of brown – that's what you are after. Like any vegetable, the sooner it is eaten the better it tastes. So although it will keep apparently cheerily in the vegetable drawer of the fridge for up to a week, you would be well advised to get it into that pan within a day or two of purchase.

COOKING If you truly love your broccoli, you will take note of the fact that the florets cook more quickly than the thicker part of the stem. And that if the stem is very thick, it will need peeling before slicing ready for cooking. That, of course, is after you've sliced the florets away at the top, like a forest of verdant bonsai treelets, and divided larger pieces into two or three. This ensures that they will cook evenly. My usual everyday way of cooking broccoli takes this into account, too. Once the salted water is **boiling**, I add the sliced stem only, bring back to the boil and then reduce the heat to let the stems simmer for, say, 2 minutes, before adding the florets and continuing to simmer gently for a further 2–3 minutes. By then both are beautifully cooked, and the florets don't get a chance to soften to mush.

Or you can **steam** your broccoli, but be warned – the colour is dulled even if the taste is full and vigorous. This is why I usually stick with the tried and tested method. Or else, if I'm prepared to stand over the pan for a few minutes, I turn to the superb Heston Blumenthal method (see overleaf).

PARTNERS Perfectly cooked broccoli is a great joy, wonderful just as it is, or with a dab of butter or a light slick of lemon olive oil. Or you might pre-cook it, then reheat in olive oil with some finely chopped garlic and a sprinkling of chilli flakes – bliss. Or try this: fry garlic and a few chopped anchovy fillets gently in olive oil over a low heat, mashing the anchovies into the oil, then toss the broccoli in this mixture until hot – another blessedly simple combination.

For broccoli served at room temperature as a salad, I would go for a simple workman-like vinaigrette as a dressing, or something sprightlier with Asian overtones. Or you might inject a spot of orange juice, or go back to those anchovies. Raw broccoli stem, peeled if the skin is tough, then sliced, is also rather good in salads.

And to finish, an obviously contradictory idea – to make the southern Italian supper dish of pasta with broccoli, add the broccoli to the pan in which the pasta is cooking some 6 minutes before it is done, then drain the whole lot together. Almost inevitably the broccoli will have softened and will be beginning to collapse. This is as it should be. Finish the pasta with some pancetta and garlic that have been fried in olive oil, or go back to those anchovies again, softened with garlic in oil. Or sauté halved cherry tomatoes in olive oil with garlic and add a handful of shredded basil as you mix tomatoes, oil and pasta. Or, if your family love tomato sauce as much as mine does, toss that in with the pasta and broccoli. Make sure there's plenty of Parmesan to sprinkle over it before eating, and there it is. Broccoli completely mis-cooked and still tasting damn fine.

SEE ALSO BROCCOLI, SPROUTING (PAGE 334).

* *

Heston Blumenthal's broccoli

A few years ago, Heston Blumenthal, Britain's most innovative and curious chef, wrote a column dedicated largely to the joys of broccoli. As you might expect, he doesn't merely boil or simmer his broccoli. Dearie me, no. His standard cooking method involves smokingly hot olive oil, butter and no water at all. And the result is so gorgeous that it had my family fighting (literally) over the last piece.

He suggests that you might vary the basic technique by adding some finely chopped chilli or chopped garlic (that's the one we like best) to the pan with the broccoli, and/or by stirring in some finely grated lemon zest at the end.

This is how it goes. Begin by cutting off all the florets of the broccoli from the central stalk. They should be fairly evenly sized, roughly 3 cm (a generous inch) across. Peel the stem only if necessary, then cut into slices around the thickness of two £1 coins. We've found that three of us gobble our way through 350–400 g (12–14 oz) of prepared broccoli with no difficulty.

Heat a few tablespoons of good olive oil (2 tablespoons for the above quantity of broccoli) in a wide, heavy-based pan over a medium heat until it just starts to smoke. Now throw in the prepared florets and clamp on the lid (which should be close fitting). Leave to cook for 2 minutes, so that, as the heat releases the water from the vegetable, it enables some steam to build up.

Remove the lid and shake the pan a bit, to make sure all the florets get a good coating with hot oil. They will already have browned a fair amount. Now season with salt and pepper – as Chef Blumenthal points out, you need far more salt than seems proper – and then add a bit of butter, 20–30g (about 1 oz) or so. Put on the lid again, and give the broccoli another 1–2 minutes on the heat. Check to see if it is cooked enough for you. If you want it a little softer, shake the broccoli around again, then replace the lid and cook for another 1–2 minutes. So good that it's worth eating all on its own.

* *

Stir-fried broccoli with oyster sauce

A hot favourite in Chinese restaurants, broccoli stir-fries well as long as the florets are kept fairly small – say around 2 cm (¾ in) across or slightly less.

Serves 3–4

400 g (14 oz) broccoli, florets separated, stem peeled and sliced
2 tablespoons sunflower or vegetable oil
3 cloves garlic, chopped
3 rashers streaky bacon, derinded and cut into thin strips

2 tablespoons oyster sauce
2 tomatoes, deseeded and finely diced
salt and pepper

Prepare the broccoli. Put the wok over a high heat and leave until it smokes. Now add the oil and garlic and stir-fry for a few seconds until lightly browned. Add the broccoli and bacon and continue to stir-fry for 4–5 minutes until crisp-tender. Stir in the oyster sauce and then the tomato dice. Taste and add salt and pepper as needed. Serve while still wok-hot, spooned over a mound of steaming rice.

* *

Broccoli with chilli and breadcrumbs

This is a quick and simple way to add zip and interest to plain boiled broccoli.

Serves 4

500g (1lb 2oz) broccoli, trimmed
4 tablespoons extra virgin olive oil
2 cloves garlic, chopped

2 red chillies, deseeded and finely chopped
25g (scant 1oz) fine stale breadcrumbs

Cut the broccoli into long slender pieces, each one including some of the flowering head and the stem. Cook lightly in salted water and drain well. Keep warm. Just before serving, heat the oil in a pan, add the garlic, chillies and breadcrumbs, and fry over a medium heat until the crumbs are brown. Scatter over the broccoli and serve forthwith.

* *

Broccoli salad with anchovy dressing

There is an undeniable affinity between anchovies and broccoli, as long as the anchovies are used with restraint.

Serves 4–6

500g (1lb 2oz) broccoli
2 teaspoons rice wine vinegar
  (or white wine vinegar)
2 tablespoons sunflower oil
salt and pepper

Dressing
6 canned anchovy fillets
1 tablespoon white wine vinegar
1 tablespoon chopped parsley
100ml (3½ floz) single cream

If using tenderstem broccoli, just trim the ends. With calabrese broccoli, choose smaller heads with plenty of stem, and cut them carefully lengthwise to give long slender pieces. Cook the broccoli in lightly salted water for 4–6 minutes until tender-crisp. Drain, run under the cold tap and then drain

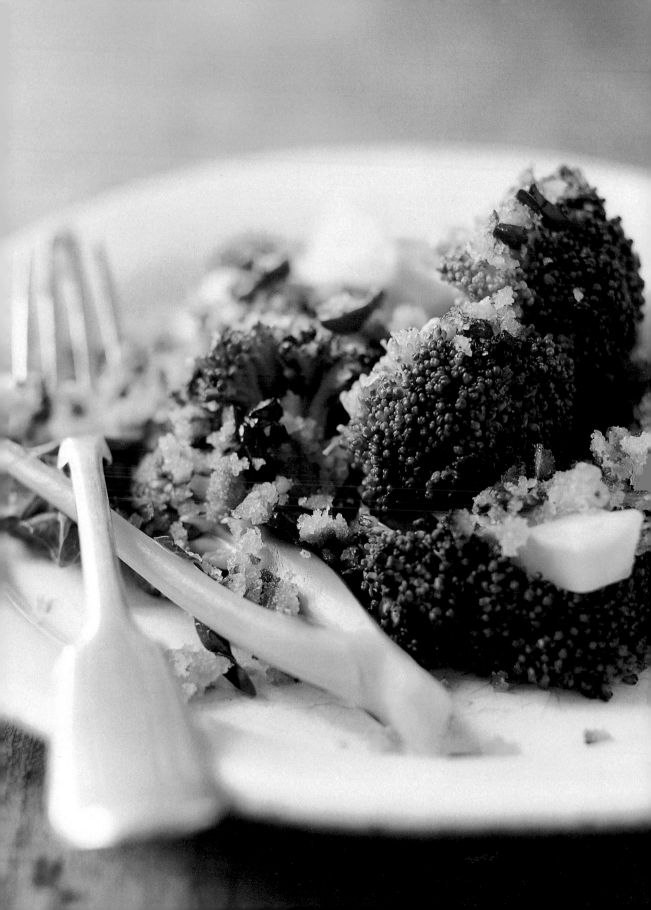

again thoroughly. Mix the rice wine vinegar with the sunflower oil, salt and pepper and toss with the broccoli, then leave to cool completely.

Put the anchovy fillets in a liquidiser with the vinegar, parsley and a little of the cream. Turn on the liquidiser and drizzle in the remaining cream as the blades whir. Taste and adjust seasoning, adding salt only if needed. Drizzle the dressing over the broccoli just before serving.

* *

Broccoli, sprouting

* * *

Sprouting broccoli is the vegetable-lover's vegetable. Not rare like turnip-rooted chervil, nor heralded like spring asparagus, it's neither funky like purple-fleshed potatoes nor fashionable like rocket. It's not even particularly versatile. And yet, and yet.... Many cooks and chefs, both professional and otherwise, rate purple sprouting broccoli as one of the great vegetables. I'm right there amongst them.

Sprouting broccoli comes in two tones: **dark, brooding purple** and **pale, yellowish white**. The former is the one most of us are familiar with. White sprouting broccoli is far less common, but no less delicious. Both have, or at least should have, a fairly short spring season, although modern techniques have stretched the season for the purple-headed stems. Even so, a long, cold, icy winter will delay the arrival of the best sprouting broccoli, grown outdoors, without cover, as it should be. One of the wonderful things about this wonderful vegetable is that it appears in late winter to relieve the tedium of our limited spectrum of home-grown produce. It's a shame that we don't give it the same kind of fanfare as the arrival of the first British asparagus, say, or tiny Jersey Royal potatoes.

White sprouting broccoli first crashed on to the Grigson radar on a visit to Leicester's large city-centre market. It was early March and I watched, open-mouthed, as customer after customer bought carrier bags full of white sprouting broccoli as if it was hurtling out of fashion. One of the many stallholders selling it explained that it is a big local delicacy, with a brief three-or-four week season. Hence the passionate enthusiasm. Is it better than purple sprouting? Maybe, maybe not – so much depends on freshness. It is certainly as good, and that, frankly is more than good enough for me. Every now and then it pops up in a greengrocer away from the Leicester area, so if you see any, grab it instantly, because you know it won't be there for long.

Practicalities

BUYING One of the characteristics I adore about sprouting broccoli is the subtle three-in-one structure. This vegetable is not just about soft florets, nor flapping leaves, nor firm stem. It is about all three, clamped together in one package. So, when you are buying look for the healthiest specimens with a good complement of substantial leaves (as usual, drooping leaves are an indicator of staleness), to balance the stalk and sprouting end. Very thick lower stems will be too tough to enjoy, but they can be cut out. Over-trimmed sprouting broccoli, on the other hand, arouses my suspicions; what is someone trying to hide? Avoid, too, any sprouting broccoli with a hint of that sulphurous scent that mars stale brassicas of all sorts.

Sure, sprouting broccoli will 'keep' for some days in the vegetable drawer of the fridge, but it's a crying shame not to get it into the pan and on to the plate as soon as you possibly can. In fact, if you want to taste it at its very best, head off to a farmers' market or good farm shop in late winter, ask for stems that have been cut within the past 24 hours, and get it cooked on the very same day. Now that's the way to treat sprouting broccoli as it deserves. Idealistic, perhaps, but there's no harm in aiming high.

COOKING There is only one way to cook incredibly fresh sprouting broccoli. Having trimmed off tougher stalk ends, plunge it into a pan of **boiling salted water** and cook it for just long enough to soften the stems without overdoing it.

I'm thinking 4–5 minutes. Drain it well, then serve hot with nothing more than an enhancing sauce or melted butter, or a little excellent olive oil and a big squeeze of lemon juice. Fabulous, fabulous stuff. Don't try to get too inventive sauce-wise. There's no point. Things that go well with sprouting broccoli are orange, lemon, anchovies, black olives, garlic, chilli, subtle spices, butter, olive oil. I love it dressed with a hollandaise scented with Seville orange juice and zest if the two seasons coincide, replaceable with the zest and juice of a blood orange, if not. Or a very lemony beurre blanc (see below). Or with a warm anchovy and garlic dressing – cook chopped garlic and anchovy fillets gently in olive oil, mashing the anchovy down to a pulp, then season with lots of pepper and, off the heat, either red wine vinegar or lemon juice. For those who cannot be persuaded that anchovies are a good thing, replace them with finely chopped red chilli.

When you have sprouting broccoli that is just a tad below perfection (or if you just fancy a change), try giving it the slow treatment. In other words, **braise it** with almost no water, for some 40 minutes or so. The result is amazingly good, with new mellow notes introduced to replace the vigour of exquisite freshness. The palate of complementary ingredients remains much the same but I'd leave butter out of this approach altogether, replacing it with a lick of olive oil.

I dare say you could get clever with sprouting broccoli – tempura, perhaps, or tartlets, or adding it to more complex dishes like a risotto – but I wouldn't do it myself. This is one great vegetable and it demands (discreetly, quietly, politely) to be treated with respect.

SEE ALSO BROCCOLI, CALABRESE (PAGE 328).

* *

Braised sprouting broccoli with garlic and chillies

I love this long gentle method of braising sprouting broccoli with a splash of wine and a helping of sliced garlic and hot chilli. Of course, you can play about with the basic premise to your heart's content. Replace the wine with water or stock if you wish. Add a handful of black olives halfway through the cooking time. My children love it braised with sun-dried tomatoes (but then they'd eat practically anything if it had sun-dried tomatoes in it). Mostly I serve broccoli cooked this way hot or warm, but if there is any left over it is excellent served next day at room temperature, with a squeeze of fresh lemon juice to sharpen.

Serves 4–6 as a side dish or first course

750 g (1 lb 10 oz) sprouting broccoli
4 tablespoons extra virgin olive oil
6 cloves garlic, sliced
2 dried red chillies, broken into small pieces
250 ml (9 fl oz) dry white wine
salt and pepper

Trim the broccoli and cut off any really thick lower stems. If necessary (to fit into the pan), cut in half.

Cover the base of a wide, deep, heavy frying pan or saucepan with a thin layer of olive oil. Cover with a thick layer of sprouting broccoli. Scatter over half the garlic, the chilli, salt and pepper and half the remaining oil. Repeat the layers. Pour over the wine. Cover and cook over a very gentle heat for 40–60 minutes until the liquid has almost all evaporated. Check and turn the broccoli occasionally and if absolutely necessary add a splash of water or more wine, to prevent burning.

Spoon the tender broccoli into a serving dish and serve swiftly.

* *

Sprouting broccoli with lemon beurre blanc

A recipe for celebrating wonderfully fresh sprouting broccoli as a course on its own. Beurre blanc is a sauce with a scary reputation which it doesn't deserve at all. It takes only minutes to make once the shallots have been softened. The trick is to get the heat just right – not too hot, but not so cool that the butter doesn't melt. I simply draw the pan on and off the heat as I whisk to keep the sauce from splitting. If it does – oily hairline streaks indicate that the worst has happened – whip the pan off the heat and plunge the base into a bowl of iced water (it's not a bad idea to have one standing by, just in case). Keep on whisking.

Serves 6

1 kg (2¼ lb) best white or purple
  sprouting broccoli, trimmed
salt

Lemon beurre blanc
40 g (1½ oz) shallots, finely chopped
2 tablespoons lemon juice
175 g (6 oz) unsalted butter, diced and chilled

Up to an hour or two before eating, put the shallots into a small pan with the lemon juice and 3 tablespoons water. Simmer gently until nearly all the liquid has evaporated, leaving behind roughly a tablespoon and a half of juice and the cooked shallots. Reserve in the pan until needed.

Bring a large pan of salted water to the boil, and add the broccoli. Bring back to the boil, then simmer for around 4 minutes until just tender. Drain well and tip into a hot serving dish. Keep warm while you finish the sauce.

Reheat the shallot mixture, adding a splash more water if necessary. Keeping the heat low, start whisking in cubes of butter, a small handful at a time. When one lot is nearly all whisked in, add the next, and then the next to make a thick, pale and creamy sauce. When all the butter is mixed in, draw off the heat and season with salt. The sauce should taste distinctly lemony to balance the other ingredients, but if you feel it is too sharp, whisk in a little more butter to balance it. Serve immediately with the broccoli.

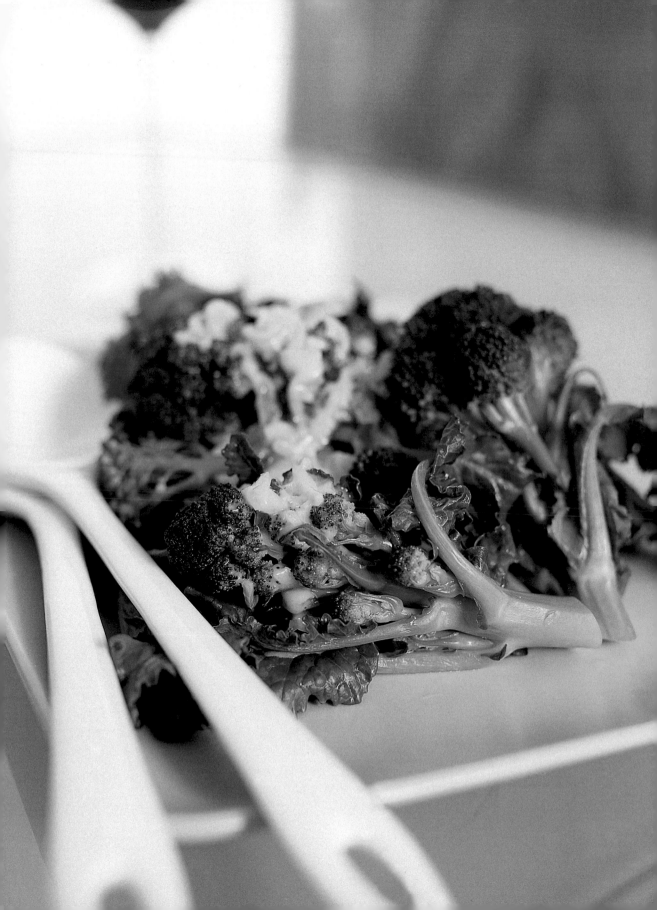

Brussels sprouts

* * *

It must be a sign of growing up – my twelve-year-old daughter has finally admitted that Brussels sprouts are okay. No more than that, but at least it's a step in the right direction. An appreciation of the humble sprout is something that comes with a degree of maturity. Some people never reach either, but most of us end up with a fondness for the Christmas vegetable incarnate, and at least an outward appearance of maturity.

Sprouts are, when you think about it, the original miniature designer vegetable. Tiny green cabbages, growing conveniently all the way up a stem. Cute, neat and compact bite-size nobbles, that luckily don't carry a designer price tag. Who could resist? The rub is that shy edge of bitterness, exacerbated all too often by overcooking. Luckily, that doesn't need to be a hindrance any more, because modern varieties of sprouts have been bred to reduce this element to no more than a comfortable balance. Freshness, naturally, is critical – that sulphur note grows with age. It can also be exacerbated by overcooking, but I'm sure that is not a crime you would commit even under the direst of circumstances. So cook sprouts with enthusiasm and cheeriness secure in the knowledge that this is one designer vegetable that has as much substance as style.

Practicalities

BUYING First choose sprouts that look lively and fresh. Not too many damaged exterior leaves, certainly not wrinkled, limp looking ones. If your sprouts have been hanging around on the shelf for an age, they will be stinky and there's not much remedying it. Smaller sprouts have more of that lovely,

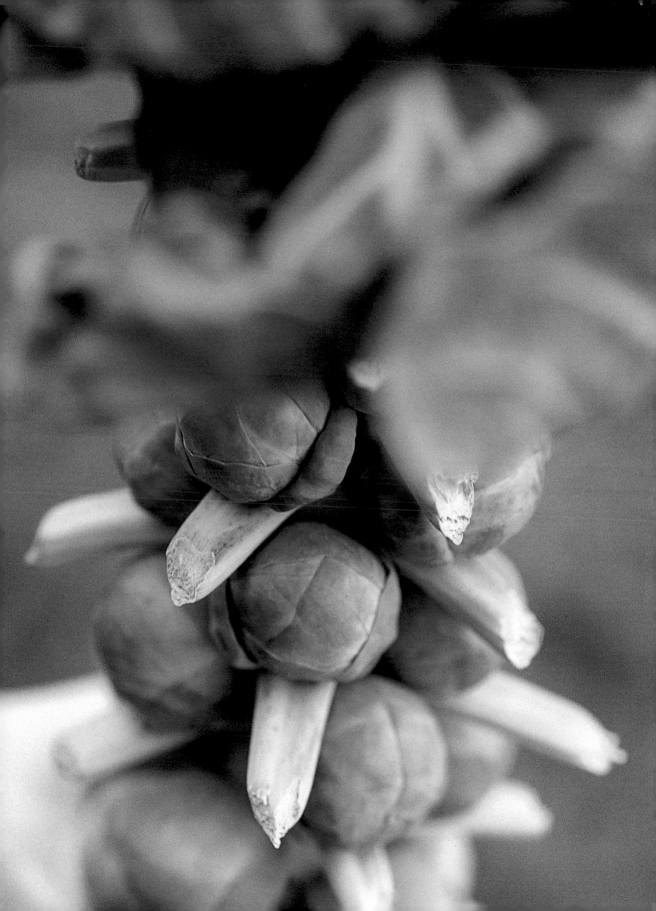

nutty taste but will take longer to prepare, pound for pound. Or kilo for kilo. Sprouts on the stem are a good buy since they stay fresher for longer, though you may pay extra for the privilege of slicing them off yourself. Sprouts should be cooked as soon as is reasonable after buying. A couple of days in the vegetable drawer of the fridge is okay. Much longer is a no-no. If you have a stem of sprouts, slice them off with a small sharp knife. Loose sprouts will need to have their bases trimmed. Remove any damaged outer leaves, then rinse the sprouts under the tap. *Don't* cut a cross in the base of each sprout. A weird, dated custom that just makes sprouts soggier than they should be.

Sprouts need relatively little time in **boiling salted water**, but it's impossible to be more precise than that about cooking times. Very small sprouts may be done in 4 minutes, but the only way to tell is to prod one with a knife and maybe cut it open and take a bite. If it is to be served straightaway, the sprout should be just tender with a touch of crispness lingering at the heart. If you intend to let them cool, and finish them in some other way, be sure to drain them when they retain some considerable crispness. It is far, far preferable to serve sprouts that are undercooked, than overcooked. In fact, raw sprouts are really rather good, so as long as sprouts are well heated through, you needn't worry.

Hot sprouts straight from the pan demand a touch of butter, or a drizzle of lemon olive oil, or perhaps a sprinkling of sesame oil. You could concoct a flavoured butter (butter, lemon zest, soft-leaved herbs, a spritz of lemon juice, all mashed together) to melt over them if you wanted to give them a small boost. Otherwise, I'd suggest that you cook sprouts a little in advance, rinse them under the cold tap as soon as they have been drained, then leave them to cool. Now they are easy to reheat with added extras that will be drawn a short way into the fabric of each sprout itself.

The best-known combination is that of chestnuts and Brussels sprouts, which is so good that it ought to be outed more than once a year on Christmas Day. For this I usually pre-cook sprouts and chestnuts (fresh if I'm in virtuous mode, vacuum-packed otherwise), then reheat them together in butter, perhaps with some shallot that has been gently fried too. The trick is to get both sprouts and chestnuts hot, hot, hot without burning the butter. A moderate to gentle heat does the business.

Why stick rigorously to the classics? You could reheat your sprouts in olive oil, with chopped garlic, dried chilli flakes and finish with a sprinkle of parsley. Or toss hot sprouts with toasted almonds, or chopped roasted hazelnuts. All excellent combinations.

Don't stop there. Brussels sprouts are also very good **sautéed** or **stir-fried** (quarter first), so that their edges catch and brown, taking on that soft-crisp texture that is so appealing. Mix them with other vegetables – peppers or strips of carrot, or a simple pile of sliced onions – and the classic ginger, garlic, chilli trio.

* *

Fried Brussels sprouts and chicory with garlic and chilli

Sprouts, but not as you know them.... Slow frying in olive oil develops an underlying sweetness that is brought to life by a hint of bitterness from the chicory and the spice of garlic and chilli. For prettiness' sake, use a head of red chicory if you find one, but if bitterness is not your cup of tea, replace the chicory with 85 g (3 oz) shredded white cabbage to give contrasting texture. The sliced sprouts soften more in the heat than the quartered ones, to vary the texture once more. Serve this as a side dish with a plainly cooked lamb chop, or a plain roast chicken, or even slices of cold turkey on Boxing Day.

Serves 3–4

500 g (1 lb 2 oz) Brussels sprouts, trimmed
1 large head chicory, sliced into discs
3 tablespoons extra virgin olive oil
2 large cloves garlic, chopped

1 dried hot red chilli, crumbled
1 tablespoon white wine vinegar
Maldon salt, or ordinary salt

Slice half the Brussels into 5 mm (¼ in) thick discs, and quarter the remainder. Heat the olive oil in a wide frying pan over a moderate heat. Add the sprouts and fry, stirring lazily, for about 4 minutes. Now add the chicory and continue with that lazy stirring for another 6 minutes or so. Scatter over the garlic and chilli, and fry for another minute or so. Season with salt, and drizzle over the vinegar. Stir once more, then taste and adjust seasoning.

* *

Gratin of Brussels sprouts with lardons, cream and almonds

This is the luxury end of the Brussels sprout spectrum, and how they love that cream. A special dish, that turns sprouts into gorgeous starlets. There is no better way to consume sprouts.

Serves 4–6

675 g (1½ lb) Brussels sprouts, trimmed
100 g (3½ oz) lardons, or back bacon
  cut into strips
15 g (½ oz) flaked almonds
15 g (½ oz) butter
1 tablespoon sunflower oil

300 ml (10 fl oz) double cream
a dash of lemon juice
4 tablespoons fresh breadcrumbs
3 tablespoons Parmesan, freshly grated
salt and pepper

Preheat the oven to 200°C/400°F/Gas 6. Simmer the sprouts in salted water until almost but not quite cooked (around 4 minutes). Drain thoroughly, and cut in half.

Sauté the lardons and almonds in the butter and oil in a wide frying pan until lightly browned. Add the sprouts and cook for a further 2–3 minutes, stirring almost constantly. Add the double cream, bring up to the boil, and let it bubble away merrily for some 2–4 minutes until reduced to a rich sauce. Season with a touch of salt and plenty of pepper.

Draw off the heat, stir in a dash of lemon juice, then spoon into a gratin dish. Mix the breadcrumbs and Parmesan, and scatter evenly over the sprouts. Bake for about 20 minutes until the top is golden brown, with the cream bubbling through seductively here and there. Serve when the cream has quietened down a little.

* *

Cabbage

* * *

Cabbage comes in multiple shapes and colours and sizes. It remains one of the most universally recognised vegetables, along with potatoes and onions and carrots. In one form or another it is part of the absolute everyday experience of practically everyone in temperate climates across the world. No wonder we take it for granted – cabbage is cheap, cabbage is good for you, cabbage is everywhere and it takes a major trip to exotic lands to escape it…

A major success story, in other words. And one that begins, for once, in Europe and our own shores. Wild cabbage is a native plant, the parent (a mere 3,000 years ago) of all the brassicas, in other words not only of cabbages, but also of broccoli and cauliflower and turnips and spring greens and numerous others. What a dynasty that wild cabbage founded.

Cabbages proper fall roughly into three overlapping, interlocking groups. There are the **hard-headed**, solid as a rock, compact cabbages of which your standard white cabbage is the most common. Then there are the looser leaved, less densely packed **green cabbages**, still round but of less use as a weapon of war. **Savoy cabbage**, with its beautiful crinkled green leaves, reigns supreme in this group. And then there are the **green pointy cabbages**, such as the spring cabbage, least densely packed of all. I've given **red cabbage** a section all to itself, though rightly it falls in with group one.

Do I have a preference? Not particularly. For coleslaw I'd always reach for a white cabbage, for roasting I prefer a looser leafed variety, and the Savoy is indisputably the looker of the family. Thereafter I'm happy with any of them as long, naturally, as it is perky and fresh. The curse of the brassica clan is that miserable stench of sulphur that intensifies as they become stale. One of the most dismaying smells I know is that of overcooked stale cabbage. Lingering in the entrance to a pub or restaurant, it proclaims loudly that this is not somewhere to come for a meal.

Practicalities

A happy, promising cabbage has firm crisp leaves showing no signs of wilting. It doesn't smell of anything but mild greenery. Odd blemishes on the outer leaves are nothing to worry about – just nature at work.

Compact white cabbages have considerable keeping power, but they won't gain anything through long storage. Quite the opposite, and of course, you won't know how long they've been kept on hold in wholesalers' and supermarkets' stores. Ergo, don't hang on to them just because you can, and just because they look as good as the day you brought them home. All cabbages benefit from being eaten sooner rather than later.

To prepare a white cabbage, slice a thin disc off the base, then quarter the whole cabbage cutting through the base. Now it is easy to cut out the central core from each quarter. Finish by shredding the cabbage by cutting across each quarter.

Leafier cabbages are prepared in similar fashion. Remove the most damaged outer leaves and discard. Pare off the browned base. Quarter the cabbage through the base. At this point, it's a good idea to rinse out insects and lingering dirt, before coring and shredding, if that's what you intend to do. With very loose-leafed cabbages, you may want to keep leaves whole – either because you like the look of them, or maybe because you want to stuff them. So, just slice off a thicker disc of base, so that the outer leaves come away at the same time, and then another, and so on, until you've progressed as far as you can. Depending on the variety of cabbage, you may or may not be left with a compact heart, which can be cooked whole, or quartered or shredded. Rinse the whole leaves after separating.

To enjoy cabbage you must either cook it briefly or for a long time. Anything in between spells disaster. By briefly, I mean a strict 3–4 minutes in **boiling salted water** or a **stew**, or up to 5 minutes in **a wok**. No more. The long time means at least 40 minutes in the oven, an hour or more of braising slowly, and so on. The results are totally different in taste, and both potentially superb.

Fresh cabbage, shredded, **blanched** for a mere 3 minutes, well drained, needs no embellishment. Now and then, however, you might like to dress it up a little just for a change. My top play on plain cabbage is to toss it in hot melted butter with a handful of caraway seeds – a popular German

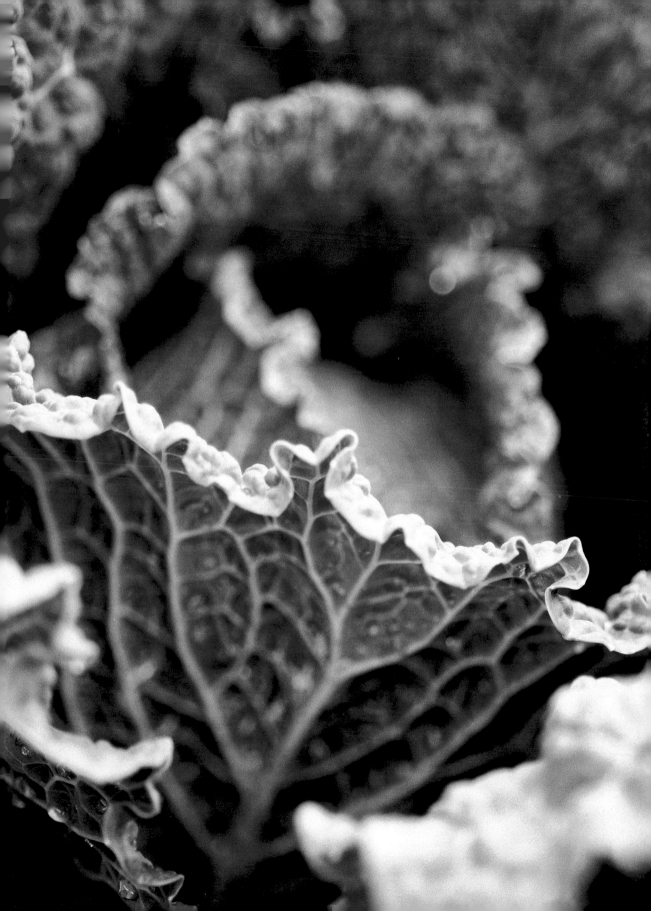

combination. Why stop there, though? Give it a citrus lift by dressing with butter and finely grated lemon or orange zest. Or take it further afield by adding a heaped teaspoonful of poppy seeds or coal-black kalonji seeds (black onion seeds) to a little hot oil, cooking for a few seconds, then tossing into the hot cabbage. For an Indian touch replace the poppy seeds with black mustard seeds and fry until they begin to pop. Quickly add cumin seeds and a spot of turmeric, then toss in the cabbage. Cabbage and bacon is always a winner – fry lardons or strips of streaky bacon and sliced shallots until the bacon is browned, then mix in the cabbage.

Shred any kind of cabbage thinly and it will **stir-fry** very nicely. You may want to keep it pure – scent the oil with chopped garlic and a touch of ginger if you wish, then toss in the cabbage and keep it moving until crisp-tender and patched here and there with brown. Alternatively, bulk it out with other vegetables – sticks of carrot, peppers in the summer, mangetout, leeks, or whatever comes to hand.

If you've never tasted **slow-cooked** cabbage, then it comes as a bit of a revelation. Like discovering a new vegetable. A sweet, nutty mellowness is exposed. I adore roasted cabbage (see below), but am equally taken with cabbage that has been braised very gently with a little stock (not even enough to cover – the cabbage will produce its own liquid), a big knob of butter, salt, pepper and nothing more. Keep the pan covered tightly, and let it burble away incredibly gently for at least 60 minutes, only adding more liquid if it threatens to burn dry (reduce the heat if you can).

It's not the usual way to tackle cabbage, but **roasting** can work spectacularly well. For this I prefer to use a slightly looser leaved cabbage – one of the spring cabbages, leaves furled snugly into a cone. All you do is quarter the cabbage lengthways into wedges (if it is large then cut into six wedges), turn in a little olive oil, season with coarse salt and roast uncovered in a hot oven (around 200°C/400°F/Gas 6) for some 40 minutes or so, turning once or twice, until the edges of the leaves are caught with brown and the stem is tender. Serve just as it is, or add a dash of sharpness in the form of a squeeze of lemon or a little balsamic or rice vinegar.

Finally, don't forget that the humble white cabbage is the essential ingredient in what has to be the most misrepresented **salad** in the world – coleslaw. Commercial coleslaw is almost invariably foul. Home-made is terrific, especially when made with real mayonnaise (see page 35) which takes no more than 3–4 minutes to knock up in a liquidiser or processor. Mix the cabbage, with grated carrot, thinly sliced onion if you like it (I use a red onion) and just enough lemony mayonnaise to coat. Eat it straightaway for a crunchy salad, or let it sit around for an hour or so to soften the cabbage – just remember to stir again before serving. I often vary my coleslaw by adding grated apple, or a handful of currants and toasted sunflower seeds, or plenty of chopped fresh parsley, chives, a modicum of tarragon and so on. To lighten it, I might replace half the mayo with yoghurt. My favourite dolled-up coleslaw, however, has to be the mango version below.

SEE ALSO RED CABBAGE AND SPRING GREENS (PAGES 362 AND 390).

* *

Mango and coriander coleslaw

This particular form of coleslaw is, I think, an outstanding success. I just love the transformation of pedestrian, everyday cabbage and carrot into a rather exotic softly spiced salad. When choosing a mango for this salad, pick a larger one that is still too firm to make the grade in the fruit salad. It's the combination of mild tartness and fruity fragrance that makes it work so well.

Serves 6–8

1 tablespoon coriander seeds
1 dessertspoon cumin seeds
¼ white cabbage
1 large carrot, coarsely grated
  (about 200 g/7 oz)
1 under-ripe mango, peeled and
  coarsely grated

2 handfuls coriander leaves, roughly
  chopped
juice of 2 limes
3 tablespoons sunflower oil
salt and pepper

Dry-fry the coriander and cumin seeds together over a moderate heat until they turn a shade or two darker and give off an intoxicating scent. Tip at once into a mortar or the bowl of your spice-grinder. Leave to cool, then grind to a fine powder.

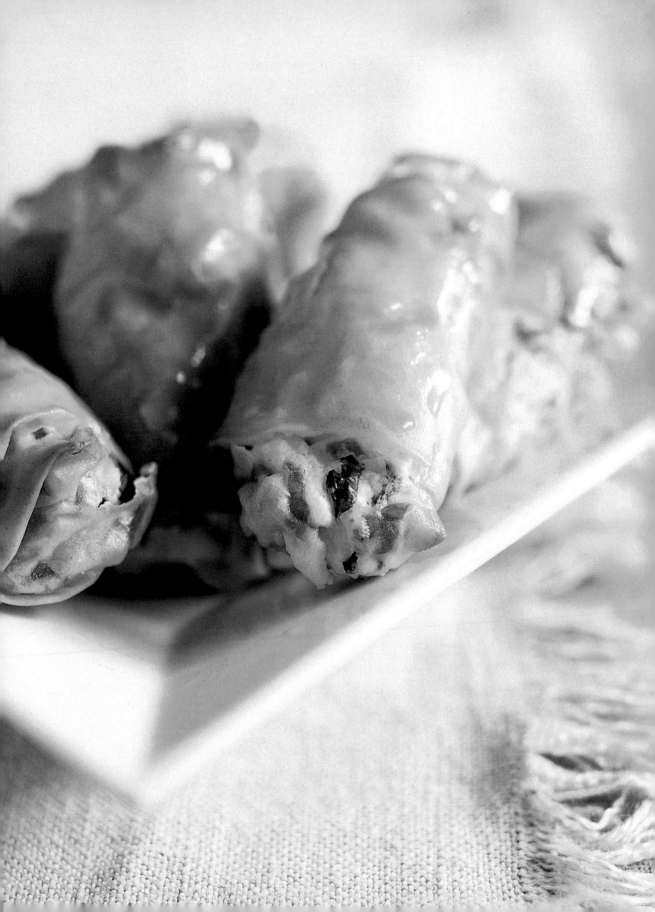

Cut out the solid wedge of stalk in the cabbage quarter then slice the remainder as thinly as you can. Mix with all the remaining ingredients adding as much of the spice mix as you like (I used it all, but there's no obligation to follow suit if you prefer a more subtle spicing). Eat within the next hour or so to enjoy the flavours at their best.

* *

Spring cabbage, feta and olive filo cigars

Crisp on the outside and melting inside, these filo pastry cigars are utterly delicious. They can be prepared several hours in advance and stored in the fridge until you are ready to bake. Serve them as a starter (two per person should be enough), or as a main course (allow three or four each, depending on appetite), accompanying them with a fresh tomato salad, and some new potatoes.

Makes 14–16

200–250g (7–9oz) filo pastry
85g (3oz) butter, melted

Filling
½ spring cabbage, trimmed of
  damaged leaves
150g (5oz) feta cheese, crumbled

85g (3oz) cream cheese
60g (2oz) black olives (weighed with
  their stones in), stoned and chopped
2 tablespoons chopped parsley
2 tablespoons chopped mint
salt and pepper

Preheat the oven to 190°C/375°F/Gas 5.

To make the filling, cut the cabbage in half lengthways, and cut out the core. Slice the leaves, then blanch in boiling salted water for about 4 minutes until tender. Drain thoroughly, then squeeze out the last of water with your hands. Chop roughly, and mix with all the remaining filling ingredients. Go carefully with the salt, as both the feta and the olives will already be quite salty.

Cut the filo pastry into strips about 15 cm (6 in) wide by around 23–30 cm (9–12 in) long – take this as a rough guide, adapting it to the size and shape of the sheets of filo. Place in a heap on the work surface, and cover with a sheet of clingfilm, covered in turn by a clean tea-towel wrung out in cold water, to prevent the filo from drying out.

Take the first strip and brush with melted butter. Place a good tablespoon of the filling at one end of the pastry. Form into a sausage shape about 10 cm (4 in) long, running parallel to one of the narrower sides. Flip the long sides of the filo over to enclose the ends, then roll up neatly. Place on a lightly buttered baking sheet. Repeat with the remaining filo and filling until all used up. Brush the tops of the 'cigars' with the last of the butter.

Bake for 10–15 minutes until golden brown. Eat hot or warm.

* *

Stir-fried Savoy cabbage with garlic and pine nuts

The natural sweetness of crinkled Savoy cabbage is brought out by stir-frying, and marrying it with sliced garlic and buttery pine nuts. Very different from your usual blanched cabbage, and barely any more effort.

Serves 3–4

½ Savoy cabbage, cut into
   1 cm (½ in) wide strips
2 tablespoons sunflower or vegetable oil
30 g (1 oz) pine nuts

4 cloves garlic, thinly sliced
2.5 cm (1 in) fresh root ginger, peeled
   and cut into matchsticks
½–1 tablespoon light soy sauce

Prepare and measure all the ingredients and arrange them in order of use, beside the hob.

Heat a roomy wok over a high heat until it begins to smoke. Add 1 table-spoon oil. Now add the pine nuts, garlic and ginger and stir-fry until the pine nuts and garlic are lightly browned. Be sure to keep everything moving so that it cooks evenly. Scrape the garlic, nuts and ginger out into a bowl.

Return the wok to the heat, and add the second tablespoon of oil. Next tip in the Savoy cabbage, and stir-fry, still over a high heat, for some 4–5 minutes until it is crisp-tender, and patched with brown here and there.

Return the cooked ingredients to the pan, add the smaller amount of soy sauce and stir for a few seconds to mix. Taste to see if the blend is salty enough and if necessary add a little more soy sauce. Serve immediately.

* *

Verzada
Slow-cooked cabbage with sausages

Cabbage and pork, pork and cabbage. Together so often you'd think they were having an affair. Proximity is at the root of this attraction – across Europe they've fed the poor for centuries, and it's only natural that they end up, time and again, in the same pot. And don't they taste good together. This northern Italian blend of slowly braised cabbage and sausages is a prime example of the coupling. Simple, cheap food to sustain the weariest soul. Serve it Italian-style with a mound of steaming, golden polenta, or go for the other natural companion, a big scoop of mashed potato.

Incidentally, like many slow-cooked dishes, this one reheats beautifully.

Serves 4

1 large white cabbage
8 Italian pork sausages, or good-quality
  British style pork sausages
30 g (1 oz) butter

1 onion, thinly sliced
85 g (3 oz) pancetta cubes or lardons
2 tablespoons white wine vinegar
salt and lots of pepper

Preheat the grill. Quarter the cabbage and discard the outer leaves. Cut the thick stalk out of each quarter, then shred the leaves into strips about 1 cm (½ in) thick. Grill the sausages swiftly, close to the heat, until browned (this is just to give them a bit of colour; they don't have to be properly cooked through at this stage).

Melt the butter in a large heavy-based pan, and add the onion and pancetta or lardons. Fry until the onion is tender but not brown. Add the cabbage and stir well so that the leaves are coated with fat. Fry for about 4 minutes then drizzle over the vinegar and season with salt and lots of pepper. Arrange the sausages on top of the cabbage, tip over any juice that they have exuded, cover the pan and cook very gently for 1 hour. Check the pan occasionally, and give it a stir once in a while. You shouldn't need to add any liquid at all, but if your lid doesn't fit too well, add a tablespoonful or two of water when necessary to prevent burning.

* *

Cauliflower

* * *

If it weren't so familiar, the cauliflower would be regarded as a bizarre-looking vegetable, hidden away inside its swaddling of green leaves. It could be a piece of petrified cloud or a fossilised cotton-wool puff, wrapped in a green silk casing. No point getting too fanciful about it though, because I doubt that I will ever convince anyone that it is a vegetable of rare distinction. Cauliflower is a handsome vegetable, a stalwart, a reliable friend of a vegetable, but no glamour-puss.

I'm fond of cauliflower, but it needs to be handled with respect. I've endured too much overcooked cauliflower in my lifetime to ever become passionate about it. That's the trouble with cauliflower, really. It's only worth eating when it is a) perfectly fresh and b) perfectly cooked (or raw). Old stinky cauliflower is shaming, and so too is disintegrating, grey, waterlogged and over-boiled cauli. Put them together and you have a recipe for disaster. No wonder they disguised it with blankets of gluey cheese sauce at school.

Cauliflower cheese was only redeemed for me when I discovered the stylish **Romanesco cauliflower**. This is the one that comes in a most fetching pale green guise, with its curds spiralling upwards in nifty designer cones.

According to my gardening books it is actually a form of broccoli, but it cooks just like cauliflower, which is why I mention it here. It also tastes much the same as standard cauliflower. Memories of the miserable cauliflower cheese of my school days were dispelled when I napped the green whorls of Romanesco with a rich cheese sauce, seasoned with Parmesan and lots of nutmeg.

Cape broccoli is another colourful cauliflower, with light purple curds instead of white. Again, the taste is pretty much the same as an ordinary cauli. Naturally, you pay for the pleasure of having colourful cauliflower, but for anyone who, like me, suffered cauliflower nightmares as a child, this may be a premium worth paying.

Practicalities

BUYING Look for cauliflowers that are still attractively cradled by green leaves. These leaves are your first clue to freshness. If they are firm and perky, then you are probably on to a winner. The curds themselves, tucked inside, should be a beautiful ivory colour – some will be whiter than others but that's more to do with variety than quality. The odd blemish is not necessarily a bad sign, but anything more than a few spots of brown is a warning that all is not as it should be. Finally, and this is more blatant on a warm day than a chilly one, sniff the air around your chosen cauli. Is there a whiff of stale, sulphurous brassica? If there is, move on and re-plan your menu with some other vegetable.

Mini-cauliflowers, those little one-portion tiddlers, are comparatively expensive. I have bought them on occasion but usually wonder why I bothered later on. There is some justification when you are cooking for one or two only and don't want to be downing cauliflower for days on end, but other than that they are an expensive frivolity.

Cauliflower should be used within a couple of days of purchase, though it will keep in an apparently unimpaired state for far longer in the vegetable drawer of your fridge. Of course, it is still edible as long as it remains firm, but staleness will be setting in, edging the cauli towards the second-rate offering that it shouldn't be.

Preparation depends on how you intend to cook the cauliflower. Most of the time you will probably want to cut and break it up into florets, for speedy cooking. So, trim off the base and remove all but the palest, smallest of leaves (which taste pretty good), then use both knife and hands to reduce the head to small, suitably sized pieces. If there are a few brown patches on the surface, just cut them off first.

When you want to cook the head whole, trim and remove leaves, then cut a cross in the base to encourage more even cooking. I make a sort of a harness for it by folding over two lengths of silver foil to form two shiny 'straps', then laying them across each other at right angles and placing the cauliflower head in the centre. By bringing the four ends of the straps up and around the cauli I can lift it safely in and out of a pan of boiling water without damage.

Florets and whole heads alike are usually cooked in **simmering salted water**. Timing is all, but varies radically in relation to size. Small florets may need no more than 2 or 3 minutes, larger ones may take up to 5. A whole head will take a good deal longer – 10–15 minutes or more, but don't leave it to chance. Cauliflower needs to be checked regularly and remember that it is far, far better to undercook than overcook. So, how do you know when it is done just so? Prodding and tasting – you should be able to push a skewer into a piece with just a modicum of pressure. If it slides in too easily, then you've overdone it. Drain quickly, run under the cold tap and assess the damage. Just too soft and it can be rescued by puréeing with a knob of butter and a little cream, then finishing with maybe a scraping of Parmesan and nutmeg. If it is collapsing, then I'd suggest chucking it straight in the bin.

When testing a whole head of cauli, remember that it will carry on cooking in its own heat for longer than small florets. In other words, the centre should still be fairly firm when you haul it out of the pan.

Steaming (or **microwaving** in small quantity) is an excellent way of cooking cauliflower, allowing a mite more room for manoeuvre on timing. It works particularly well if you are cooking the whole head.

Broken into pieces – fairly large ones – cauliflower is surprisingly good **roasted** in a hot oven. Toss it with a little olive oil and a few sprigs of thyme or a couple of bay leaves and give it around 30 minutes at 220°C/425°F/Gas 7 until browned and tender. I'm not too keen on marrying garlic with cauliflower, but the addition of a little chilli won't go amiss.

As long as the florets are cut pretty small, cauliflower can also be successfully **stir-fried**, either mixed with other vegetables (lovely with mangetouts and cashew nuts, for instance) or on its own, finished with a handful of sliced spring onion and a drizzle of lemon olive oil, or Middle Eastern sumac when you can get it.

PARTNERS Matching cauliflower with other flavours is more hazardous than with many vegetables. It's one of the rare vegetables that isn't enormously enhanced by garlic, although there are exceptions to this rule. I wouldn't at all mind settling down to a helping of lightly cooked cauliflower embellished with brown-fried garlic and chilli sizzled in olive oil, for instance, but I don't think it should go anywhere near cauliflower cheese, or roasted cauliflower.

And that brings me to cheese, which is a natural friend to any cauliflower. When making cauliflower cheese, don't skimp on the sauce. Give it plenty of time to simmer to a caressing richness and flavour it with lots of Parmesan and a little bit of mature Cheddar or vintage Gruyère so that the sauce is not too heavy. Nutmeg is important, too, and you might also add a couple of spoonfuls of mustard. When you haven't time to make a good white sauce, try dolloping a generous amount of crème fraîche on to the cauliflower packed snugly in a shallow heatproof dish, then sprinkling a thick layer of grated cheese over the top and sliding it straight under the grill. The result is excellent, though rather richer than the traditional dish.

Cauliflower goes well with nuts, particularly almonds (a scattering of toasted or fried flaked almonds is a pleasing way to dress up plain cauliflower), and with poppy seeds in which case just fry them briefly in a little oil or butter before spooning over. Herbs like tarragon, mint and parsley all work well, but the more perfumed fragrance of basil is overwhelming.

Perhaps one of the most delicious ways of eating cauliflower is in a salad, either raw (make the florets small) or lightly blanched to soften them slightly. Dress blanched cauliflower while still warm so that it absorbs some of the dressing as it cools. My friend Annabel makes a lovely cauliflower salad, tossing the lightly blanched cauliflower first in a little vinaigrette, then in mayonnaise once cooled, along with toasted almond flakes and chopped parsley. To this you might add pieces of tomato, deseeded and cut into thick slices, or a tumble of watercress or rocket, or some crisp croûtons.

* *

Deep-fried cauliflower with sweet, sour and hot dressing

Definitely first-course material, this – utterly unexpected and utterly delicious. If you have never eaten deep-fried cauliflower before then you will be amazed at how good and how different it tastes. I met it first in one of Oxford's surprisingly large collection of Lebanese restaurants, but in this recipe it is partnered with a vibrant South-East Asian hot, sour and sweet dipping sauce. Using the whole lime adds a note of bitterness to the sauce which I love, as well as blending in the fragrant essential oils from the zest. If whole chunks of lime fail to tempt, then just use the juice to make a less complex blend.

Serves 4

½ large cauliflower, or a whole small
  cauliflower
sunflower or vegetable oil for deep-frying
salt

Dressing
1 clove garlic, roughly chopped
2 hot red chillies, deseeded and roughly
  chopped
a small handful of mint leaves
2 tablespoons caster sugar
1 lime, quartered then cut into small pieces
2 tablespoons fish sauce
1 tablespoon water

To make the dressing, pound the garlic, chillies and mint with the sugar until you have a smooth paste. Now add the lime pieces, and pound vigorously to squeeze out all the lime and break up the skin. Mix in the fish sauce and water. Taste and adjust seasoning.

Break the cauliflower into florets and blanch in boiling salted water for 5 minutes. Drain well, and dry on kitchen paper. Heat a pan of oil to a temperature of around 180°C/350°F. Test by dropping a small piece of cauliflower into the oil; it should fizzle and bubble around it and the cauliflower should brown within about 45 seconds to a minute. Deep-fry the remaining cauliflower in batches, draining on kitchen paper for a few seconds, before serving with the dipping sauce on the side.

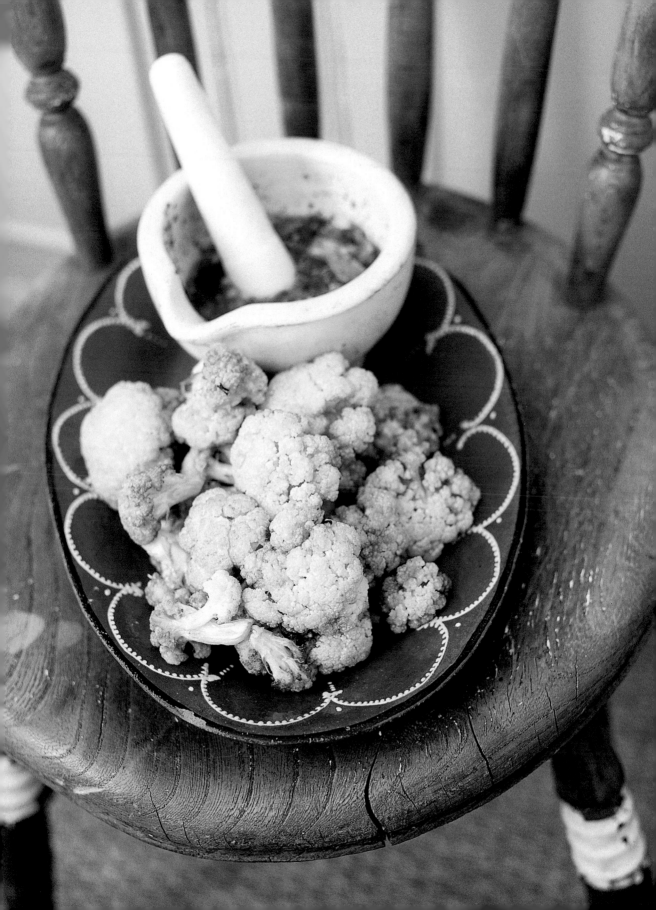

* *

Smoked cauliflower cheese soup

It may have crossed my path before, but the only memorable cauliflower cheese soup I've savoured in recent years was served up in the grand hall at Christchurch College in Oxford. Until, that is, I made my own version using a slab of particularly fine smoked Cheddar that I'd been hoarding for a suitable occasion.

If you want to make the soup in advance and reheat it, stop at the point where the vegetables and stock are liquidised. Only stir in the cheese just before serving.

Serves 6

1 cauliflower, broken into florets
1 large onion
1 medium floury potato, peeled and
  cut into cubes
2 cloves garlic, sliced
1 bouquet garni (2 sprigs parsley, 1 bay leaf,
  1 generous sprig thyme, tied together
  with string)
30 g (1 oz) butter
1 litre (1¾ pints) chicken or
  vegetable stock

100 g (3½ oz) smoked Cheddar,
  coarsely grated
salt and pepper

To serve
1–2 of the following: a shake of cayenne
  pepper, chopped parsley or chives,
  croûtons, or a dollop of soured cream

Sweat the vegetables, garlic and bouquet garni with the butter in a covered pan over a low heat for 10 minutes, stirring once or twice. Add the stock, a little salt and loads and loads of pepper and bring up to the boil. Simmer until the cauliflower and potato are just tender and no more. Remove the bouquet garni and liquidise the soup, adding more stock or a little milk to thin it down as necessary.

Just before serving, reheat thoroughly, but keep the soup just short of a boil. Stir in two-thirds of the cheese, taste and see if you think it needs more. Add it if it does. Taste one more time and if you are satisfied, proceed to serve the soup with cayenne, parsley, chives, croutons or cream as circumstances suggest.

* *

Potato and cauliflower curry

Stranded in Delhi airport, I eventually found my way to a small canteen somewhere down a long grey corridor. The only item on the menu? Potato and cauliflower curry. It did a great job of consoling me in the face of a flightless future. Eventually, I made it back home, and ever since I've had a big soft spot for this Indian favourite.

Serves 4

1 onion, chopped
3 cloves garlic, chopped
4 cm (1½ in) piece fresh root ginger, roughly
  chopped
2 red chillies, deseeded and roughly
  chopped
3 tablespoons sunflower or vegetable oil
500 g (1 lb 2 oz) potatoes, cut into 2–3 cm
  (1–1¼ in) cubes
1 cauliflower, broken into florets

1 teaspoon brown mustard seeds
1 teaspoon ground cumin
1 level teaspoon turmeric
2 teaspoons ground coriander
6 tablespoons tomato passata
salt

To serve
4 tablespoons thick Greek yoghurt (optional)
a handful of coriander leaves

Grind the onion with the garlic, ginger, chilli and 3 tablespoons water in a processor until smooth. Reserve.

Heat the oil in a frying pan large enough to take the potato and cauliflower in one single layer with a little room to spare (but not too much). Fry the potato and cauliflower until beginning to catch here and there. Lift out of the pan and reserve. Now add the mustard seeds to the oil in the pan. As soon as the mustard seeds start to pop and dance, add the onion mixture and fry over a moderate heat, stirring constantly, until thickened – some 3–4 minutes. Stir in the remaining spices and stir for a minute or two more.

Now stir in the tomato passata, 600 ml (1 pint) water and salt. Bring up to the boil, return the potatoes and cauliflower to the pan and then half cover and leave to simmer quietly for 10 minutes or so until both are tender, and the sauce is much reduced.

Serve topped with the yoghurt, if using, and a big flurry of coriander.

* *

Cauliflower and garlic purée

Garlic and cauliflower are poached in milk to produce a pale, delicate, unctuous purée that partners fish particularly well.

Serves 4

1 head garlic, cloves separated
1 small cauliflower, broken into small
  florets
about 400–450 ml (14–15 fl oz) milk

30 g (1 oz) butter
freshly grated nutmeg
a few chopped chives
salt

Blanch the peeled cloves of garlic in boiling water for 4 minutes, then drain. Put in a pan with the cauliflower florets, season with salt and add enough milk to nearly cover. Bring gently up to the boil, then turn the heat down very low and simmer for around 7–8 minutes until both cauli and garlic are tender, but not yet totally collapsing.

With a slotted spoon, transfer cauliflower and garlic to a processor and add a few nice slurps of the milk, the butter, and some nutmeg. Process until smooth adding more milk as needed, to form a thick purée. Taste and adjust the seasoning. Serve sprinkled with a few snippets of chive for colour.

* *

Red cabbage

* * *

There's a good deal to be said for a spot of colour. Design-wise it changes the way we think about so many things, vegetables included. Green in all its many hues indicates fresh, healthy, lively, active and, for some, a dismaying lack of indulgence. Dark purple, on the other hand, is the colour of royalty, mystery, hidden secrets, sophistication and discretion. In vegetables, purple also indicates the presence of anthocyanins. These are amongst that great and good group of antioxidants found in virtually all vegetables. Not only do they bring sensational colour, they also help protect against a variety of ailments, most notably cancer and heart disease. The tragedy is that anthocyanins are water soluble, and have a nasty habit of transmuting when heated to a corpsy grey-blue, or in some cases sombre black-green. And that, my friends, is why no normal human being eats plain boiled red cabbage with any hint of pleasure. If you want to get a spot of brooding royal colour on the plate, you have to be clever about it.

Red cabbage is not merely white cabbage with attitude. It's a different vegetable altogether and has its own rulebook.

Practicalities

BUYING There is no obvious way of judging when a red cabbage is peachy fresh and newly cut. That hefty globe of solid leafage is built to last. Inevitably time saps flavour to some degree, there's no getting away from that, but here is one vegetable where spoilage is slow. When you are buying red cabbage, check for the obvious signs of decrepitude – flabbiness, sulphurous smell, soft patches and so on – but there's no need to get too het up about über-freshness, as you should, say, with spring greens. When I see rather small red cabbages I do question whether someone has hacked off vast quantities of outer leaves that have seen better days, but of course they could just be genuinely small. In such cases I take a second sniff to see if I can detect any telltale malodours.

Assuming you've purchased a fine, healthy, fresh red cabbage, it will keep pretty well for a couple of weeks in a cool, dry place – but no more than that.

Preparation is standard. Trim off the base and peel off the outer layer of leaves, then grab your biggest knife and cut your cannonball of a cabbage in four, through the stem. Slice out the thick stem in each quarter and discard, then slice the hunk of cabbage thinly across the grain, to produce strips of finer or coarser width, according to taste and recipe.

COOKING **Raw** red cabbage, thinly shredded, is a good addition to a **salad** in mid-winter – crisp and juicy, but sometimes rather hard to load smoothly on a fork. To soften it just enough to make it more malleable, but not enough to lose its crispness, I **blanch** it for a minute but no more, with a dash of vinegar or lemon in the water, then drain and refresh in cold water to prevent further cooking. Only the brevity of this procedure makes it acceptable (see introduction). When you have more time on your hands, you could, alternatively, toss the shredded cabbage with salt and lemon or lime, then set it aside for an hour before finishing the salad – this has a similar physical effect, with the added bonus of adding flavour at the same time. The process will draw water from the cabbage, which may need to be drained off. Taste before you add more salt or sharpness in the form of a dressing.

Astute readers will have remarked that both processes involve the addition of an acid component. In fact, nearly all red cabbage recipes include vinegar or lemon or something of this sort. It's not only to do with taste. The acid reacts with the purple anthocyanins, setting the colour. Without it, the cabbage will bleach to a peculiar grey, and in some instances may even turn a quite alarming sludge blue. It's still edible, but not enticing.

When it comes to cooking proper, red cabbage likes either a brief slap of high heat (**stir-frying** is ideal, and you can use it in the recipe on page 352 instead of Savoy) or extreme gentle, lengthy **braising**. Sweet and sour oven-braised red cabbage has become something of a classic. Though it originates in Germany, the practice of adding apple and sugar and vinegar, along with other ingredients, then letting the whole lot mulch down over a period of hours to a fabulous tenderness has become part and parcel of our own culinary repertoire. The variations are numerous, but the theme is constant, and vastly preferable to pickling red cabbage in vats of malt vinegar – a heinous crime, that is, I'm delighted to say, less common than it used to be.

PARTNERS Classic partners to red cabbage include not just apple, but also orange, both zest and juice. It takes well to warm spicing – cinnamon, cloves in moderation, star anise, caraway, nutmeg and so on. And a shot of red wine, red wine vinegar, port, Madeira or Marsala, or anything of a similar hue and nature, rarely goes amiss. The other strong contender is pork, in practically any form. Try burying thick strips of belly pork, slabs of bacon, sausages or pork chops (brown all of them first) in amongst red cabbage that is to be braised. At the end of the cooking time the flavours will be superlative.

When stir-frying, add plenty of ginger and garlic, soy sauce or kecap manis (Indonesian sweet soy sauce), and finish with a spritz of lime or lemon to invigorate. I often add black olives to stir-fried cabbage or salads, and a handful of currants and toasted pine nuts will also bring either to life. Herbs are not exempt, either. Parsley is an obvious herb to add, but think about a touch of fresh dill or lemon thyme, warming marjoram or spicier oregano.

SEE ALSO CABBAGE (PAGE 345).

* *

Red cabbage, avocado and orange salad

This is an excellent salad for the winter months, when green leaves feel insubstantial and unseasonal.

Serves 4

½ red cabbage, halved, cored and
  finely shredded
juice of ½ lemon
2 avocadoes, halved, stoned and
  sliced
2 large or 3 small oranges, segmented
60g (2oz) flaked almonds, toasted
salt and pepper

Dressing
½ teaspoon runny honey
½ tablespoon white wine vinegar
3 tablespoons sunflower oil
2 teaspoons toasted sesame oil

Blanch the red cabbage in boiling, lightly salted water, acidulated with a squeeze of the lemon juice, for 1 minute, then drain thoroughly.

To make the dressing, whisk the honey with the vinegar, salt and pepper, then whisk in the oils. Taste and adjust seasonings. Toss the hot red cabbage in half the dressing, then leave to cool.

Turn the avocado slices in the remaining lemon juice as you prepare them to prevent browning. Mix with the red cabbage, oranges, almonds and more dressing, to taste, just before serving.

* *

Braised red cabbage with apple and red wine

This is the absolute classic, unbeatable way with red cabbage. It's inherited from Germany and Austria, and has become part of our tradition, too. It is a malleable recipe to which you can make all kind of additions, subtractions or substitutions. I certainly do. If I haven't got an open bottle of red wine, then I substitute port, or even orange juice. I've used cooking apples instead of eating (reduce the vinegar a little to compensate for additional sourness), added strips of orange or lemon zest, increased the onions, and done without onions altogether. Changing the spicing is probably what yields the biggest variations: caraway, coriander, cumin, nutmeg or allspice are spices to try.

Serves 6

1 large red cabbage
1 large onion, halved and sliced
2 eating apples, cored and roughly chopped
100 ml (3½ fl oz) red wine (or port)
4 tablespoons caster sugar
2 tablespoons red wine vinegar

4 cloves
2 cinnamon sticks
1 blade of mace
40 g (1½ oz) unsalted or lightly salted butter
salt and pepper

Preheat the oven to 150°C/300°F/Gas 2.

Quarter the red cabbage, then core and slice finely. Mix in a capacious casserole dish with all the remaining ingredients except the butter. Dot the butter over the top. If the casserole is flameproof, bring up to the boil on top of the hob – not absolutely necessary, but it does give the cabbage a beginner's boost, thereby marginally abbreviating a lengthy cooking time. Transfer the casserole, covered, to the oven (or just put it straight in there from cold) and leave to cook down gently for 3–3½ hours. Stir after about 1 hour, and then again every 40 minutes or so. The cabbage will eventually cook down to a sublime melting tenderness, having absorbed most of the liquid.

Taste and adjust seasoning and either serve at once or reheat thoroughly when the next meal comes along.

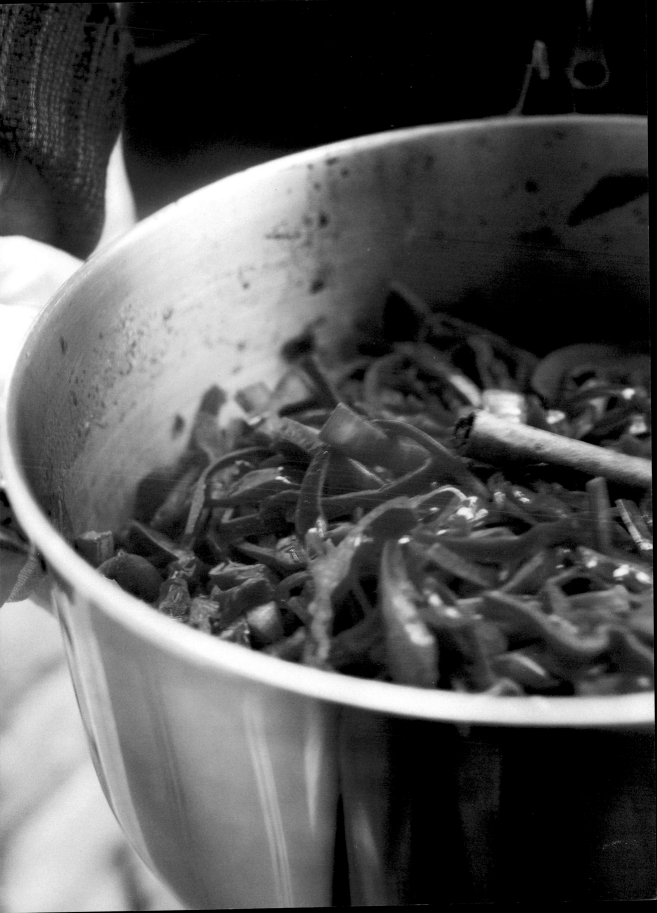

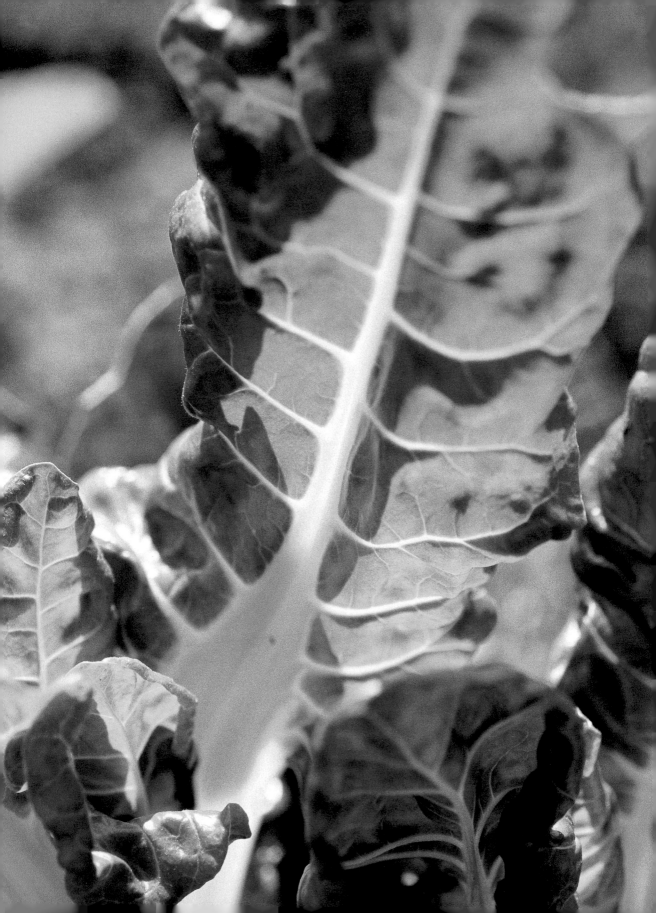

Green and leafy

* *

Curly kale and Cavolo nero
Pak choi Spinach
Spring greens Swiss chard

* *

Curly kale and Cavolo nero

* * *

With its dark slate-green, frilly leaves, kale is one of the handsomest of all our vegetable greens, and also one of the most ancient. Those leaves are quite remarkable when you take a good look at them – like some wild can-can skirt frothing in and out with the beat, or the white head of a roller hurtling, breaking and frothing on the sea shore. You will no doubt have read from this that I like curly kale. It is not, I am sad to say, a universal liking, but perhaps that comes from over-enthusiastic insistence that 'eating your greens is good for you' or just over-enthusiastic and negligent cooking of stale kale. One of the problems with vegetables that keep their appearance impressively well, especially brassicas, is that the pristine exterior belies its suitability for the pot and the table. Old kale is second-rate kale, I say. Nothing to like there.

Kale is not, however, only fit for cattle feed as at least one of my friends would have it. For all her disdain she still managed to down seconds of the sausage and kale risotto (see below) that I'd cooked, so perhaps she was prepared to revise her opinion. By then conversation had moved on to matters more critical, so I've never discovered.

Kale's rich, deep, almost meaty flavour allied to that firm texture is what marks it out amongst greens, though in fact the term kale is a broad umbrella. **Curly kale** is what most of us think of as kale. However, in the States, **collard greens** are a form of uncurly kale, while if you ever holiday closer to home on the island of Jersey (assuming you don't live there, in which case skip the rest of this sentence) you may catch sight of a field of curious cabbages on strong and very long stems – these are the famous **walking-stick cabbages**, also known as **giant Jersey kale**. And if you want a fashionable kale, look no further than the sexy **cavolo nero** from Tuscany, with its elegant, curving Prince-of-Wales'-feather leaves. The taste is distinctly similar to that of curly kale, though I am sure devotees would insist that the latter is more refined. Perhaps. Lovers of Portuguese food will be familiar with 'caldo verde', the ubiquitous Portuguese soup which is made with **'couve'** – yet another form of kale.

The corollary of this is that we can get away with substituting one for the other in many classic recipes. So, you want to make a proper Tuscan 'ribollita' and there's no cavolo nero springing up round you? No problems – grab a bag of curly kale and you're away. Want to create that down-home, soul food feeling in your own backyard? You won't find collard greens for sale easily, so turn straight to that wonderfully cheap bag of kale. What a brilliantly cosmopolitan vegetable it is.

Practicalities

BUYING
Whether it is curly kale or cavolo nero you are buying, the leaves should be firm and bouncy and verging on tough. These are the butch gang of the cabbage clan, despite the frilly petticoat look, with sturdy, thick leaves that hold their shape well. Check the ends of the stems. Overly brown or slimy ends are the clear sign of too-long storage.

Kale of any kind, but particularly curly kale, needs to be rinsed well. There's no shortage of dirt hiding amongst the folds, not to mention the occasional insect. So swish the leaves around in two changes of water to be sure, and check each one as well as you can before draining and drying.

COOKING
Cut out the tougher, thicker stems before cooking, then cut leaves into broad ribbons. Kales need longer in **simmering** water than most brassicas – say 5–6 minutes to soften the leaves. And, of course, it needs to be totally and thoroughly drained before serving. Plainly cooked curly kale benefits from a touch of melting butter to give it an air of luxury, but as long as it was fresh in the first place, that's all you need add to make it a warmly welcome side dish.

Cavolo nero or kale are also good Italian style, in other words cooked until tender, then served with a little olive oil and lots of freshly squeezed lemon juice over them – most greens of whatever sort take to this with considerable ease. Or you could toss the cooked kale in olive oil that has had roughly chopped anchovies and garlic fried in it.

In Florence's central market a seller of cavolo nero once told me that she **blanched** the shredded leaves, then dressed them with olive oil and lemon, piled them on to griddled pieces of bread that had been rubbed with raw garlic and topped them with shaved Parmesan, to make fetching bruschettas. It's an idea that I've appropriated with enthusiasm.

For a more northerly approach, try cooking curly kale with bacon. **Fry** bacon and onion together, adding a touch of lard if the bacon does not produce enough fat, then pack in prepared kale, add pepper, a touch of salt and a splash of water, cover tightly and cook over a medium heat, stirring occasionally, until the kale is just tender – add a little more water if necessary.

Although I haven't tried it, my friend Manuela tells me that she often uses half kale and half marrow in her torta verde on page 210, instead of the courgette, and that it tastes fabulous.

SEE ALSO BRASSICAS (PAGE 326).

* *

Sausage and kale risotto

No doubt about it, this is definitely a winter risotto, with its flavour coming from butch kale and nuggets of sausage browned to a sizzling mess. Make it when the wind howls or the rain pelts down, to stave off the cold weather blues.

If you can buy good real Italian sausages in a deli near you, then that's what you should choose for this recipe. Failing that, any relatively high-meat, high-quality pork sausage will act as an admirable stand-in.

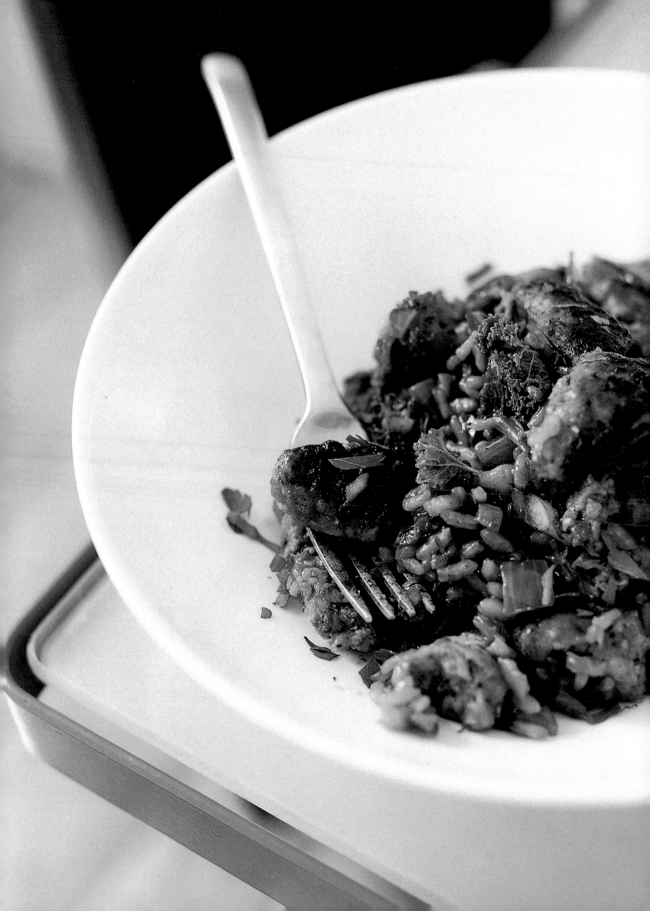

Serves 4

400 g (14 oz) meaty, first-class pork sausages
900 ml–1.2 litres (1½–2 pints) chicken stock
45 g (1½ oz) butter
1 onion, chopped
3 cloves garlic, chopped
1–2 medium-hot red chillies, deseeded
  and chopped
225 g (8 oz) risotto rice

150 ml (5 fl oz) red wine
200 g (7 oz) canned chopped tomatoes
2 tablespoons chopped parsley
lots of freshly grated nutmeg
150 g (5 oz) kale, trimmed and
  coarsely shredded
30 g (1 oz) Parmesan, freshly grated
salt and pepper

Place a frying pan over a medium heat until good and hot. Meanwhile, cut your sausages in half lengthways (don't worry that this is messy and inexact – they are going to be broken up anyway). Lay the sausages, cut-side down, in the hot pan and sizzle until browned. Turn over and brown the other side (they'll curl up but that's okay). Pull the meat away from the skins (which can be discarded), break up roughly and return to the hot pan for a few more minutes for a spot more sizzling and browning – sausage meat has a tiresome leaning towards greyness if not browned properly. Scoop all the sausage chunks out of the pan and reserve.

Pour the stock into a saucepan and heat up slowly on a back burner. When it gets to boiling point, turn the heat right down low, so that the stock stays hot but doesn't boil away.

Meanwhile, melt half the butter in a wide, shallow saucepan. Add the onion, garlic and chillies and fry gently until the onion is tender and translucent, without browning. Now add the rice and stir around for a minute until each grain is coated with butter. Pour in the wine and carry on stirring until it has nearly all disappeared. Now add the tomatoes, half the parsley, salt, lots of pepper and a generous grating of fresh nutmeg. Pour in a ladleful of hot stock and carry right on stirring. Once this batch of liquid has all but boiled away, add another mega slurp of hot stock, and stir and so on. After some 10–15 minutes of this stirring business, stir in the prepared kale, then go right back to stirring and adding stock as and when required.

After 15–20 minutes, the rice should be almost al dente. Stir in the sausage and more stock (or a spot of hot water), then stir for a couple more minutes until the rice is perfectly al dente. Draw off the heat.

Stir in the remaining butter and the Parmesan, and taste and adjust seasonings. Sprinkle with the last of the parsley and serve.

* *

Curly kale (or cavolo nero) with rosemary and chilli

Slowly steam-fried with sweet onion and hot chilli, kale becomes a rather sexy beast in a vegetably sort of a way. It intensifies that deep, savoury flavour. It's probably too powerful to serve with most fish, but would be excellent with roast free-range chicken, or just piled on top of a small bowlful of rice.
It makes a brilliant topping for bruschetta, too – griddle slices of good bread, rub with raw garlic, top with the cooked kale and then finish with a spoonful of mild, creamy young goat's cheese – as a chic vegetarian starter.

Serves 4

250 g (9 oz) curly kale or cavolo nero
3 tablespoons extra virgin olive oil
1 large onion, sliced
2 sprigs rosemary

1 medium or hot fresh red chilli, deseeded
  and thinly sliced
4 garlic cloves, sliced
salt and pepper

Trim the kale or cavolo nero, removing the tough stems. Rinse well, then cut into shreds roughly 1 cm (½ in) thick. Shake off excess water, but don't attempt to dry.

Heat the olive oil in a wide, deep frying pan with a heavy base over a medium heat. Add the onion, turn down the heat and fry gently until very tender. Now add the rosemary, chilli and garlic and fry for 1 more minute.

Pack in the kale or cavolo nero, and season with salt. Cover with a tight-fitting lid (mine doesn't fit too well, so I put a bowl on top to hold it snugly in place), reduce the heat to its absolute minimum and leave to cook gently for about 20 minutes. Stir once after 5 minutes, then again 10 minutes later. Chuck out the bedraggled rosemary stalks, then taste and adjust seasoning. Serve at once.

* *

Casarecce pasta with cavolo nero and olives

That sturdy quality of cavolo nero remains even when it is finely shredded, as here, giving the sauce more substance than you might expect. This is not glamour pasta, but it won't let you down on a winter's night.

Serves 4–5

500 g (1 lb 2 oz) casarecce or fusilli
  or other pasta shapes
salt
150 g (5 oz) soft, mild goat's cheese
freshly grated Parmesan or pecorino
  to serve

Sauce
1 onion, chopped
2 cloves garlic, chopped
3 tablespoons extra virgin olive oil

650 g (1 lb 7 oz) ripe tomatoes, skinned,
  deseeded and roughly chopped,
  or 2 x 400 g cans chopped tomatoes
1 tablespoon tomato purée
1–2 hot dried chillies, crumbled
1 teaspoon caster sugar
125 g (4½ oz) cavolo nero leaves,
  finely shredded
80 g (scant 3 oz) green olives, stoned
  and sliced
salt and pepper

To make the sauce, fry the onion and garlic in the olive oil until tender – allow a good 10 minutes for this. While they are frying, put a large pan of salted water on to heat up. Once it is boiling add the pasta, bring back to the boil and cook until the pasta is al dente (check packet for timings).

When the onion and garlic are ready, add the tomatoes, tomato purée, chillies, caster sugar, salt and pepper. Bring up to the boil, then simmer for 10 minutes. Stir in the cavolo nero and keep on simmering for 5 minutes or so before adding the olives. Let them heat through for a minute or so. Taste and adjust seasoning. Keep the sauce warm, if necessary, until the pasta is ready.

When the pasta has been drained, return to the pan and toss with the sauce. Serve and top each helping with a spoonful of the soft goat's cheese. Sprinkle with freshly grated Parmesan or pecorino before eating.

Pak choi

* * *

Pak choi sounds exotic and in some ways it is. It has been grown in China for at least two millennia, yet has waited until relatively recently to make a break for our shores. Of the many oriental greens, it is the one that has made the most impact on the general market. Like the European Swiss chard it is a two-in-one vegetable: the broad white stems are the main substance, crisp and juicy with a sweetish scent; the green leaves taste harmoniously different and, perhaps more importantly, provide a tender, leafy contrast in texture. Unlike chard, they are usually cooked together, largely because of the form of the vegetable. It's the way it grows, stems gathered together at the base in a snug bunch, yet not so tightly clutched together as, say, a cabbage.

And talking of cabbage, we come to the less exotic side of pak choi. In fact it is nothing more than another member of the vast group of edible brassicas. Just a fancy form of familiar, unexotic cabbage. To be fair, the taste is more delicate, but that hint of sulphury brassica lingers lightly.

As well as the usual version of pak choi (incidentally, this is the same thing as pak soi or bok choi), you will find a whole host of related greens in Chinese supermarkets, all of them good for stir-frying or steaming or blanching. The prettiest of these has to be **tat soi** (a.k.a. **tah tsai**), which grows in a ground-clinging flattish rosette of leaves.

Practicalities

BUYING Firm, dark green leaves must be the priority. Though they are not as stiff as the leaves of chard, say, there is no way that they should be shrivelling up. Medium-sized 'heads' of pak choi give you the best of both worlds. More flavour than the really small ones, but still small enough to cook either whole, or halved lengthways. Big, big pak choi need to be divided into individual leaves and stems, in other words more work and little gain.

Pak choi are not capital keepers. That greenery has a tendency to wilt, so store in the vegetable drawer of the fridge and use them within a couple of days of purchase. Before cooking, rinse pak choi well and glance through the leaves as well as you can to check for insect life. Remove. Shake as much water as you can from the leaves and stems. Now remove any damaged stems or leaves (often the outer ribs will be bruised, having protected the inner leaves in transit), and cut a thin slice from the base of each clump. There are two main methods for cooking pak choi: **blanching** in boiling water or **stir-frying**. Pak choi cooks in a surprisingly brief time, either way.

Small whole pak choi, or halved or quartered larger ones, need little more than 2–3 minutes in boiling salted water. More than that and they become slimy and soft. Ideally, the ribs will retain a notion of crispness to contrast with the leaf. So, cook quickly, drain extra well and then serve the pak choi as a side dish, with a knob of butter or a drizzle of lemon olive oil, or for a more oriental touch, a few splashes of sesame oil and soy sauce. For an extra lift, fry chopped garlic and chilli in a little sunflower oil, and spoon over the hot drained pak choi, together with soy sauce or kecap manis (Indonesian sweet soy sauce) and a teaspoon or so of sesame oil. Incidentally, sesame oil should always be used as a condiment; it's strong and a little goes a long way. When overheated it loses much of its deep flavour.

Which is why you should never stir-fry in sesame oil. To **stir-fry** pak choi, first slice across the head, cutting the ribs and greens into pieces some 1–2cm (1/2–1in) broad. Dry on a clean tea-towel, or in a salad spinner. Heat a wok over a high heat until smoking, add a tablespoon of sunflower or vegetable oil, garlic, ginger, chilli or any other flavourings, and then follow with the stem pieces. Stir-fry for around 2–3 minutes before adding the leafy strips, and continue for a further 2 minutes until wilted. That's it. Season with soy sauce, fish sauce, sesame oil, lime juice or just serve as they are.

There is no reason why you shouldn't treat pak choi in a European way – perhaps stealing from the recipes for Swiss chard – but somehow it doesn't seem right. Pak choi doesn't possess the depth of flavour of chard, for instance. It craves big, bold companion flavours: chilli, ginger, garlic, spices, coriander, mint, and all the rest of the Asian gang.

SEE ALSO BRASSICAS (PAGE 326).

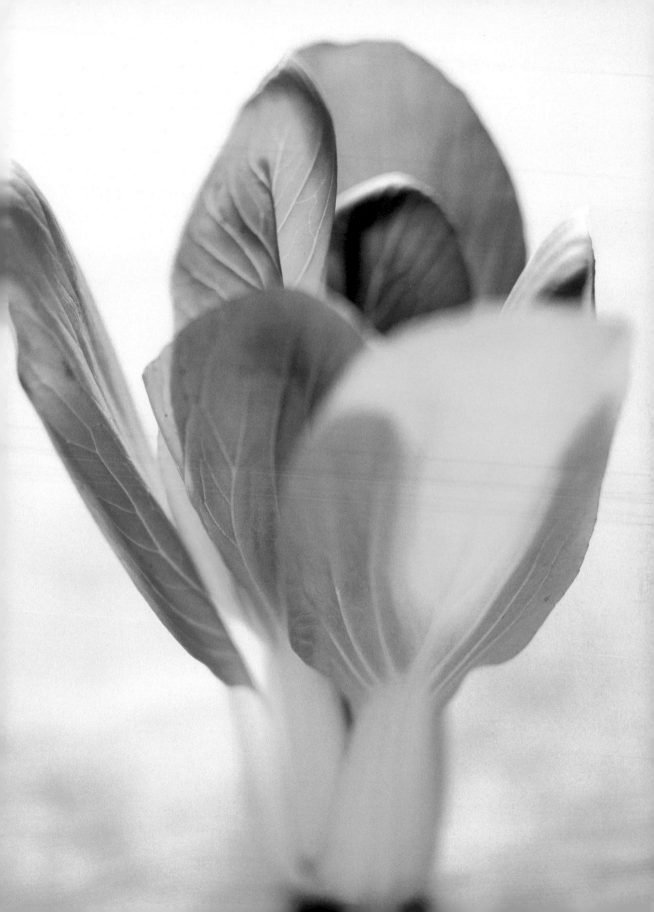

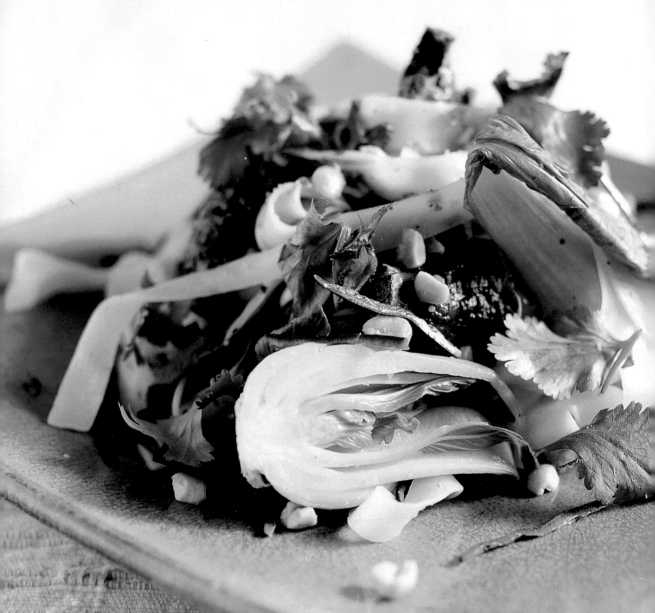

* *

Warm rice noodle, beef and pak choi salad with toasted peanuts

What better way to show off pak choi than tossed with slithery rice noodles or rice sticks, rare roast beef and a jumping chilli hot dressing?

Serves 4

60 g (2 oz) shelled peanuts
400 g (14 oz) sirloin steak(s)
a little sunflower oil
6 pak choi, halved or quartered lengthways, depending on size
250 g (9 oz) medium rice noodles
a handful of coriander leaves
1 medium or hot red chilli, deseeded and finely sliced

Dressing
1 large clove garlic, quartered
1 cm ($\frac{1}{2}$ in) piece fresh root ginger, roughly chopped
1–2 hot red chillies, deseeded and roughly chopped
1$\frac{1}{2}$ tablespoons caster sugar
juice of 1$\frac{1}{2}$ limes
3 tablespoons fish sauce

Make the dressing first. Put the garlic, ginger and chilli in a mortar and add the sugar. Pound to a paste. Work in the lime juice, the fish sauce and 3 tablespoons water. Reserve.

Roast the peanuts in a moderately hot oven (around 200°C/400°F/Gas 6) for 5 minutes or so until browned. Chop roughly.

Shortly before you wish to serve the salad, bring a large pan of water to the boil and put a griddle pan on to heat up thoroughly. As soon as the griddle pan is good and hot, brush the sirloin steak with a little oil and lay it on the griddle, giving it 3–4 minutes on each side. As soon as it is done, transfer to a warm plate and keep it warm while you get everything else sorted (around 3–5 minutes ideally, so that the steak has time to rest).

As you turn the steak, drop the pak choi into the simmering water. Cook for 2 minutes, then add the noodles, turn off the heat and leave to stand for 3 minutes. Drain both well, pressing excess water out of the pak choi. Toss in the dressing, together with the coriander leaves.

Slice the steak. Divide the noodles and pak choi between serving plates. Top with steak, scatter plentifully with peanuts and chilli, and serve quickly.

* *

Spinach

* * *

One of the best vegetable jokes I know: Everyone believes that spinach is chock-a-block full of iron but the truth is that the original researcher was having an off day and inserted the decimal point in the wrong place, thus multiplying the traces of iron tenfold. Or was it the secretary typing up the notes? Or the printer? Doesn't matter. The thrust is that spinach then gained an enviable reputation as being incredibly loaded with iron, and thus Popeye was born. Much as I admire Popeye as an early attempt to encourage children to eat their greens, the shame was that his fortifying spinach came out of a tin. Tinned spinach is not a pleasant experience and quite unlike fresh or even frozen. These days it's not much in evidence, thank heavens. So much for Popeye's long-term influence.

Cartoon characters aside, spinach still excites passionate like and dislike. And even if the decimal point saga is complete bunkum, there's no doubting that spinach is good for you. I think spinach is terrific and cook it often. It's a perfect side-kick to fish and chicken and meat and cheese dishes and eggs and practically anything else you care to mention. It's also a well-behaved and welcome ingredient in any number of composite dishes from the brilliant spinach-laden Greek spanakopitta (see page 388) to the Italian green pasta. Any recipe with the word 'Florentine' in its name, e.g. eggs Florentine, includes spinach. Spinach even freezes well. It is, in short, an all-rounder.

Practicalities

BUYING Totally fresh spinach has firm, squeaky leaves bursting with energy.
I'm talking in particular about **mature spinach** with larger leaves.
Shamefully, this is getting harder to come by. At least it is in supermarkets.
To find it at its best, turn to farmers' markets and farm shops and the
increasingly rare independent greengrocers. Mature spinach leaves have

a richer, deeper flavour than the little tiddlers and will cost far less. **Baby leaf spinach**, fine for salads, has a tendency to arrive washed and neatly packaged, ready for use. This is seductive but don't always let yourself be seduced. For most spinach recipes you are going to need big helpings of raw leaves, so it's worth buying mature leaves, which cost less and deliver more.

Remember, too, that visual perfection has its limitations. Sure, the presence of yellowing leaves, or over-dark, semi-translucent, decaying leaves is a bad thing. In practice these are more likely to appear in an enclosed plastic pack than loose spinach. Wilting is not good either. BUT a few small holes here and there and the odd blemish is nothing to worry about.

Before cooking spinach, be sure to rinse it. Unless, of course, it has been pre-washed. A mouthful of gritty spinach is deeply unpleasant. So, tip the spinach into a sink or bowl filled with cold water and swish it around a bit. Then give it a minute or so for the grit to settle. Check leaves as you transfer them from water to colander, and remove the thickest stems and any damaged spots. Repeat the process once more, but this time you can dispense with all that checking. Shake off excess water.

COOKING The first thing you need to know about cooking spinach, large or small leaf, is that it exudes lakes of green water, collapsing to a fraction of its original volume. To put enough cooked spinach on the plates of four people, as an accompaniment, you will need to begin with around 400–500g (14–18oz) fresh spinach. The second is that spinach needs very little cooking – the less time in the pan the better.

The normal way to cook spinach is to cram it, still damp from rinsing, into a big, deep, wide pan, slam on the lid and **simmer** it over a moderate heat. After around 3 minutes, remove the lid and turn the spinach so that the still firm leaves on the top have a chance to meet the heat. Replace the lid and let the spinach finish cooking – another 1–2 minutes. Now drain in a sieve, pressing down gently to squeeze out more water, before serving with a knob of butter. When the spinach is to be used as an ingredient, let it cool slightly then squeeze out as much water as you can with your hands. This diminishes the volume still further, but is essential if you are to avoid soggy pastry, or over-damp doughs, or watery purées. Only if you are making a spinach soup (what a good idea) should you skip this stage.

I think you get better results, especially if you are serving the spinach as an accompaniment, from **stir-frying** it, which takes, literally, seconds. You will need a big roomy wok, so that much of the internal moisture of the spinach sizzles away instantly. Have a warm serving dish standing by. Blot as much water as you can off the spinach with kitchen towels or a clean tea-towel. Heat the wok until it smokes, then add a tablespoon of sunflower or vegetable oil (and chopped garlic, ginger and so on if you wish). Pile spinach into the wok – it will sizzle and spit as it hits the oil. Stir-fry until the leaves just begin to collapse but still retain a bright green colour. Scoop out the cooked spinach into the warm dish, then stir-fry a second batch if needed.

Frozen leaf spinach is a permanent inhabitant of my freezer. Spinach freezes well and makes a fine standby when you can't get fresh. It has already been cooked, so merely needs thawing out and draining before use. To serve as a vegetable it is just a matter of reheating and seasoning, but it really shines as an ingredient in composite recipes, such as the spinach gnocchi below. Remember, though, that like fresh spinach all that liquid will need to be squeezed out before mixing.

PARTNERS Pasta and spinach are soul mates, and so easy to bring together. Cook pasta as normal until al dente, turn off the heat, then stir the raw spinach leaves (shredded if they are large) into the hot water with the pasta. By the time you've taken the pan to the sink to drain it, the spinach will be perfectly cooked and pasta and greens ready to take whatever other sauce you are adding. In other words, you might just fancy stirring in a large knob of butter, freshly grated nutmeg and lots of Parmesan. Or a few spoonfuls of tomato sauce, a touch of olive oil and some cubes of mozzarella to half melt in the heat of the pasta. Or add prawns that have been sizzled in olive oil with garlic, chilli and fennel seeds, then spritz with lemon juice to lift or enrich with a touch of cream. Or add a fully fledged slow-cooked bolognaise sauce. And so on and so forth – the permutations are endless.

And so too is the list of recipes that bring spinach into play. It is a great vegetable, ready to harmonise with a vast array of other ingredients. Those that spring immediately to mind include nutmeg (a great friend), orange, Parmesan, feta and other lively cheeses, anchovy, tomato, eggs, cream, nuts and many, many more. Two favourite quick ways with spinach: the first is the Catalan/Italian combining of spinach with pine nuts, raisins and sometimes anchovies, the second is enriched with cream, nutmeg and orange juice,

384

preferably Seville orange juice. To make the first, get out your wok, heat until it smokes, then throw in lots of chopped garlic and a handful of pine nuts, and if you wish, some chopped canned anchovy fillets. Stir-fry for a few seconds, before adding a small mountain of spinach. Stir-fry until wilted and there it is – ready to go. The second requires cooked spinach (or thawed frozen spinach), water squeezed out, roughly chopped. Return it to the pan with the juice of half a large orange, or a whole small one and a knob of butter, salt and nutmeg. Stir for a few minutes until most of the orange juice has been absorbed, then stir in a generous slug of double cream. Simmer until thick and pulpy, taste and adjust seasoning and serve. Excellent with fish. If you want something less rich, sprinkle a tablespoon or so of flour over the spinach as it simmers with the orange, stir in, along with a glass of milk. Again let it simmer until thickened, with no lingering taste of raw flour.

* *

Spinach with walnuts and crème fraîche

This Bulgarian way of pairing spinach with walnuts and tart, rich cream is extremely good. It is lovely served alongside grilled or poached fish (especially smoked haddock), or plain roast chicken.

Serves 5–6

500 g (1 lb 2 oz) spinach, cooked and drained
1 onion, chopped
30 g (1 oz) butter
2 cloves garlic, finely chopped

60 g (2 oz) shelled walnuts, roughly chopped
200 g (7 oz) crème fraîche
3 tablespoons freshly grated Parmesan
salt and pepper

Squeeze out as much water as you can from the spinach. Fry the onion gently in the butter until translucent and tender, then add the garlic and walnuts. Fry for another minute. Add the spinach, cream, salt and pepper and stir well. Simmer for a few minutes until the cream has thickened a little. Stir in the Parmesan. Taste, adjust seasoning and serve.

Gnocchi di spinaci e ricotta

A classic of Italian cooking, spinach and ricotta gnocchi bear scant resemblance to the better-known potato gnocchi. Lighter and prettier and easier to make, they have a fabulous flavour and pretensions to healthiness, what with all that spinach.

Serves 4

either 500 g (1 lb 2 oz) frozen spinach
  or 650 g (1 lb 7 oz) fresh spinach
250 g (9 oz) ricotta cheese
100 g (3½ oz) Parmesan, freshly grated
150 g (5 oz) plain flour, plus extra for rolling
  the gnocchi
2 eggs
freshly grated nutmeg
salt and pepper

Sauce
1 medium onion, chopped
1 carrot, finely diced
2 tablespoons extra virgin olive oil
2 cloves garlic, chopped
2 x 400 g cans chopped tomato
2 tablespoons tomato purée
1 teaspoon caster sugar
1 bouquet garni (3 generous sprigs thyme,
  2 bay leaves, 2 big sprigs parsley,
    tied together with string)
salt and pepper

If using frozen spinach just let it thaw then tip into a sieve. If using fresh spinach cook lightly (either by stir-frying with a small splash of oil in a wok, or by the more traditional method of stuffing the whole lot into a saucepan, with only the water it was washed in clinging to the leaves, covering and cooking over a moderate heat for a few minutes until wilting). Once cooked, tip into a sieve to start draining.

With either sort of spinach, the key thing now is to squeeze out as much water as possible. And it is quite phenomenal how much water comes out of a pile of spinach, and what a distressingly small amount of greenery you end up with. Never mind – the best is still there. Weigh it to be on the safe side, though – you will need 250 g (9 oz) of fiercely squeezed spinach for the gnocchi. Chop it up finely.

Beat the ricotta until smooth. Add the spinach, Parmesan, flour, eggs, plenty of nutmeg and plenty of salt and pepper too. Mix the whole lot together with your hands, making sure it is evenly blended. Cover and leave

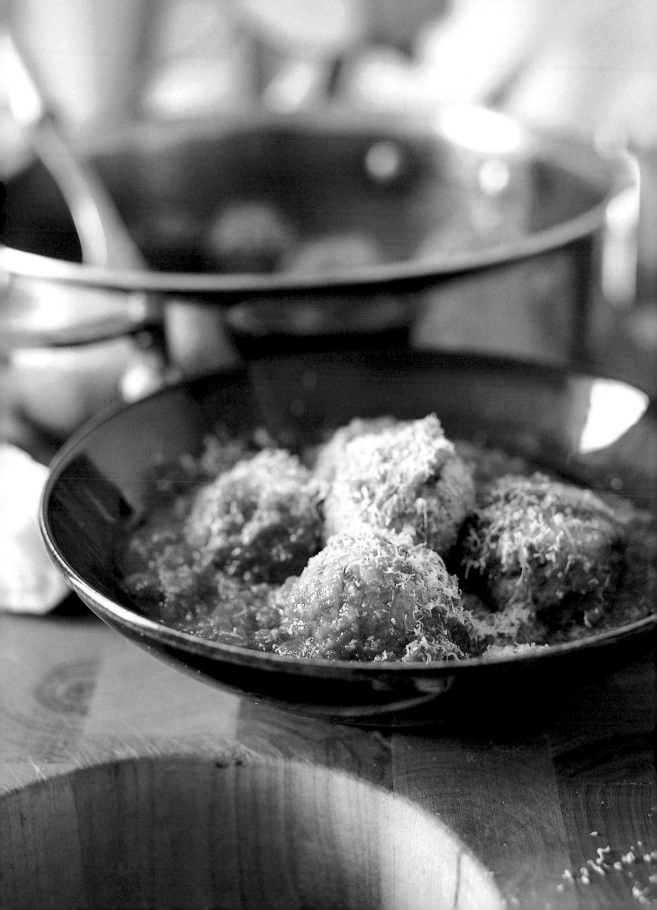

in the fridge for an hour or more before moving on to the next step.

To make the sauce, fry the onion and carrot slowly in the oil until tender. Now add the garlic and cook for another minute. Tip in the tomatoes and tomato purée, the caster sugar and the bouquet garni, then season with salt and pepper. Leave to simmer vaguely for about 30 minutes, stirring frequently to prevent catching on the bottom, even adding a splash of water if necessary. Cool slightly, remove the bouquet garni and liquidise. Return to the pan and reheat when needed.

Dredge a large plate with mountains of flour. Take dessertspoons of the chilled ricotta mixture, roll into neat balls, then roll in the flour. Place on a floured tray. Set aside until needed.

Shortly before you intend to scoff the gnocchi, bring a wide, shallow pan of water to the boil, then turn the heat down to a more peaceful simmer. Carefully add your gnocchi to the pan, taking care not to overcrowd, and poach for some 10–15 minutes, turning occasionally. Whilst they are cooking, reheat the tomato sauce.

Once done lift the gnocchi out with a draining spoon, carefully letting all the water drip back into the pan. Arrange on warm plates, or in one shallow serving dish, and nap with tomato sauce. Pass the Parmesan around too.

* *

Spanakopitta

Every bakery and snack bar in Athens, and for all I know the rest of Greece, can be relied upon to sell 'green pies' of some type. The commonest is spinach pie, with or without feta. How lucky they are to have this as their standard snack. When it is properly made and freshly baked, this is perhaps the best of all recipes for spinach – a true celebration of a vegetable that doesn't always get the praise and treatment it rightly deserves. Serve it with a ripe tomato and black olive salad and you have a small bit of Greek heaven on the plate.

Serves 8 as a main course

950g (2lb 2oz) fresh spinach
1 large onion, chopped
8 spring onions, thinly sliced
2 tablespoons extra virgin olive oil
4 tablespoons chopped parsley

4 tablespoons chopped dill
350g (12oz) feta cheese, crumbled
3–4 large eggs
300–350g (11–12oz) filo pastry
100g (3½oz) unsalted butter, melted

Preheat the oven to 190°C/375°F/Gas 5. Rinse the spinach and shake off excess water. Shred thickly if using large-leaved spinach, or if using baby spinach leaves leave as they are.

Fry the onion gently in the olive oil in a big, deep saucepan. When tender, add the spring onions and cook for another minute. Cram as much of the spinach as you can into the pan, then cover tightly and leave to cook for about 3 minutes. Turn the spinach carefully – there should be room now for the rest of the spinach to go in. Clamp the lid back on, and cook for another 3 minutes, then turn and stir – by now the spinach should be cooked and the firmer leaves at the top will shrink as you stir. Tip the mixture into a colander to drain and cool while you start layering the filo pastry.

Unroll your filo pastry and lay flat on the work surface, then cover with a sheet of clingfilm. This keeps the pastry from drying out. Brush a 33 x 25 x 5cm (13 x 10 x 2in) deep roasting tin (or thereabouts) with a little melted butter. Take the first sheet of filo from the pile, and brush with butter. Lay in the base of the dish. Repeat with a second sheet, overlapping with the first, so that the base is covered. Now butter another couple of sheets and lay them at right angles to the first two, overlapping again, and folding excess pastry over on to itself so that it fits neatly. Repeat with another 8 sheets (by my reckoning that's 12 so far).

Tip the drained spinach mixture into a bowl and add the herbs, feta, eggs, salt (not too much as the feta is salty) and pepper. Mix well and spread evenly over the pastry. Repeat the whole buttering and layering of pastry sheets over the spinach mixture, using another 12 sheets in total. Brush the top with the remaining butter. Take a sharp knife and cut the top layers of filo only into squares. Dip your fingers in cold water and scatter a few drops of water lightly over the pastry to stop the edges curling up.

Bake for 30–40 minutes until golden brown. Let it settle for 5–10 minutes, then cut into squares. Eat warm or cold.

Spring greens

I've just fallen in love with spring greens all over again. Humble amongst vegetables, it's true, but at their best they taste as spectacularly good as many a leaf with a far heftier price tag attached. My new love affair began with a delivery of organic greens, picked fresh that morning. I cooked them in the most basic of ways – shredded broadly, plunged into boiling salted water for 3 minutes, drained and plonked on the table just as they were. Wow. We could have eaten double. Any slight reservations with the first helping were dissipated within seconds. We fought, politely, over the last few ribbons of green. One friend, an excellent cook, even asked for the recipe.

Was it the freshness? Undoubtedly. And was it the organic-ness? Possibly, though it's harder to be sure, since I don't know that I've ever eaten non-organic spring greens so soon after they were picked. What I have learned for sure, though, is that I shan't be buying spring greens from large retailers ever again.

Spring greens are a form of **loose-leafed cabbage**, easy and comparatively quick to grow. They probably existed long before tightly hearted cabbages came on the scene, and have certainly had a long, long and troublesome history dividing families along the 'eat-your-greens/shan't' lines. My mother, the late Jane Grigson, had endured this as a child. Spring greens rarely featured on the menu as I was growing up and nor did kale. If you own, or come across, a copy of her wonderful *Vegetable Book* it doesn't take much reading between the lines to tell that she only cooked these 'nastier aspects of the cabbage clan' under duress. On spring greens '…cabbages that have failed to develop a heart. Heartlessness is never a desirable quality…'. Her dislike and their virtual absence on the plates of my childhood have, ironically, ensured that I adore both vegetables.

If you have suffered in the way that my mother suffered, it may be that you will never feel the same, but please try just one more time. Wait until you find them in prime freshness at a farmers' market or a farm shop or in a vegetable box, and cook them lightly. You might find that you too will fall in love with these humble leaves.

Practicalities

Spring greens are only worth buying when they are impeccably fresh – in other words a maximum of 48 hours since they were plucked from the ground and preferably less. The trouble is that it is not so easy to tell at a glance as the leaves hold their shape well for some time. So peer detective-like at the stalks – can you find any evidence of browning or sliminess at the bases? Yes? Then avoid them like the plague. I'd suggest, too, that you only buy spring greens when you can quiz someone connected with the growing process. In other words, buy from farmers' markets or from farm shops. Or blag them from an acquaintance who grows their own. Or grow them yourself. And if you are sure that you have acquired impeccably fresh greens, don't ruin them by holding them hostage. Prepare and cook them that day or the next if you want to get the most out of them.

Before cooking wash them well – grit spoils even the freshest of greens. Cut out the tougher stems and discard any leaves that are damaged or look past their best. For basic cooking it is easiest to cut the leaves into wide strips, then plunge them into a pan of **boiling salted water** for a mere 3–4 minutes, before draining well. Very fresh greens need nothing more, though of course you might like to enrich them a little with a knob of butter. If you don't want to be draining big pans of water at the last minute, you could pre-cook them lightly (3 minutes max), drain, run under the cold tap to halt cooking, then drain again. Just before serving toss them in hot melted butter, perhaps with a sprinkling of caraway seeds, which go delectably well with most leafy vegetables. Or sizzle a little chopped garlic in olive oil, then toss the spring greens in that until good and hot.

Spring greens are excellent **stir-fried** for just long enough to soften them and bring out their brightest green – we're talking around 3 minutes again. You may want to keep them pure by just heating a tablespoon of sunflower oil in the smoking wok before tossing in the greens, or scent the oil with

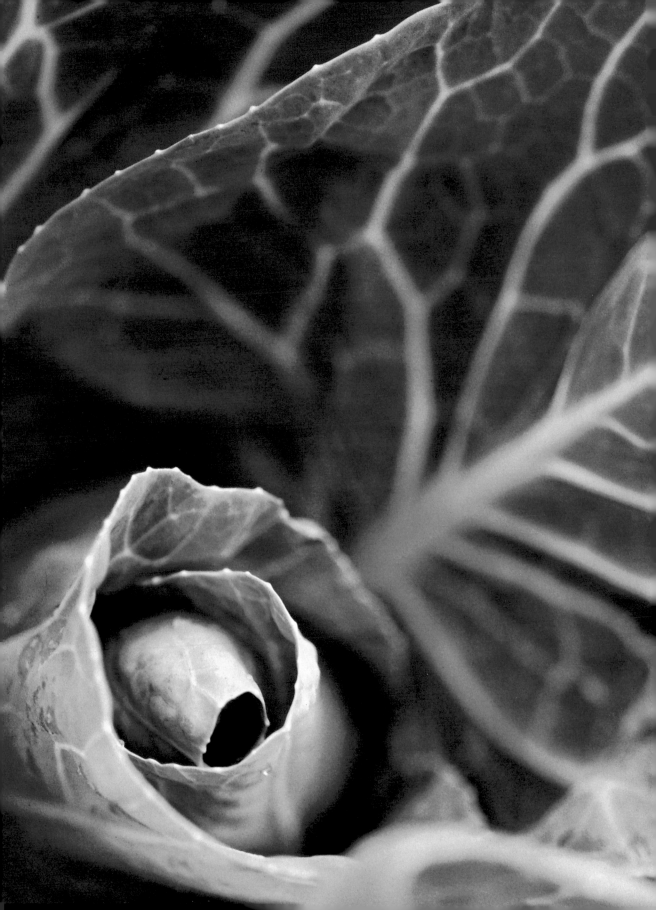

chopped garlic, ginger and, for a kick, a chopped hot red chilli or two. One colleague of mine loves them simply stir-fried (or blanched), then flavoured with a spoonful of Dijon mustard – another way to inject a quick lift and tingle on the tongue.

The Chinese **deep-fry** very finely shredded spring greens (and other greens, too) for split seconds in hot oil to produce 'seaweed'. In restaurants it is usually finished with a sprinkling of sweet-salt powdered dried shrimp, but at home it is easiest to season the mass of crisp deep-fried greens with a sprinkling of sugar and salt.

To change the taste of the greens radically, cook them slowly for some time. You could substitute spring greens for the kale in the recipe for kale with rosemary and chilli on page 375, for instance. Or simply cook them gently in the oven with a knob of butter and a ladle of decent home-made stock. To this you could, naturally, add all kinds of little extras, from a handful of chopped ham or cooked pork and fried onion to lemon zest and lemon juice, or garlic, chilli, ginger, soy sauce, fish sauce and so on.

As a last-minute addition to soups and stews, they add substance as well as contrasting flavour. And if you have any lightly cooked spring greens left over, chop them roughly next day and stir into buttery mash, or make bubble and squeak with them.

SEE ALSO BRASSICAS (PAGE 326).

* *

Chicken and chickpea stew with spring greens

This is a showcase for spring greens at their very best, cooked in two ways to show off their often overlooked versatility. The red of the stew sets off the lightly cooked greens in its sauce, while the thatch of crisp deep-fried 'seaweed' offers a wonderful contrast of textures. The stew can be made in advance, to the point where the greens are added, but leave the deep-frying until the last possible moment.

Serves 4

8 chicken thighs (bone in and skin on)
2 tablespoons extra virgin olive oil
2 cloves garlic, sliced
1 teaspoon fennel seeds
1 bay leaf
500 g (1 lb 2 oz) tomato passata
1 tablespoon tomato purée
1 teaspoon caster sugar

2 x 410 g cans chickpeas, drained and rinsed
175 g (6 oz) spring greens, roughly chopped
salt and pepper

To garnish
6 leaves spring greens
sunflower or vegetable oil for deep-frying

Brown the chicken thighs all over in hot olive oil in a wide frying pan. Remove from the pan and reserve. Reduce the heat, and fry the garlic, fennel seeds and bay until the garlic is just beginning to brown. Quickly add the tomato passata, tomato purée and sugar, and bring up to the boil, stirring in the residues from frying. Return the chicken to the pan, add enough water to just cover and season generously. Cover and simmer gently for 30 minutes until the chicken is cooked through.

Place about 2 ladlefuls of the sauce and about one-third of the chickpeas in a liquidiser, together with a ladleful of water, and liquidise, adding a little more water if necessary. Stir this back into the stew, then add the spring greens and remaining chickpeas. Simmer for a further 5 minutes. Taste and adjust seasonings.

While the stew is cooking, take the spring greens for garnishing and snip out thick stalks, so that all you have left is tender green leaves. Pile them on top of each other, roll up tightly and cut across the roll to give shreds as fine as grass. Heat up a pan of sunflower or vegetable oil to 180°C/350°F (when a cube of bread is dropped into the oil, it should fizz energetically and brown within 20–30 seconds). Deep-fry a handful of spring greens at a time, dropping them into the oil at arm's length. The oil will immediately boil up and splutter angrily, but don't panic – this is meant to happen. Scoop the fried greens out as soon as the spluttering and bubbling dies back – some 10–20 seconds is all it will take. Drain the greens on kitchen paper, and season with salt.

To serve the stew, ladle into big bowls and top each one with a thatch of deep-fried spring greens. Serve immediately, before the contrast of textures is lost.

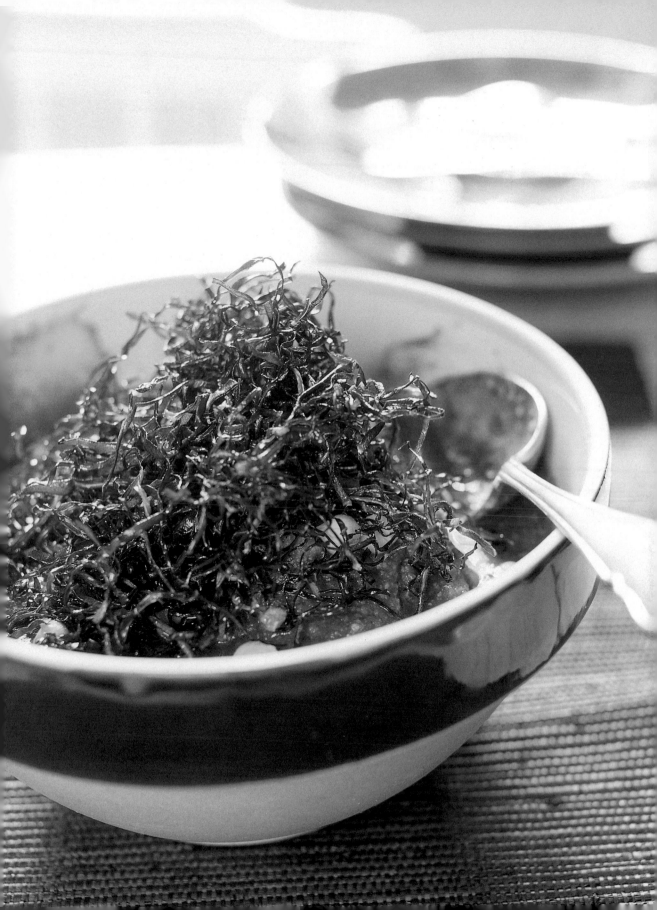

Swiss chard

* * *

With its broad ivory ribs and dark, springy green leaves, Swiss chard is a rare two-in-one vegetable. In modern parlance, it could almost be termed a BOGOF* vegetable, except that this smacks of bargain basement and loss leaders, and Swiss chard is far too sophisticated for that. The sweet, crisply juicy nature of the ribs is a nicely judged contrast to the deeper, more savoury stance of the leaves – yet again, Mother Nature, aided by a long line of gardening gurus and patient plantsmen, gets it just right.

The name itself is something of an oddity. 'Chard' comes from the French 'chardon', a thistle, which Swiss chard isn't. The broad ribs do have a loose resemblance to the stems of the cardoon (see page 122), which is. There's the etymological connection. The bigger question is what does Swiss chard have to do with Switzerland? Not a great deal apparently. The full name first appears in 19th-century seed catalogues, with no discernible rhyme or reason to it. Swiss chard does rhyme with Swiss guard but I suspect that's just a catchy coincidence.

Beautiful chard is the glamorous cousin of more humble beetroot, and musters in as probably the most tasty of a clutch of beet leaves that are all edible. None of the others are blessed with the wide rib, nor for that matter have they been bred to provide a multitude of kaleidoscope colours. Glowing **ruby chard** (or **rhubarb chard** in the States) is the red-stemmed version of Swiss chard, with fabulous vivid ribs, designed to stand out ornamentally in the vegetable garden as much as on the plate. Then there is **yellow-ribbed chard**, almost as pretty, and even a **blue-stemmed chard**. Whether the colorations make for variations in flavour is open to debate – I think that there is a distinguishing creamy, nutty subtlety to ruby chard, but having

* buy one get one free

never tasted ruby and white side by side, I wouldn't stake my life on being able to tell them apart blindfold. What is incontrovertible, however, is that they both taste superb.

Practicalities

Squeaky fresh is what you are after. Those dusky green leaves with a hint of blue buried in them must be imbued with vigour and verve. Ideally the ribs will be broad – a good 2.5 cm (1 in) across at their widest, offering generous contrast to the leaves. In younger smaller-leaved chard this may not be so. It's no slur, but you lose out on what marks chard out from so many other vegetables. Very small juvenile leaves, almost totally devoid of rib, are sometimes included in salad mixes, and very nice too.

As with all green and leafy vegetables, the sooner you cook and eat them the better. So, stash the leaves in the vegetable drawer of the fridge, but don't leave them there for more than a day or two.

When you are in a tearing rush, you can get away with minimal preparation – a quick rinse, then just cutting the leaves into wide ribbons, before **steaming, braising or blanching** in boiling salted water. The better option is to separate the broad rib from the green leaf (use a sharp knife or a pair of scissors) as they cook at different rates. In fact you might even decide to cook them and serve them separately as two completely different vegetables. Think about it. For everyday eating, it makes sense to cut the leaves into broad strips before cooking. Although that wide expanse of firm greenery does suggest wrapping possibilities. More of that below.

Ribs too are easiest sliced thickly, though it is not mandatory. If you want to keep them long and they will fit into the pan, fine. When I'm serving chard as a plain accompaniment to the meal, I take a wide, shallow pan, pour in just enough water to cover the base, and add either a knob of butter or a dash of extra virgin olive oil. As soon as it is simmering, in go the chard ribs, salt and on goes the lid. The heat is low. After 2 minutes, I pack in the dark green leaves, jam the lid back on and cook for a further 2–3 minutes. Then I check the veg to see if they are done, turning them to mix together and drain off any excess liquid. That's it. Serve them just as they are, or embellish with another knob of butter, or a drizzle of fresh, best olive oil or scented lemon olive oil, and maybe a big squeeze of lemon or Seville orange juice.

Both stem and leaf also respond beautifully to a few minutes **in a hot wok** – as soon as it is smoking, add a tablespoon of sunflower or vegetable oil, a little chopped garlic, ginger, or chilli if you wish, or a handful of thinly sliced shallots (or all four), stir once, then in with the sliced ribs. After a minute or so's stir-frying, it's time to add the leaves. Stir-fry for a couple of minutes more until they are tender enough, and voilà, they are ready to eat.

Remember those big leaves? Obvious candidates for a spot of stuffing and rolling and wrapping, which is exactly how they are often used in France, Italy, Switzerland and other countries with a strong love of chard. You could, perhaps, replace vine leaves with chard leaves in traditional Greek dolmades (stuffed vine leaves) recipes, or fill them, more French style, with a mix of minced pork or veal, breadcrumbs, raisins and pine nuts, or take a more innovative touch and mash some cooked potato or sweet potato with lots of parsley and thyme, an egg, heaps of grated Parmesan, chopped spring onions and use that as a filling. Before you begin you will need to blanch the leaves in boiling water for the shortest of times (think seconds not minutes) then drain and lay out flat on a cloth to dry out. Once filled and rolled, tuck them neatly into an oiled heavy-based pan, cover with stock or water and aromatics, salt and pepper, then cook very gently, covered, for some 40 minutes or so (longer for raw meat fillings – say an hour or more), checking occasionally and adding a little more liquid if necessary.

That deep almost meaty flavour of the leaves has inspired cooks for centuries, especially during fast days, when meat was not on the menu. It appears in pies (Manuela suggests replacing courgettes with raw chard in her Ligurian pie on page 210), rolled and stuffed with rice, herbs and tomatoes in Greece and Switzerland, in stuffings for fish, on Spanish 'cocas', the Catalan equivalent of pizzas, or in Italian frittatas. Blanched and chopped fine,
they are an important ingredient in farces for filled pastas, too. In France, especially the south, 'blettes' are employed with relish in a multitude of dishes. Most unexpected of all are the 'tourtes de blettes', sweet chard tarts from Provence, studded with raisins and nuts – jangling on the untutored palate at first, but once over the initial impact, really quite delicious.

Swiss chard with avgolemono sauce

Greek avgolemono sauce, made with eggs and lemon juice, is a joy with practically any lightly cooked greens you care to mention, but it does have a particular affinity with Swiss chard. Here I've suggested cooking and serving both leaves and rib with the sauce, but you could just dish up the ribs, cooked separately, with the avgolemono sauce, and save the greens to stir-fry with a main course.

Serves 4

500 g (1 lb 2 oz) Swiss chard
1 level teaspoon cornflour
juice of 1 large lemon

2 egg yolks
300 ml (10 fl oz) vegetable or chicken stock
salt and pepper

Prepare the chard, separating the green leaves from the ribs. Cut the leaves into wide ribbons. Slice the ribs diagonally into diamonds. Mix the cornflour with enough of the lemon juice to form a paste, then stir in the remainder along with the egg yolks.

Bring the stock up to the boil, then reduce the heat to a gentle simmer. Season with salt and pepper. Add the ribs and simmer for 2 minutes, then add the leaves and continue cooking for a further 3 minutes or so until just tender. Drain the chard, returning the hot stock to the pan. Keep the chard warm while you finish the sauce. Bring the stock back to the boil, then draw off the heat. Gradually pour into the egg and lemon mixture, whisking continuously.

Return the chard to the pan, pour over the lemon and egg mixture and shake over a gentle heat until the sauce thickens slightly. Do not let it boil. Taste and add more salt and lemon juice if needed, then serve immediately.

Gratin of chard and new potatoes

Olives and chard go together particularly well. In this gratin the olives are blended with anchovies and sun-dried tomatoes to give a salty, piquant dressing to lift the chard and waxy little potatoes. Serve it as a first course, or a side dish with grilled chicken, or perhaps just on its own with a fresh tomato salad and good bread on the side.

Serves 4–6

450 g (1 lb) ruby or Swiss chard
5 tablespoons olive oil
400 g (14 oz) new potatoes, scrubbed
60 g (2 oz) black olives, stoned
2 canned anchovy fillets, chopped
2 pieces sun-dried tomato, chopped

½ tablespoon capers, drained and rinsed
1 tablespoon chopped parsley
60 g (2 oz) Gruyère cheese, grated
30 g (1 oz) Parmesan, freshly grated
salt and pepper

Preheat the oven to 190°C/375°F/Gas 5.

Pile up several chard leaves and stems at a time and snip off the leaves with a pair of scissors or a sharp knife. Shred the leaves and cut the broad ribs into 1 cm (½ in) pieces. Warm 2 tablespoons olive oil in a wide pan and add the ribs. Stir, then cover and cook over a low heat for 4 minutes, stirring occasionally. Now add the leaves, stir, then cover again and cook for a further 5 minutes until just tender. Season with salt and pepper.

Cook the new potatoes in lightly salted water until just tender, then slice thinly.

Put the olives, anchovies, sun-dried tomato, capers, parsley and 2 tablespoons olive oil into the blender, and process to form a paste.

Oil a 30 cm (12 in) gratin dish. Layer the cooked chard (with any cooking juices) and potatoes, spreading a little of the processed mixture between each layer and seasoning with pepper. Finish with a layer of chard. Mix the Gruyère and Parmesan and sprinkle over the top. Drizzle over the remaining oil and then bake for about 25–30 minutes, until the cheese is browned and sizzling. Serve hot or warm.

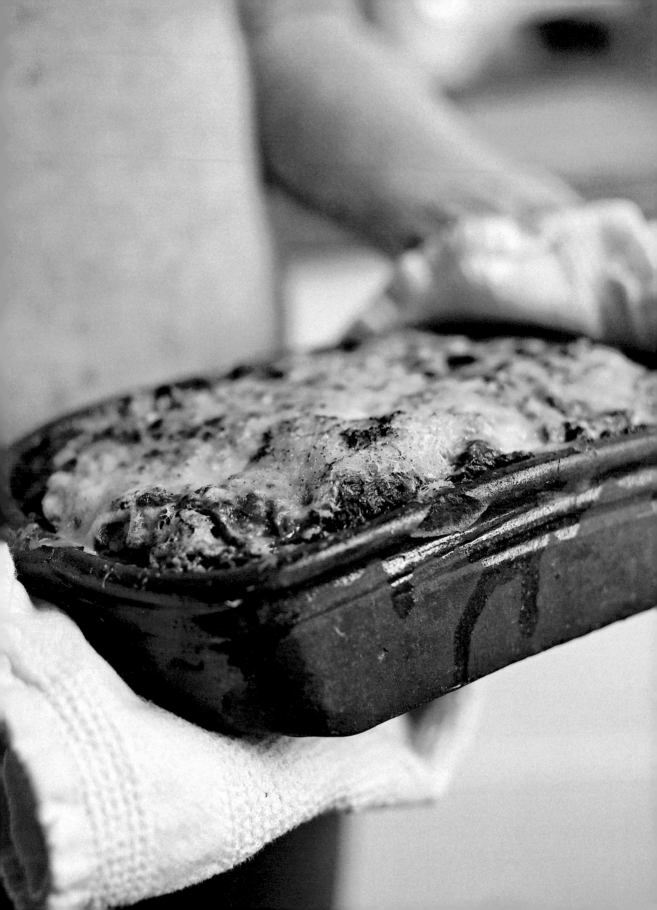

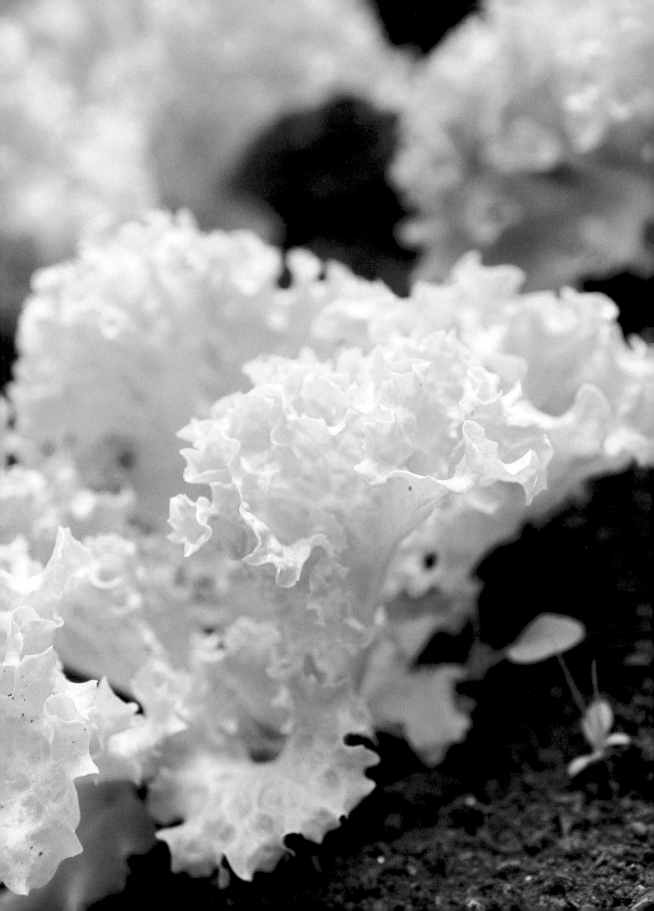

Salad leaves

* *

Chicory Chinese cabbage
Lettuces Purslane
Radicchio Rocket **Sorrel**
Watercress and land cress

Chicory

* * *

The things you have to do for TV. Back in the early 1990s I found myself
stuffing green sticks up heads of chicory in order to 'plant' them in neat rows
in a box of compost in an expert's airing cupboard. It was a lie, I admit. Those
perfect-looking spears of chicory that emerged from the dark on screen had
come from the supermarket that morning. Well, we were desperate, hurtling
towards the end of our shooting schedule, and you just can't rush forcing.
Witloof chicory is not a plant that takes kindly to chivvying.

Growing chicory is a two-tier job. The first centres about root-production,
out in the open earth, in a perfectly standard fashion, i.e. plant seed, rely on
Mother Nature to feed and water if possible, admire green foliage as it
emerges from the ground, fingers crossed that root is forming, dig up muddy
root. So far so good, except that that healthy green foliage is unbearably
bitter, so has to go. Stored correctly the muddy roots can then hang around
for a while, waiting to go back into action.

Tier two is where we called in too late. As the winter cold sets in (we're
talking old-fashioned methods here – modern chicory cultivation no doubt
dispenses entirely with connections to tiresome weather conditions), roots
are replanted in succession, in cosy, snug, dark, duvet conditions (hence the
airing cupboard) where they swing back into action, thrusting forth shoots
that reach upward in search of light. A handsome bullet-shaped spear of
closely wrapped leaves develops. Lo and behold, when at last you get to see
their ghostly forms they are pale, pale ivory white, with leaf edges and tips
of pale acid yellow.

The miracle is that this time around the leaves taste so good. Juicy, firm,
and a brilliant balance of sweetness and a trace of character-building
bitterness. Chicory is the ultimate winter salad leaf, but also doubles as a
uniquely delicious vegetable when cooked. Bitterness is an odd gift in food,

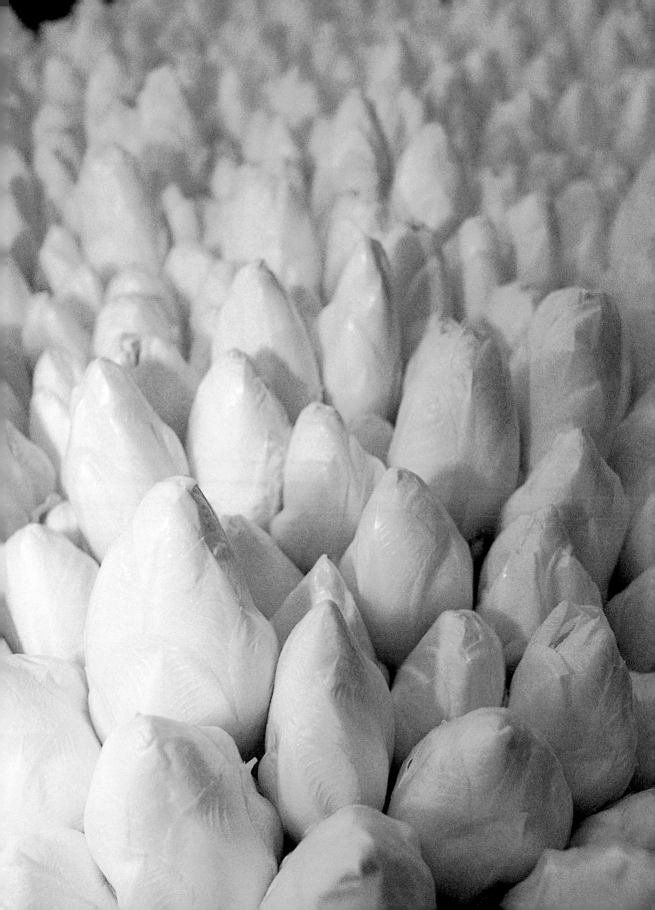

not dissimilar in some ways to chilli heat. Some people adore it and long for more, more, more, whilst others can never see the point of it, rejecting it out of hand. The trick with chicory is not to let it get out of hand. From the second it sees the light, bitterness begins to build in those handsome 'chicons'. In the past, growers lovingly protected each one with a wrap of purple, light-excluding tissue paper, but it's rare to see that kind of attention doled out to any vegetable these days. The point is though, that if you are to enjoy chicory at its finest and most subtle, you must learn how to buy the best. More than most, this is not a vegetable with a static flavour.

Practicalities

BUYING The first things to check when buying chicory are the colours. What you are hoping to see are white, almost opalescent leaves edged with the palest, purest yellow. The more delicate the colouring, the milder the bitter notes will be. The slightest hint of green creeping in along the edges is a warning. It's saying, 'I have been exposed to light for too long and I'm fast recreating my true bitterness.' Block your ears and walk away.

With correct colour should come tightly curved, plump leaves, clinging around each other and tapering off to a soft point. Chicory that is flabby or with drying leaf edges is old, even if it has been stored away from light. Avoid, too, chicons with bruised outer leaves – bad handling somewhere along the line, one suspects.

The corollary of all this is that one shouldn't keep chicory lurking around in the vegetable drawer of the fridge for too long. Keep it in the dark, and use it within a couple of days at most. Kept for longer than that, it may still look pretty good, but will be gathering bitterness quietly. Fine if you like that kind of taste (I do, in fact, but it's not everyone's cup of tea), but not ideal when you are sharing.

Chicory preparation is minimal. Those tightly curled leaves keep dirt out, so all you really need do is slice off the oxidised brown base. The bitterest part of the chicon is the basal cone and so, if you wish, cut this out with the tip of a narrow-bladed sharp knife. That's it for the basics. Next steps depend on how you intend to use your chicory. For salads, it is enough just to slice it across the chicon into strips around 5 mm–1 cm (¼–½ in) wide. Or for whole leaves to dip into this or that, or to carry a cargo of some sort, just cut off another slice of base, so that the leaves come away easily. When chicory is to be cooked, it is usually left whole, just as it is.

When it comes to chicory in salads, I veer instantly to what was, I believe, my mother's favourite winter salad – sliced curls of chicory, handfuls of peppery watercress, and chunks of sweet juicy orange, dressed lightly with a simple white wine vinegar or lemon vinaigrette. It is a sublime combination and almost impossible to improve on. Still, there's no reason to be stick in the mud. Unless you are a passionate chicory lover, it's probably best considered as a contributor rather than a mainstay of a salad. So, you might well like to toss it with a few handfuls of rocket, some prawns, halved cherry tomatoes, chopped parsley and a lemon and olive oil dressing, to form a fresh starter. Or add cooked chickpeas (canned are fine), shredded sweet cos lettuce, strips of grilled pepper (from a can in winter), and dress the whole lot with a warm dressing made by sizzling chorizo in olive oil with chopped garlic, then finishing with lots of lemon juice. Think too, in terms of adding black olives, crab, toasted almonds, Parma ham, papaya, mango, or mixing (another classic this) with apple, walnuts and mayonnaise to make a Waldorf salad (see page 129).

Chicory leaves are nature's edible scoops. Which makes them great party animals. Arrange them in a glass beside some utterly lovely dip, or arrange them in circles on a serving plate and pile something equally lovely in the lower curve. When short on time, but yearning for a touch of luxury, try a blob of crème fraîche or soured cream, surmounted by a small spoonful of caviar – for most of us that means the excellent and affordable herring roe caviar that you can now buy in fishmongers and supermarkets, but if you feel like splashing out, the real thing will go down a storm. Or make a cream of Roquefort with a touch of mayonnaise and load that in, perhaps with a little diced tomato on top for colour and sweetness. Or go South American and mix finely diced mango, tomato, shallot, chilli, season with salt, pepper, lime juice and oodles of fine chopped coriander. And so on and so forth.

Cooked chicory demands an altogether more restrained, classical touch. Softening the chicons in boiling water, or roasting them in the oven, emphasises the bitterness. In this enhanced state, they naturally gravitate towards the caressing presence of cream or butter. At the most elemental, blanch whole chicory spears for just long enough to soften (around 8–10 minutes), drain assiduously (water gets trapped in the layers), then serve while still hot with a knob of butter melting over them. Nicer still, blanch them, drain and leave to cool, then reheat by frying gently in butter, with a sprinkle of parsley. You could also try drizzling on some orange juice, or a little honey, or both. Or, blanch, cut in half lengthways, drain, then reheat with a small knob of butter, finishing with a good slug of double cream simmering until almost all absorbed, and finally sharpening with a squeeze of lemon juice. So good.

In similar vein, make a chicory gratin: pack the chicons tightly in an ovenproof dish, smear with crème fraîche, season and top with freshly grated Parmesan or vintage Gruyère, then whip into a hot oven for 20–30 minutes until bubbling and sizzling. Which brings me to the best of all chicory dishes, the French 'endives au jambon'. 'Endive' is the French for chicory; 'jambon', as you know, is ham. Lightly cooked spears of endive, wrapped in good-quality slices of cooked ham, laid side by side in a gratin dish, covered with a mustardy white sauce, a flourish of cheese and baked until browned. Chicory as main course and quite unbeatable. For quantities and detail see the parsnip and ham gratin on page 59, and replace parsnip with heads of chicory.

* *

Chicory, pear and watercress salad with walnut dressing

Light and fresh and ideal for late autumn or early winter when all of the ingredients are at their best. If you have nasturtiums in the garden, replace some or all of the watercress with peppery nasturtium leaves.

If you would like to serve the salad as a starter, you might like to perch a slice of blue cheese (Roquefort, Stilton or Gorgonzola all work well) on top of each helping, or embellish them with a few slices of cured raw ham. Serrano or Parma ham will do very nicely indeed.

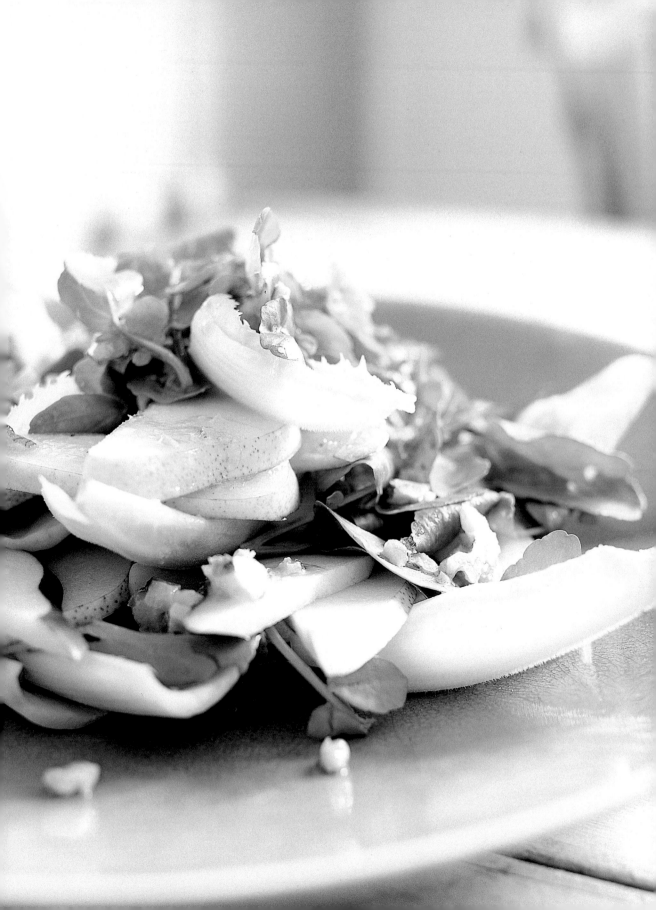

Serves 4–6

2 ripe pears
juice of ½ lemon
2 heads chicory, trimmed and sliced
a big handful of watercress or rocket leaves

Dressing
60 g (2 oz) shelled walnuts, toasted
½ tablespoon white wine vinegar
¼ teaspoon Dijon mustard
3 tablespoons walnut oil
salt and pepper

Prepare the dressing first. Chop the toasted walnuts finely. Whisk the vinegar with the mustard, salt and pepper, then gradually whisk in the oil. Stir in the walnuts.

Not too long before serving, peel the pears if they have a thick, grainy skin. Quarter, core and then slice thinly. Toss with lemon juice to prevent browning. Mix with the chicory and watercress or rocket. Spoon the dressing over them, then toss at the table. Serve straightaway.

* *

Caramelised chicory

If you have any fondness for chicory, then try this at once. It is just divine. So good in fact that I ate half of it at one sitting, though in theory one chicon alone should be enough per person. Serve hot or warm.

Serves 4 (or 2 chicory aficionados)

4 heads chicory
20 g (¾ oz) butter
2 teaspoons runny honey
juice of ½ large orange
salt and pepper

Preheat the oven to 180°C/350°F/Gas 4.

Trim the chicory and cut in half lengthways. Rub half the butter thickly over the bottom of an ovenproof dish, and pack the chicory halves, in a single layer, into the dish. Drizzle over the honey and orange juice and season with salt and pepper. Dot with the remaining butter. Roast, uncovered, for about 1 hour, turning and basting the chicory every 15 minutes. Keep a close eye on proceedings towards the end of the cooking time and take the dish out of the oven when the juices have reduced to a few spoonfuls of thick syrup and the chicory is looking suitably caramelised.

* *

Chinese cabbage

* * *

Many of the oriental brassicas are beautiful, with their whorls of white and green, or elegant jagged-edged foliage, all conspiring to promote a mildly exotic yet unintimidating attractiveness. **Chinese cabbage** is the exception. Neither its other western names, **Chinese leaf** and **Peking cabbage**, nor the Chinese pe-tsai, can disguise the fact that it is big and bulky and solid. I have read that it can swell up to a whopping 27 kg (60 lb), which seems quite extraordinary. Just imagine lugging that home with the shopping.

The Chinese cabbages sold here weigh in at a more comfortable 1 kg (2¼ lb) a piece, give or take. They are one of the mildest tasting of all the oriental brassicas. They have no more than a delicate whiff of cabbaginess and detractors might suggest that they are insipid. In reality, it is their texture that gives them their major appeal. Crisp, juicy broad ribs slip away to delicate yellow/green frilled edges. This combination of taste and texture makes them ideal carriers for bigger, butch flavourings, and there's no better example of this than the Korean kimchi, searingly hot, fermented Chinese cabbage pickles that lie at the heart of the country's cuisine. It also means that they are a natural winner in the salad stakes, contributing a succulence that is rare in most salad leaves, and again, working as a natural base for additional, showier ingredients.

Practicalities

Whilst Chinese cabbage is sometimes sold in supermarkets, it's a safer bet to head to an oriental supermarket to search it out (probably cheaper, too). Ideally, your chosen cabbage will be heavy and solid, with broad outer leaves of clean white, tapering off to a pale green or yellow edge.

Like our own cannonballs of white cabbage, the sheer density of this vegetable ensures that it keeps for a fair amount of time, but it will be at its best in the early days. The downside of this is that it is easy to disguise a not-so-fresh Chinese cabbage, simply by trimming off the outer leaves and base to reveal pristine inner leaves. It is best to buy them, therefore, from a busy, popular shop where the turnover is likely to be speedy. Sniff the cabbage discreetly before popping into your shopping basket. It shouldn't smell of anything much, so if there is a distinct sulphurous whiff, it would be advisable to re-plan your menu.

At home, store the Chinese cabbage in the vegetable drawer of the fridge, where it can hang out happily for up to 5 days, if needs must. The easiest way to prepare it is to remove any damaged outer leaves, then simply slice off whatever you need, cutting across the leaves to produce narrow or broad ribbons as required. Rinse after cutting if necessary, and return the remainder of the cabbage to the fridge.

Whilst it is undoubtedly true that Chinese cabbage makes brilliant pickles, I've always left these to the professionals (i.e. bought jars of kimchi at the same time as the fresh Chinese cabbage). One of these days I will have a go at making my own, but for now, **salads** and **stir-fries** are where Chinese cabbage goes in our household.

Though it slides quite nicely into mixed green salads and the like, Chinese cabbage becomes a more interesting proposition when it is enlivened with a whizzy Asian dressing, blessed with chilli, garlic, lime, soy or fish sauce, sesame oil and the like. With that in hand, you can then add any number of other ingredients, prawns, slices of griddled chicken or steak, coriander, basil and mint, tomatoes, shreds of carrots, chopped toasted nuts, slices of tart, under-ripe mango, grapefruit or pomelo, and more.

Likewise, it benefits from bold eastern seasonings when stir-fried. Garlic, chilli and ginger, of course, soy sauce, fish sauce, kecap manis (Indonesian sweet soy sauce), sesame oil, a final garnish of chopped spring onions.

Lighter Chinese styles, with the juices thickened with cornflour remind me of invalid food, emphasising nothing but the lack of emphatic taste. Best avoided, I think.

* *

Stir-fried Chinese leaf with dried shrimps

Adding a handful of dried shrimps to a simple stir-fry of Chinese leaf gives it an enormous lift. I guess it's the umami factor – those shrimps have plenty of the deep savoury flavour that you find in bacon or mature cheese. You don't need a lot, but it makes a big difference.

You can buy them in any Chinese grocery store – sometimes they are tiny, but for this I prefer the medium-sized shrimp, about as big as the tip of your thumbnail. Those that you don't use can be stored for several months in an airtight container in the fridge – try adding them to a stir-fry of Savoy cabbage or courgettes.

Serves 4

30 g (1 oz) Chinese dried shrimps
2 tablespoons sunflower or vegetable oil
4 cloves garlic, chopped

1 cm (½ in) piece fresh root ginger, chopped
1 head Chinese leaf, thickly shredded
4 spring onions, thinly sliced
salt

Soak the dried shrimps in 4 tablespoons water for half an hour. Drain, reserving the soaking water.

Heat a roomy wok over a high heat until it smokes. Add the oil, swirl once, then add the garlic and ginger. Stir-fry for a few seconds, then add the shrimps and stir-fry for a few seconds longer. Now quickly tip in the cabbage and stir-fry for about 2 minutes. Pour in the reserved soaking water and season with salt, then cover and leave to cook for another 1–2 minutes, until the cabbage is crisp-tender. Stir in the spring onions, and serve immediately.

* *

Pink grapefruit and Chinese leaf salad with beetroot threads

I defy anyone not to feel scintillatingly healthy and revived by this salad. The fresh instant-impact taste of the ingredients works mini-miracles. It looks drop-dead gorgeous, too.

One small word of warning. Grating raw beetroot is messy, though less messy than handling cooked. Do not be tempted to toss the beetroot into the salad with the dressing – it will bleed left, right and centre. Be content with piling it on top.

Serves 2–3

1 pink or red-fleshed grapefruit
1/4 Chinese cabbage
1/2 medium raw beetroot, peeled and
  coarsely grated
15–20 g (1/2–3/4 oz) toasted coconut flakes or
  toasted almonds

Dressing
2 tablespoons rice wine vinegar
1/2 teaspoon finely grated fresh root ginger
2 teaspoons sesame oil
1/2 teaspoon caster sugar
salt and pepper

To make the dressing just whisk all the ingredients together.

Peel the grapefruit. If the segments of your grapefruit are firm, use a small sharp knife to separate them: cut down close to the thin membrane that separates one segment from another, on both sides of each segment, so that it falls out on to the board. Many grapefruits are too soft for this to work sensibly, so just separate the segments and pull off the translucent skin on each one, trying to keep the skinned segments whole. Reserve the segments and any juice that has oozed out.

Just before serving, tear or cut the Chinese cabbage leaves up roughly and mix with the grapefruit segments, the coconut or almonds and the dressing. Scatter the shreds of beetroot on top and serve.

Lettuces

* * *

Life moves on, and we barely notice the little things that disappear as technology propels us forward. On the whole, this is a good thing, and affords us the pleasure of nostalgia. Whenever I remember it, which admittedly is not often, I think warmly of my mother's wire salad basket. As household tasks go, being sent outside to swing the water off newly washed salad leaves was one of the better ones. It was fun to stand, legs firmly braced, swinging the basket round and round, centrifugal forces tugging at my arm and sending an arc of water droplets shooting out.

Arm and basket have now been replaced by the ugly but effective plastic salad spinners that take up so much space in the cupboard. Redundant rusting salad baskets are relegated to the status of quaint egg-holders in photos of idealised country living. Funny how things pan out in the end.

If we are not careful, it may even come to the point when the plastic salad spinner teeters on the verge of extinction. The dominance of pouched salad mixes marches on. I use them, and so do most of us, but it's all too easy to come to believe that every salad we ever eat either has to be a pile of rocket, or a mix of eight different dwarf-sized salad leaves of multiple shape and hue. In fact, the best lettuce salad of all, the height of perfection, is the salad that is made out of a single lettuce picked that day from the garden and taken straight to the kitchen to be washed, spun and dressed. No need for designer leaves, for contrasts and cleverness, for inspirational frolics, for fancy dressings, not when you have a sparkling, fresh bowlful of green lettuce leaves. That's when you understand the real point of eating salad.

Are you muttering that we can't all be perfect gardeners as well as cooks, parents, workers, and everything else expected of us these days? I agree. I don't grow my own lettuces, either. I've tried in a casual way in the past, but when, miraculously, rabbits and slugs have failed to demolish my nascent

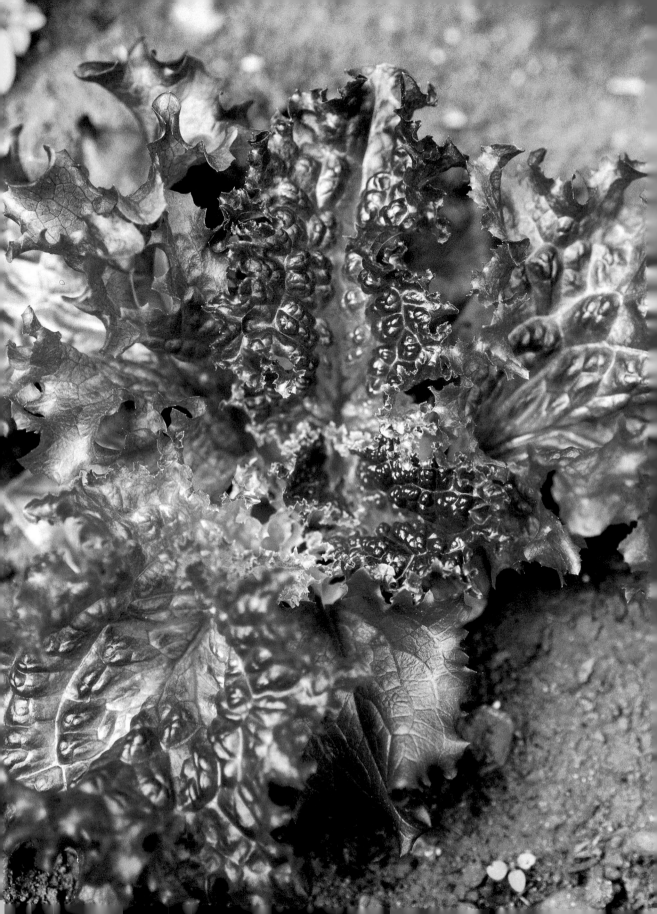

greenery, the mature lettuces bolt to bitter heights the second I turn my back. However, I do know a good lettuce when I see one, and they are one of the most pleasing sights of a summer month, ranged in verdant finery on a market stall, or nestling cosily next to the carrots in my vegetable box. It genuinely doesn't take up much time to wash and spin dry a fresh lettuce. Not something to do every day, perhaps, but at the weekend it can become a positive pleasure, even with a garish plastic salad spinner.

Practicalities

BUYING So many lettuces, so little time. A pouch of **prepared salad leaves** in the fridge means you can toss together a salad at the drop of a hat. It means that you can enjoy the taste of two or three different types of leaf without wasting the remainder of two or three whole lettuces. Always give the bag a gentle shake before buying, so that you can assess the state of the leaves within. In their enclosed atmosphere they are not so likely to wilt before the sell-by-date, but you may spot leaves whose colour is darkening damply to a slimy state, or stalk ends that are browner than they should be. Do not waste your money on them.

Back home keep bagged salads in the salad crisper drawer of the fridge, and use as soon as possible, certainly within a day or two once the bag is opened.

With unbagged whole lettuces, it is a doddle to assess freshness. A glance is enough. Does it look bright and lively and enticing? Or floppy and miserable and lacking self-esteem? Even that most ordinary of British lettuces, the **soft-leaved butterhead**, should exhibit clear signs of jaunty character if it is newly arrived from the field. As for the beauties of the lettuce world, a burnished, exuberant **Batavia**, for instance...well, there's no doubting when they're fresh as daisies.

With freshness being the burning issue with whole lettuces, it would be foolish not to eat them as soon as possible. That day, or at the very most within 48 hours. Even if you're not going to use more than, say, half the lettuce at first go, it still makes sense to wash and pick over the whole thing at once. That way the remainder can sit in a plastic bag in the vegetable drawer or salad crisper drawer of your fridge, as convenient as any pre-prepared bagged salad, waiting for you to grab whatever you need whenever you need it. The method is undemanding – cut off the base, throw out any outer leaves that are badly damaged or too keenly perforated with slug holes, then drop the remaining leaves into a bowl or sink of cold water. Swish them around gently, then take the leaves out one by one, rinsing off any clingy dirt and removing unwelcome wildlife. Spin, in several batches if needs be, until more or less dry. Job done.

Lettuce can be cooked. Not all lettuces take to it brilliantly, but some are quite amenable to heat, though they will, without fail, diminish to a fraction of their original volume. Tightly furled lettuces, like **little gem**, are good cooked whole. You will need one per person – blanch for a minute or so in boiling salted water then drain and press out trapped water, before tossing with melted butter and fresh chervil or chives. Or halve or quarter heads, toss with a vinaigrette and roast in a hot oven for 10 minutes, or grill just like radicchio (see page 430). Or you could stir broadly shredded lettuce into a small amount of bubbling double cream, sharpen with a squeeze of lemon and finish with a grating of nutmeg.

Perhaps easier to deal with as a concept is lettuce soup. Usually combined with other summer vegetables (e.g. courgettes or peas), lettuce contributes a unique, sweet, subtle scent. One of the most famous lettuce dishes is petits pois à la française (see page 265) where the lettuce almost melts into the peas in a delicate enhancing fashion. Although it barely qualifies as cooking, shredded lettuce leaves are lovely tossed into hot pasta, together with lots of diced tomato, capers and fresh herbs, and olive oil. In the time it takes to mix and dish up the pasta, the heat will have softened the lettuce to just the right degree. Italians do a great line in lightly cooked **frisée**, also known as **curly endive** (technically it's a form of chicory, like radicchio, as is Batavia), which has a mild bitter taste, more pronounced in the greener outer leaves, diminishing as you work in towards the golden heart. Try blanching the stronger outer leaves in boiling water for seconds, then draining well, before sautéing in olive oil with chopped garlic and chilli.

Enough of hot lettuce. Good though it can be, everyone knows that the rightful destiny of a lettuce is the salad bowl. A great green salad is a joy. To make it you need a perfectly fresh lettuce, washed and dried (wet lettuce dilutes the dressing), and just the right amount of vinaigrette (see below) made from first-class oils and vinegar or lemon. With the occasional rarest of exceptions, bottled dressings are anathema to a proper salad. A bottle of the best extra virgin olive oil you can afford and another of good wine vinegar, or a simple lemon, salt and pepper are all you need to make a handsome dressing that fits the salad (for a potato or rice salad, for instance, a sharper dressing is required than for a green salad). You can add to it and improve it and play with flavourings in a way that you can't with a bottled dressing.

Never dress a lettuce salad until you are on the verge of eating it. The oil in the dressing wilts the leaves prematurely. I find that the easiest procedure, especially when I have guests as well as family, is to whisk up the dressing directly in the salad bowl in advance, then to cross the salad servers in the bowl over the dressing. The washed lettuce leaves stay in the fridge until some 20–30 minutes before serving, at which point they are piled on top of the salad servers. This way they have time to lose their chill, and only a few minor leaves will tumble down into the dressing. The majority stay clear, ready to toss when we reach the right stage of the meal.

Although salads go well alongside so many main courses, or can be built up to make a starter or a main dish, I love nothing better than to settle, French-style, to a helping of salad, alongside a wedge of good cheese, before fruit or a pudding. Green salad and cheese – a moment of everyday magic.

Cooks and chefs through the ages have inevitably codified rules and regulations about creating an ideal mixed green salad. Forget them. Take the best of what is available and do your own thing with it. Contrasting textures and tastes can be fabulous – mix pale green **feuille de chêne** lettuce with crisp frisée and peppery **rocket**, for instance – but so too is a mix of sweet lettuces, like torn-up leaves of cos partnered with **mâche (lamb's lettuce)** and frilly **lollo biondo**. Or stretch the original concept of a green salad to include leaves, green salad vegetables (celery, cucumber, thin shreds of fennel, raw fresh peas, avocado) and soft-leaved herbs (flat-leafed parsley, basil, coriander, chervil, chives and others).

One could fill pages with ideas for lettuce-based salads, but instead I shall limit myself to just two broad forays into the myriad possibilities. The first is to point out the blessed affinity between nuts and salad leaves. One of the easiest ways of bringing a touch of effortless class to a humble salad is to add toasted nuts and replace the olive oil with the corresponding nut oil where possible. Top of my list would be a bowl of cos or **Webb's wonder**, tossed with a generous handful of newly toasted and cooled walnut halves and a dressing made with walnut oil. A small touch of heaven, especially when served with goat's cheese. Hazelnuts and hazelnut oil are excellent with mâche. Match toasted pine nuts (be careful – they burn extra quickly) with an avocado oil and so on.

The second is to remind you how appealing warm salads can be. They were all the rage some 15 years ago, but have lost out more recently. You need a fairly robust lettuce or salad leaf (e.g. cos, Webb's wonder, rocket, frisée) to withstand the heat. With the lettuce ready and waiting, the method runs something like this: heat 3 or 4 tablespoons of olive oil in a frying pan and add chopped garlic, strips of bacon, cubes of chorizo, cubes of slightly stale bread, or thinly sliced chicken or salmon, fry until browned/cooked through, take off the heat, wait a few seconds for the temperature to fall slightly then stir in a tablespoon or so of wine vinegar, some Dijon or coarse-grain mustard if you wish, salt and pepper. Quickly pour over the lettuce while still hot. Toss briefly and eat at once.

Iceberg lettuce became the darling of the catering world because it keeps so well (unnaturally well, you might say), has very little taste to lose, is deeply inoffensive, whilst being juicy and crunchy. For these same reasons, many non-caterers have dismissed it as being a pointless addition to the lettuce world. I want to put my hand up and say that I quite like iceberg in moderation, but it has to be thinly sliced and mixed with other things, most importantly an extremely appetising dressing. Childishly, I also like it because of a little trick I was taught years ago. To remove the central core of an iceberg lettuce, clasp it firmly with both hands, then bang the stem end down firmly on the work surface three times. Now turn the iceberg upside down and you should be able to twist the stem cone out in one easy movement. Neat, huh?

Now halve or quarter the iceberg, wrap what you aren't using immediately in clingfilm and return to the fridge. It's worth noting, whilst I'm on the subject, that fat ribbons of iceberg make a rather good last-few-seconds addition to a stir-fry.

* *

French dressing or vinaigrette

These are synonyms for the standard European salad dressing, that stands or falls by the quality and balance of its simple ingredients. It can be varied hugely, widely, wisely or indeed inadvisably. Sharpness will need to be adjusted to fit the main ingredients of the salad and personal taste, but should not be so strong that it disguises their taste.

Enough dressing for 2 green salads for 3–4 people

1 tablespoon good-quality red or white wine
   vinegar or lemon juice
½ teaspoon Dijon mustard
a pinch or two of caster sugar (optional)
4–5 tablespoons extra virgin olive oil or
   groundnut oil
salt and pepper

Method 1 Whisk the vinegar or lemon juice with the mustard, sugar, salt and pepper. Gradually whisk in the oil a tablespoon at a time. Taste and adjust the ratio of sharp to smooth to salt. Set aside until needed, then whisk again briefly if necessary.

   Method 2 Put all ingredients into a jam jar. Seal tightly and shake until evenly mixed. Taste and adjust the ratio of sharp to smooth to salt. Set aside until needed, then shake again briefly if necessary.

* *

Italian curly endive and bean soup

I love the blend of earthy beans with the mild bitterness of curly endive
(or frisée) in this Italian soup. It's the perfect reassuring rustic dish for those
unwelcome overcast summer days, when the temperature is not what you
think it should be. Of course, if the day turns out to be unexpectedly hot,
change the menu instantly by making a salad with the curly endive, and
a separate salad with beans, celery and diced tomato.

Serves 6

1 large onion, chopped
2 sticks celery, chopped
4 cloves garlic, chopped
2 tablespoons extra virgin olive oil, plus a
    little extra for serving
400 g (14 oz) shelled fresh borlotti or haricot
    beans or 300 g (11 oz) dried haricot or
    borlotti beans, soaked overnight

1 bouquet garni (1 bay leaf, 2 sprigs thyme,
    2 parsley stalks, tied together with string)
2 litres (3½ pints) chicken or vegetable
    stock
1 head curly endive or frisée lettuce, well
    rinsed, damaged leaves removed
salt and pepper

Fry the onion, celery and garlic gently in the olive oil in a large saucepan
until very tender, without browning. Now add the beans, bouquet garni and
the stock. If using dried beans, add an extra 200 ml (7 fl oz) of water as they'll
need longer cooking. Bring up to the boil and simmer until the beans are so
tender they are beginning to collapse.

Take off the heat and discard the bundle of herbs. Liquidise enough of
the beans to thicken the soup but leave some chunky – I use a hand-held
liquidiser wand which plunges straight into the pan, and makes it easier
to judge when the soup is thick enough for my taste.

Meanwhile, bring a pan of water up to the boil. Set aside a few sprigs of
frisée, then plunge the rest into the boiling water. Bring back to the boil then
drain immediately. Chop roughly.

10 minutes before you are ready to eat, reheat the soup, thinning down
a little if necessary, and stir in the frisée, salt and pepper. Simmer for 1–2
minutes, then serve, drizzling each bowlful with a trickle of olive oil, and
garnishing with small frisée sprigs.

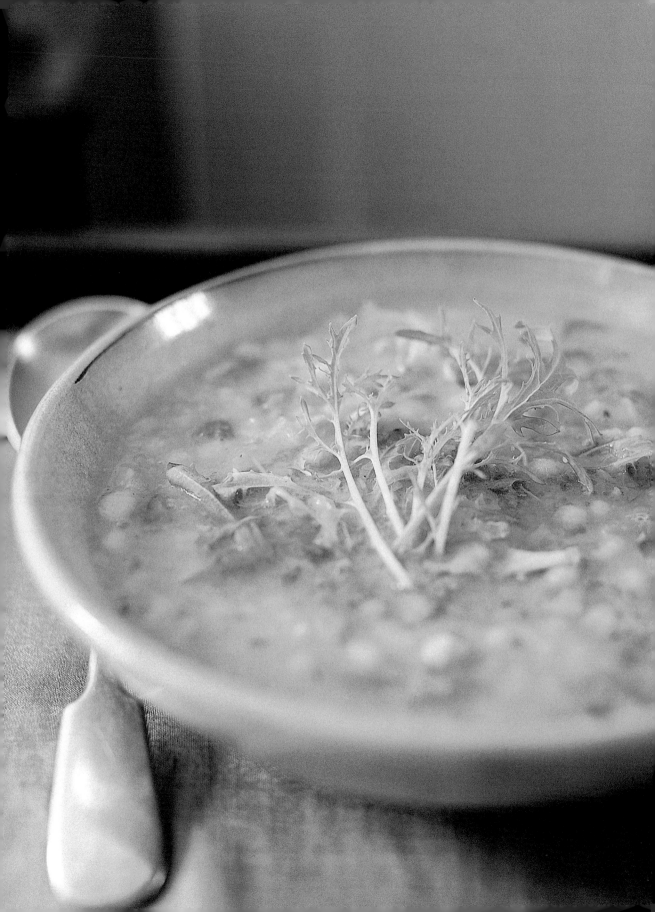

Couronne niçoise

This is the summer luncheon version of salade niçoise in a roll. The roll is replaced with a large ring of crisp choux pastry. It looks pretty, tastes divine.

The choux ring, by the way, can be cooked 24 hours in advance, but don't fill it until just before serving.

Serves 6

Choux paste
300 ml (10 fl oz) water
115 g (4 oz) unsalted butter, diced
150 g (5 oz) plain flour
½ teaspoon salt
4 eggs
60 g (2 oz) Gruyère cheese, grated
1 teaspoon kalonji seeds (black onion seeds)
   or poppy seeds

Filling
1 x 185 g can tuna, drained and flaked
3 heaped tablespoons mayonnaise

1 tablespoon rinsed capers, chopped
3 canned anchovy fillets, chopped
2 hard-boiled eggs, chopped
4 spring onions, thinly sliced
2 handfuls frisée or 4 leaves cos lettuce,
   torn into small pieces
100 g (3½ oz) cooked green beans
120 g (generous 4 oz) cherry tomatoes, sliced
8 black olives, stoned and roughly chopped
3 tablespoons vinaigrette (see page 421)
1 grilled, skinned red or orange pepper,
   deseeded and cut into strips
salt and pepper

To make the choux pastry ring, preheat the oven to 230°C/450°F/Gas 8, and line a large baking tray with non-stick baking parchment. Using a dinner plate or saucepan lid as a template, mark out a circle of around 28–30 cm (11–12 in) in diameter. Turn the paper over so that the outline is still visible, but you are not actually getting the ink/graphite into your food.

Heat the water and the butter gently until the butter has melted, without letting the water boil. Once the butter has completely melted, bring up to a rolling boil. Immediately tip the flour and salt into the pan. Turn the heat down low. Beat the flour into the butter and water mixture until it forms a loose ball. Take off the heat.

Now break in the first egg and beat in thoroughly. Beat in the second egg, and then the third. Break the last egg into a bowl and whisk lightly, then beat in dribbles of the egg until the paste reaches a fairly stiff dropping consistency, and has a glossy sheen to it.

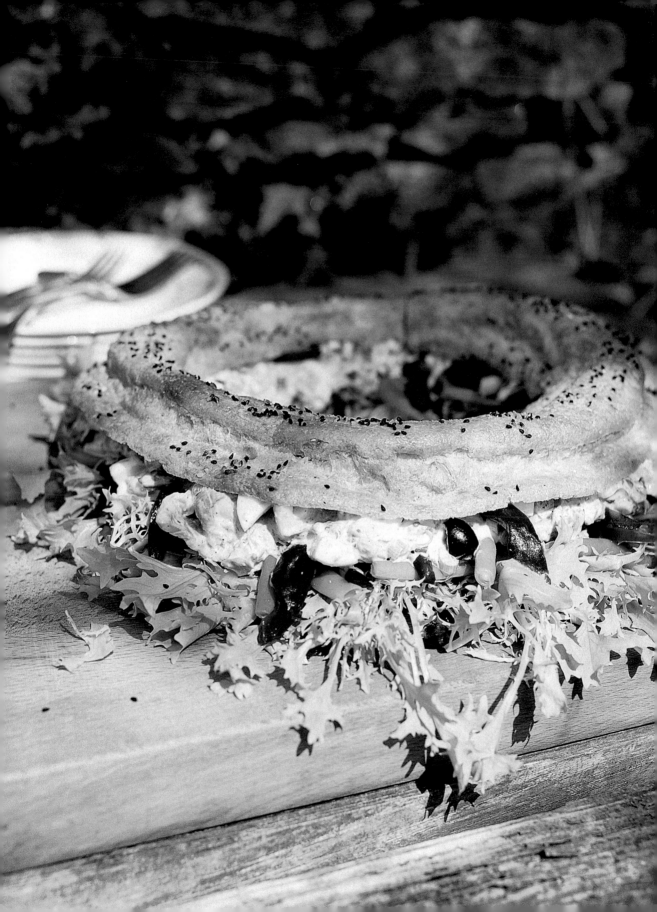

Fit a piping bag with a 1 cm (½ in) nozzle. Fill the bag with the choux paste and pipe a circle of warm dough over the guideline. Now pipe a second circle just inside the first, cheek to cheek. Finish with a third circle sitting on top of the first two.

Sprinkle the choux pastry with cheese and seeds then slide into the preheated oven. Bake for 15 minutes until well puffed. Now reduce the heat to 200°C/400°F/Gas 6 and bake for a further 10 minutes. Make holes in the sides of the ring with a skewer to release the steam, then return to the oven, reduced to a mere 180°C/350°F/Gas 4 and cook for a further 10 minutes. Turn off the oven, leave the door ajar and leave to cool down in the oven. Once cool, carefully slice in half horizontally.

While the choux ring is cooking and drying out, turn to the filling. Mash the tuna up with the mayonnaise, then stir in the capers, anchovies, hard-boiled eggs and spring onions. Season to taste (it may need no more than a good measure of pepper).

Make a bed of frisée in the base of the pastry ring, then top with green beans, tomato slices and olives. Drizzle over the vinaigrette. Top with spoonfuls of the tuna mixture, then finish with strips of grilled pepper. Serve swiftly, before the pastry goes soggy.

* *

Purslane

* * *

I wish we saw more of purslane. It's an exceptional salad leaf, quite unlike any other, with fleshy lobes, crisp stem and a unique mildly astringent taste. It grows well enough in colder climates, but is better known in northern Africa and parts of Italy and France, where it takes a regular place in salads. This popularity ensures that there are several different forms of what is essentially the same plant, so it's hard to be precise with descriptions.

I've bought handsome **red-stemmed purslane** with fat-lip leaves no bigger than my thumb nail, and larger-leaved **golden purslane.**

If you are not a vegetable grower, you will have to head to a Middle Eastern or possibly Turkish food store to track down purslane. Its naturally botoxed leaves are easy to recognise, try it if the opportunity arises.

Practicalities

BUYING
Whatever sort of purslane you find, the leaves should be smooth skinned and fleshy. Wrinkles mean that it is drying out so there's little point in buying it. Keep it in the fridge and eat within a couple of days. To prepare, simply pick over and discard any damaged leaves and stems, and throw out fatter, stringier lower stems. Then nibble a leaf to assess the degree of astringency. Large-leafed purslane can be too strong for comfort. Either cook it, or chop finely and add to a salad with lots of other ingredients, as a seasoning rather than a main element.

COOKING
To cook stronger purslane, blanch for a minute in boiling water, then drain and serve warm dressed with finest olive oil and a squeeze of lemon. Or you could toss it in hot butter or olive oil for a few minutes until tender and less powerful. I like it with tomato, too – perhaps some chopped deseeded pieces mixed in for the last few seconds so that they warm through, but don't disintegrate.

Purslane with a more restrained astringency should be taken straight to the salad bowl, where it makes a handsome addition to any mixed green salad, and is lovely in a grilled pepper salad. One of my favourites is the Middle Eastern 'fattoush'. This salad, with its vast quantities of herbs (parsley, mint, and corriander), is wonderfully refreshing in summer. Based on cucumber, tomatoes and onion – with added triangles of toasted pitta – it is good without the purslane, but even nicer with as the purslane adds a slight edge to the mixture of vegetables and greenery.

* *

Radicchio

* * *

Radicchio had its 15 minutes of fame some time ago, back in the late 1980s and 1990s, when designer salads were all the rage. The fall-out left rocket at the top of the heap, the great survivor, and radicchio relegated to a few shredded leaves tossed into mixed packs of continental salads, more for colour than for taste. It is now almost impossible to buy whole heads of radicchio in supermarkets. For this you must head to a smart greengrocer.

Although I regret this, I have to admit that it is not so surprising. The bitterness of radicchio leaves is not to everyone's taste. Just because I love it does not mean that money can be made from selling it in every food shop in the land. The ironic thing is that radicchio is merely a form of chicory, and its alter-ego, witloof chicory forced in the dark, seems increasingly popular.

Those of us who have a taste for the fresh bitterness of radicchio leaves must learn to stick together and celebrate this increasingly rare vegetable. Pilgrimages to Treviso in the north-east of Italy should be organised to sample it at its freshest and finest, in all its several forms. For yes, there are many radicchios, not just the purple ball we know and admire. Aficionados will delight in the discovery of long-leaved **Treviso radicchio**, the open rosettes of **Chioggia radicchio** or the stunningly beautiful red-speckled, yellow leaves of **Castelfranco radicchio** amongst others.

From Italy, we should take our inspiration for using radicchio not merely as a salad leaf, delightful though that is, but also as an ingredient in cooked dishes. Grilled, braised, sautéed, deep-fried – you name it, radicchio will take them all on board with extraordinary aplomb for a mere has-been salad leaf.

Practicalities

BUYING Whilst it is fair enough to expect the outer leaves of a ball of radicchio to have sustained the odd bit of damage, they should still be firm and richly

428

coloured (not brown). Not so long ago a greengrocer who shall remain nameless tried (and failed) to convince me that floppy-leaved radicchio was in good order. It wasn't and never would be. Whilst radicchio is not as crisp as, say, iceberg lettuce, its leaves should hold their shape without flopping or flapping. Always cast a glance at the base of the ball – if it is dark brown, or slimy, then ask for fresher radicchio if it is available. When you get it home, slip it into the vegetable drawer of the fridge, where it will keep for 4 or 5 days assuming it was in good shape to start with.

Basic preparation consists merely of slicing a thin disc off the base, and removing the outer leaves unless they are in pristine order. Thereafter, preparation depends on end use. For salads you may need no more than a few leaves to add a note of bitterness and colour amongst the sweeter greenery. In this case, just remove a few leaves and shred or tear up as you fancy. For larger quantities, simply slice across the whole head of radicchio to release broad ribbons of red.

But don't relegate radicchio to a mere note amongst other salad leaves. It has far more potential than that. For a start, those crisp leaves that hold their shape so well make superb containers. You could look to Asia for ideas for fillings – there are superb mixtures of fried minced chicken flavoured with coriander, chilli and lemongrass, for instance, which are usually parcelled up in ordinary lettuce leaves or soft rice-paper wrappers, but are possibly even better in radicchio. Or you might try rice-based fillings, enlivened with plenty of herbs and a lively dressing, diced tomato or cheese or a pile of couscous, mixed with sautéed pine nuts, diced dried apricots and onion, and enriched with spices and coriander.

COOKING Heating emphasises the bitterness of radicchio. A good, gentle introduction to this is to serve **deep-fried** breaded radicchio leaves. Sounds odd, but they make a handsome, and unexpected starter. Take individual leaves, dust them with flour, dip into beaten egg, then coat in breadcrumbs and deep-fry until golden brown. Serve them with tzatziki (see page 208), or with goat's cheese cream (mash goat's cheese with soured cream and stir in plenty of chopped chives, salt and pepper), or on top of a mound of rocket and grilled pepper or tomatoes, dressed with a brisk vinaigrette.

Radicchio **risotto** is another winner, which can be made mildly bitter or boosted according to preference. Follow a basic risotto recipe, or the one on page 325 omitting the wild garlic and potatoes, then stir in shredded radicchio when the rice is a mere thread away from al dente. For more substance add raw prawns with the radicchio, so that they are both perfectly cooked but no more when the risotto is placed on the table.

Radicchio takes to the frying pan or wok with grace. Those who love the bitterness will simply **sauté** lots of radicchio in olive oil or butter, perhaps with garlic, then eat it straight. Others may prefer to mix it with balancing ingredients. If you've never tried sautéed potatoes with radicchio, then give it a go – when your potatoes are all but done, add a handful of shredded radicchio to the pan for the final burst of cooking. Or sauté them with sliced chicken breast and shallot or onion to pile into tortillas together with soured cream, avocado and a tomato salsa. A touch of sweetness in the frying pan won't go amiss, either. Sauté radicchio with pine nuts and raisins then finish with a drizzle of honey and a shake of red wine vinegar. And when you are **stir-frying**, include radicchio amongst the last batch of veg to go into the wok so that it softens but doesn't lose all firmness in the intense heat.

The best-known way to cook radicchio, however, is to **grill** it. Sounds odd, but it is actually pretty straightforward. The head of radicchio is quartered, cutting through the base so that the wedges of purple hold together. It is then tossed in oil or a vinaigrette (I prefer the latter) and cooked for a few minutes under a thoroughly preheated grill. That's it. And pretty damn fine it is, too.

* *

Grilled radicchio with pear and Camembert

This is a fantastic quick and delicious first course, balancing the natural bitterness of radicchio with a touch of sweetness from the warm pear and the melting, sizzling cheese. 10 minutes from start to plate.

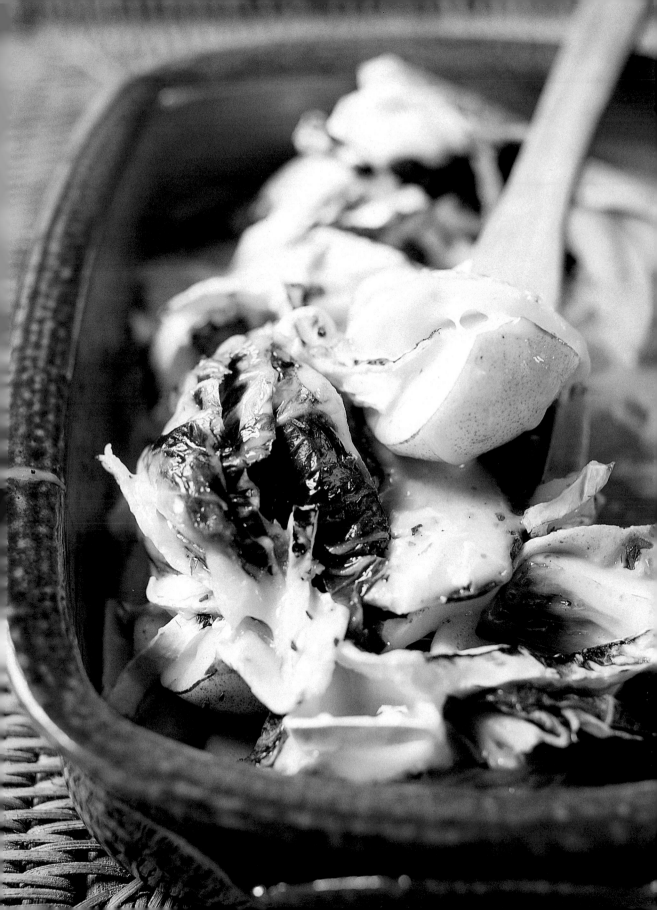

Serves 4 as a first course, 2 as a light main course

1 head radicchio	**Dressing**
1 ripe pear	½ tablespoon red wine vinegar
125 g (4½ oz) Camembert cheese, thinly sliced	½ teaspoon dried Greek rigani, or dried oregano
	1½ tablespoons extra virgin olive oil
	salt and pepper

Preheat the grill. Cut the radicchio into quarters, right through the stem end so that each wedge holds together. Whisk the vinegar with rigani, salt and pepper and gradually whisk in the oil. Quarter and core the pear, then immediately turn in the dressing to prevent premature browning. Turn the radicchio quarters in the dressing too.

Arrange the pears and radicchio in a heatproof dish and pour over the last of the dressing. Slide under the grill, and grill for about 5–6 minutes, turning the pieces once or twice, until browned outside.

Lay the slices of Camembert over the radicchio and pear, and return to the grill for a few minutes until the cheese is oozing and runny. Eat while still hot and sizzling.

* *

Rocket

* * *

The 1980s saw the second coming of rocket, riding into town with a host of acolytes. They rode under a new banner, that of 'Designer Salads'. At first they were all incredibly popular, everyone adored cuties like lollo rosso, then gradually the supremacy of rocket was established once and for all. It was no stranger to British dinner plates, having been recorded as growing in gardens in the Elizabethan era, but this time it took firm control, muscling other leaves from our meals, overshadowing our own humble peppery watercress, letting everyone know that no other leaf could compare. Gifted with charisma, good looks, presence and charm, it made its mark with consummate ease. Long live Lord Rocket, still going strong some 20 years later.

I have no problems pledging my allegiance. I adore rocket, not to the exclusion of all other salad leaves, but it's one that I never tire of. There's a peppery robustness, a firm texture of substance, and a surprising ability to get on handsomely with so many other savoury flavours. What's not to love?

Mizuna, mibuna, tat soi and a handful of other lesser leaves are recent latecomers to the designer salad scene. Like rocket they have a bolder character than many other salad leaves, and make for the basis of a more substantial salad. They are all included from time to time in bags of mixed salad leaves, where they meld into the general mass, but if you can buy them loose, at a farm shop, say, they are worth giving more of a show-case position, using them in much the same way as you would rocket.

Practicalities

BUYING There are three distinct sorts of rocket, as far as a cook is concerned. There is your **standard rocket or 'roquette'** which is what turns up most of the time, and is also known by Americans and Italians as **'arugula'**. Then there is **'wild rocket'**, which is no more wild than my cat Ginger, snoozing in front of the fire. It is cultivated, of course, but has thinner, whippier leaves, more jagged, and a slightly raunchier flavour than ordinary rocket. Finally, there is what is often sold as **'rokka'**, especially in Greek/Turkish food stores. About half the price of supermarket rocket, it has large wide leaves, and a stronger flavour than either of the other two. It's excellent in mixed salads, or in sandwiches, or cooked rocket dishes, but too powerful on its own for all but the most addicted rocket-lovers.

Only buy rocket if it looks firm-leaved, and has a healthy vigour to it. Limp rocket is past its best, and won't live up to expectations. If you have been lucky enough to buy rocket loose, rinse well as soon as you get home, spin dry, then store in a plastic bag in the fridge. Use it within a day or two to enjoy it at its finest. The same goes for pouched rocket.

When I write salad recipes, I have to consciously restrain myself from using rocket in every one. It's such an amenable salad leaf, offering a great base for any one of hundreds of other ingredients, and so easy to use. That's why it appears on the menu in every restaurant throughout the land, or so it seems. It adds colour and taste and rarely clashes. A neat rocket salad, dressed with no more than lemon, olive oil, salt and pepper, is delicious, and a great partner with a grilled steak, with a slab of salmon fillet, with a slice of cheese on toast, with a wedge of frittata, and so on and on and on. Start adding to the basic salad and the permutations are infinite. Right now I've got a bit of taste for rocket, roast tomato and feta salad, but it might just as well be rocket, chickpeas and prawns, or rocket, fried pitta bread triangles and roast red onions, or rocket with silvery marinated anchovies and halved cherry tomatoes, or a more classic mix of rocket with Parma ham and shavings of Parmesan, embellished perhaps with slices of ripe pear.

As well as straight salads, rocket is a winner in sandwiches, again of all sorts from beef paste to chicken tikka (if you must), and I just love it packed into warm pitta bread with tomato and cubes of grilled lamb slid straight from a hot skewer, all finished with a slick of thick Greek yoghurt.

Rocket pesto (see overleaf) is a halfway house between raw and cooked rocket, as the heat of pasta will semi-cook it. It is good tossed with spaghetti on its own, but even nicer, I think, with shellfish or salmon added as well. I love it drizzled over roast slices of winter squash. Also appetising are roughly chopped rocket leaves, tossed with pasta and tomato sauce, perhaps with a few teaspoons of capers for piquancy. Piling a loose mound of rocket leaves on a pizza steaming hot from the oven is an easy way to induce a touch of style, and the beauty of it is that the rocket ends up partially softened, without losing all of its raw pepperiness.

COOKING As it cooks, rocket loses much of its bulk. Therefore I would suggest that you don't try rocket soups (very good incidentally) or the like with the more expensive, more refined forms of rocket. This is where 'rokka' comes to the fore. Since anything more than a few seconds of heat will kill off most of the pepperiness of the rokka, no-one will be offended by it.

* *

Grilled chicken skewers with rocket pesto and soured cream

With amazing effectiveness, a home-made pesto elevates the most ordinary of suppers and this is a case in point. Under the grill, or out on the barbecue, chicken kebabs become twice as nice served with rocket pesto and a spot of soured cream.

You'll have more pesto than you need for one sitting, but the remainder can be stored in an airtight container in the fridge for 3 or 4 days, and used on pasta, or swirled into a soup, or spread in a sandwich instead of butter.

Serves 4 generously

4 chicken breasts or 8 chicken thighs, boned and skinned
2 cloves garlic, crushed
juice of 1 lemon
2 tablespoons extra virgin olive oil
24 cherry tomatoes
4 tablespoons soured cream or crème fraîche to serve
salt and pepper

Pesto
100g (3½ oz) rocket leaves, roughly torn up
60g (2oz) shelled cashew nuts, lightly toasted
2 cloves garlic, roughly chopped
60g (2oz) pecorino or Parmesan, roughly broken into chunks
100ml (3½ fl oz) extra virgin olive oil

To make the pesto, put all the ingredients bar the olive oil into the bowl of the processor, and process to a paste. Gradually trickle in the oil until you have a thick cream. Season with some pepper, and scrape into a small bowl.

Cut the chicken into 4cm (1½ in) chunks and marinate with the crushed garlic, lemon juice, olive oil and salt and pepper for at least half an hour, but better still a couple of hours or even overnight.

Preheat the grill or barbecue thoroughly. Thread the pieces of chicken on to skewers, interspersing here and there with a cherry tomato. Grill or barbecue for about 7–8 minutes, turning occasionally, until the chicken is just cooked through.

Serve immediately, passing the pesto and cream around the table for people to help themselves.

Sorrel

Sorrel perches on the tri-cusp (if there is such a word) of salad leaf, herb and tart relish. It is none of these exactly, yet all of them simultaneously. It is a multi-skilling leaf, one that treads its own path.

You wouldn't want to, and indeed probably couldn't, eat a plateful of sorrel salad. It's too sharply mouth puckering, too charged with oxalic acid for comfort or health. On the other hand, a few leaves (torn up if they are of the larger **garden or French sorrel**, left untouched if they are the handsome, small shield-shaped **buckler sorrel**) tossed into a mixed green salad brings a clear lemony note. Verging on herbal, it can be chopped up fine and added to stuffings and egg dishes with good effect. Its outstanding skill, however, comes as relish, for want of a better word. Cooked, it dissolves to a dark delicious sludge that is just brilliant with fish and eggs in particular, and makes one of the best of all spring soups.

The only sensible way to get hold of garden sorrel in sufficient quantities to make it worthwhile is to grow it yourself. The price, on the rare occasion that I've seen it for sale in shops, is outrageous. One small plant of garden or French sorrel, purchased in a garden centre, will keep you in sorrel for years to come at practically no effort beyond digging a hole and popping the root ball into it. It grows merrily out in the garden, or in a pot by the kitchen door, or in a window box surrounded by traffic fumes. Once established, sorrel just goes from strength to strength. The only time my sorrel has ever failed is when my cats took to weeing on it, but otherwise it is pretty much indestructible. Cut out the towering flowering stems regularly throughout the summer, and it will go on pushing out leaves well into the autumn.

If you only have room for one sort of sorrel in your garden/window box, go for the big-leaved garden sorrel. Buckler leaf sorrel is less useful.

Practicalities

BUYING Assuming that you are growing your own sorrel, or that a mate has been kind enough to let you raid theirs, it's worth pointing out that you need to harvest it by the handful. Other than in a salad, a mere leaf or two will barely register. You would need to buy at least three average supermarket packs of sorrel to make, say, a sorrel soup for four with a noticeable tang to it.

To prepare, swish the sorrel leaves around in a bowl or sink of cold water and snap off and discard the thicker, tougher stalks. Dry in a salad spinner, or a clean tea-towel. For a salad, tear or shred leaves just before serving. For cooking, you are most likely to need a 'chiffonade' of leaves. This is just a fancy way of saying fine ribbons. Pile 4–5 leaves up on top of each other, then roll them up tightly like a cigar. Slice across the cigar, and there you are – a perfect chiffonade of sorrel.

COOKING Your basic sorrel sludge is made by cooking plenty of sorrel ribbons in a little butter over a low heat until it collapses and darkens. It can be used as it is, but looks unattractive, so you might, for instance, spoon some on to a plate and sit a slice of poached or baked fish on top of it. Or spread it thickly in the base of a savoury tartlet, or on a slice of griddled bread and top with a poached egg, or creamy scrambled egg.

A little sorrel sludge spooned into a hot ramekin, topped with an egg and a spoonful of cream, then rushed back into the oven to bake, makes an old-fashioned but delicious first course or supper dish. To make a sorrel omelette, soften a little sorrel in butter in your omelette pan, before pouring in the whisked eggs, so that the sorrel is cooked right in. Alternatively, you may prefer to pile a handful of finely shredded sorrel on to the almost cooked omelette, then flip the hot sides over the sorrel so that it softens in the omelette's own heat.

For the easiest sauce, to partner fish, stir double cream into the sorrel sludge, bring up to the boil and simmer for a couple of minutes to thicken before seasoning. Sorted. Some of the cream can be replaced with a little stock, for a lighter effect.

Sorrel soup

One of the best tonics on a chilly spring day, this soup with its bright sorrel sharpness is always welcome. Later on, when the temperature rises, serve it chilled.

Serves 6

3 big handfuls large-leaved sorrel
2 tablespoons extra virgin olive oil
1 onion, chopped
400 g (14 oz) potatoes, peeled and diced
1 bouquet garni (1 bay leaf, 2 sprigs parsley,
  2 sprigs thyme, tied together with string)

1.5 litres (2 ¾ pints) light chicken or
  vegetable stock
6 tablespoons double cream (optional)
salt and pepper

Cut out and discard the larger tougher stems of the sorrel, then shred the leaves roughly. Warm the oil in a large saucepan and add the onion, potatoes and bouquet garni. Stir to coat in oil, then cover and sweat over a very low heat for 10 minutes or so.

Uncover and pour in the stock, then season with salt and pepper. Bring up to the boil and simmer for 15 minutes or so until the potato is very tender. Take off the heat, remove the bouquet garni, then stir in the sorrel. Liquidise in batches and return to the pan. Reheat when required, stir in the cream if using, then taste and adjust seasoning. Serve straightaway.

Sorrel and new potato frittata

Italian frittatas can be thin or thick and sturdy like this one, but either way they are brilliant for supper or lunch or even for a picnic, as they are as good cold as hot. Serve big wedges of the frittata with tomato and green salads in summer, or with generous helpings of spinach or spring greens in winter.

Serves 4–6

6 eggs
2 tablespoons freshly grated Parmesan
freshly grated nutmeg
1 large onion, sliced
3 tablespoons extra virgin olive oil

400 g (14 oz) new potatoes, cooked and
  halved or thickly sliced
60 g (2 oz) sorrel leaves, finely shredded
120 g (4½ oz) Comté, fontina or Taleggio
  cheese, thinly sliced
salt and pepper

Preheat the grill. Beat the eggs with the Parmesan, salt, pepper and nutmeg.

Fry the onion gently in the oil until tender, then turn up the heat and add the new potatoes and continue frying until both are patched with brown. Stir in the sorrel. Pour over the egg mixture, and turn the heat down a little. Let it cook undisturbed for about 5 minutes, or until cooked about two-thirds of the way through. Now lay the cheese slices on top, and slide the frittata under the grill until the cheese has melted and the top is lightly browned.

Serve the frittata hot, warm or at room temperature, cut into wedges.

* *

Sweet sorrel turnovers

Well, who'da thought it? These turnovers are just dandy. If you grow your own sorrel, then you've got to try them. They taste something like a French 'chausson aux pommes' (apple turnover), but with a thinner layer of filling. They were once a simple home treat both in Lancashire and Cornwall where they are known as 'sour sauce pasties'.

Makes 4

125 g (4½ oz) sorrel leaves, chopped
85 g (3 oz) light muscovado sugar
250 g (9 oz) puff pastry

1 egg, beaten
caster sugar for sprinkling

Preheat the oven to 220°C/425°F/Gas 7. Roll the pastry out to a thickness of 5 mm (¼ in). Cut out four 13 cm (5 in) circles.

Mix the sorrel with the brown sugar and divide between the pastry circles quickly before the sugar starts to draw out the juices. Brush the edges of the pastry with a little egg, then fold over to enclose the filling. Press the edges together firmly then knock up with the back of a knife. Brush with egg, sprinkle with caster sugar and bake in the preheated oven for 15–20 minutes until golden brown. Serve warm.

* *

Watercress and Land cress

* * *

Of all the characterful salad leaves, **watercress** comes top in my kitchen. Yup, it beats rocket, radicchio, curly endive, mizuna and all the rest. It's not merely that it feels so absolutely British in a way which the others don't. It's as much to do with the peppery taste, with textures (crisp stem, soft leaves) and with the colour and look of the plant.

And it reminds me of my childhood. Supper in front of the television was a rare treat to be savoured. As often as not, it consisted of big bowls of soup, followed by watercress sandwiches, of which both my parents were inordinately fond. Quite rightly, for when they are made with thick soft slices of first-class white bread, spread with salty butter and then packed as full as can be with watercress, they are unbeatable. I still rate watercress sandwiches among my favourite things.

Land cress is similar to watercress in taste, though more powerfully peppery. For a gardener the advantage is that it does not require running water to grow. It does very nicely, thank you, in an ordinary patch of earth.

Practicalities

BUYING Reasons why I like to buy watercress in bunches, not in plastic pouches:

1) you can tell at a glance how fresh it is – there's no hiding yellowing or wilting leaves;

2) it will only look fresh if it has been recently picked;

3) leaves can be rinsed quickly under the tap, then slashed off in one flash of the blade, leaving the stems (good for soup);

4) It's easier to keep lively (more on this below).

So, assuming that you too have perfect bunches of gorgeous watercress, the best way to keep them at the peak of perfection is to plunge them, leaves downward, stems waggling upwards, into a bowl of cold water, and place it in the fridge. This does not seem at all logical, but believe me, it works far better than standing the stems in the water. Like this, it will keep for several days. Bagged loose sprigs of watercress, once opened, need using up fast.

Watercress adds a much appreciated bite to any green salad, and many more mixed salads. There are few better examples than the blend of watercress with sweet slices or chunks of orange and the bitter touch of chicory, perhaps lifted with a sprinkling of toasted flaked almonds – one of the great winter salads. Watercress does go particularly well with the sweetness of fruit – toss sprigs of watercress with wedges of ripe pear, crumbled blue cheese, toasted walnuts and a lemony dressing for an autumn starter or buffet, for instance, or partner watercress with late summer peaches or nectarines and shredded cooked chicken. One pleasing British tradition is to embellish roast pheasant or other feathered game, with small posies of watercress – the heat of the meat softens the watercress, releasing more of its flavour without destroying the pepperiness. I like this idea, and use it more widely, making a bed of fresh watercress leaves to cushion roast or grilled chicken, lamb or pork, or roast fillets of salmon or other fish.

Direct heat changes watercress, doing away with much of its delicious spry pepperiness. As a result, watercress soup and watercress sauce can turn out a touch disappointing. The answer is to make the base sauce or soup with the stems of the watercress, then to liquidise with the uncooked leaves (or simply chop them finely and stir in) just seconds before serving. That way you get the best of both worlds, as well as a pretty speckledy green colour.

* *

Twice-baked watercress soufflés

These are the most user-friendly sort of soufflés. Made and baked in advance, they then just head back into the oven, drenched with cream, to reheat and brown a few minutes before serving. They are devastatingly rich.

Makes 6–8, depending on the capacity of the ramekins

45 g (1½ oz) butter, plus extra for greasing
45 g (1½ oz) plain flour
300 ml (10 fl oz) milk
2 tablespoons freshly grated Parmesan
60 g (2 oz) Gruyère cheese, grated
freshly grated nutmeg
85 g (3 oz) watercress, very finely chopped

3 eggs, separated
salt and pepper

To finish
200 ml (7 fl oz) double cream
1½ tablespoons freshly grated Parmesan
a bunch of fresh watercress sprigs

Preheat the oven to 200°C/400°F/Gas 6. Melt the butter and stir in the flour. Stir for a minute without letting it colour. Take off the heat and start stirring in the milk, a little at a time, until the sauce is creamy. Then start adding it in bigger sloshes, stirring in well each time. Return the sauce to the heat and bring back to a gentle simmer, stirring constantly for 2 minutes. Take off the heat, and stir in the cheeses and seasoning. Then beat in the chopped watercress and the egg yolks.

Grease 6–8 ramekins or small pudding moulds generously, and stand in a roasting tin. Whisk the egg whites to stiff peaks. Stir a tablespoon of the whites into the watercress mixture, then fold in the remainder. Divide the mixture between the prepared ramekins, filling almost to the brim. Pour enough boiling water into the roasting tin to come about 2–3 cm (1 in) up the sides of the moulds. Bake in the oven for 15–20 minutes.

Take the ramekins out of the water and cool. When quite cold, run a knife around the edge of each to loosen, then turn out. Grease an ovenproof dish lightly and arrange the soufflés in it, browned sides up. Cover and chill until almost ready to serve. To finish, preheat the oven to 220°C/425°F/Gas 7. Season the cream with salt and pepper and pour over the soufflés. Sprinkle with Parmesan. Bake for 15 minutes, until browned and bubbling. Serve hot.

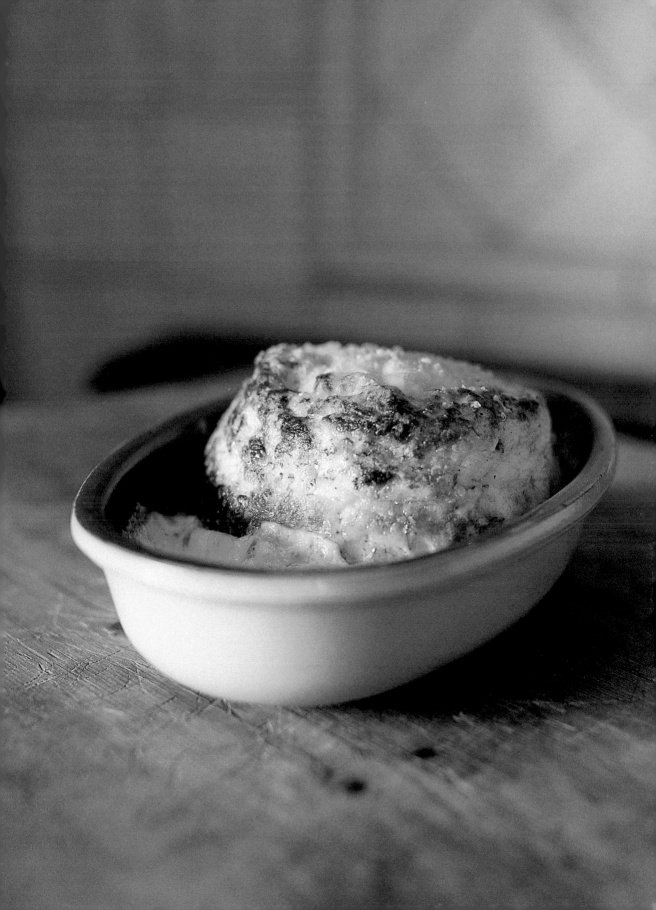

Index